Physical Edu

for People with Visual Impairments and Deafblindness

Foundations of Instruction

Lauren J. Lieberman, Paul E. Ponchillia, and Susan V. Ponchillia

AFB PRESS
American Foundation for the Blind

Printed in the United States of America

Library of Congress Cataloging-in-Publication Data

Lieberman, Lauren J., 1965-

Physical education and sports for people with visual impairments and deafblindness : foundations of instruction / Lauren J. Lieberman, Paul E. Ponchillia, and Susan V. Ponchillia.

p. cm.

Includes bibliographical references and index.

ISBN 978-0-89128-454-3 (pbk. : alk. paper) — ISBN 978-0-89128-455-0 (ascii download) — ISBN 978-0-89128-553-3 (online subscription) — ISBN 978-0-89128-554-0 (epub) — ISBN 978-0-89128-555-7 (mobi) 1. Physical education for the blind. 2. Physical education for the deaf. I. Ponchillia, Paul E. II. Ponchillia, Susan Kay Vlahas. III. Title.

HV1767.L55 2013

613.7'10871–dc23

2012031897

The American Foundation for the Blind removes barriers, creates solutions, and expands possibilities so people with vision loss can achieve their full potential.

This book is dedicated to Dr. Susan V. Ponchillia, who herself was one of the most dedicated professionals the field of work with people with visual impairments has known. Dr. Ponchillia passed away during the writing of this manuscript, but she contributed much, much more than the one-third portion of the work we expected of her. As in all other aspects of her life, she allowed nothing to interfere with either the amount or the quality of the work she did on behalf of people with visual impairment; it was simply more important to her than anything else, so she went about it regardless of how she felt or of her knowledge of what the future held for her.

Susan's first part-time job in the field was as a recreation assistant at the Michigan Commission for the Blind's Training Center (MCBTC). Her own interests in sports and active recreation, coupled with the experience she obtained at MCBTC, led her to pursue a line of research on sports and recreation for people with visual impairments during her 25-year tenure at the Department of Blindness and Low Vision Studies at Western Michigan University. During that 25 year period, she also co-directed the Sports Education Camps for Students with Visual Impairments, co-directed the United States Association of Blind Athletes Midwest Regional Goalball Tournament, and volunteered for virtually every local recreational activity for people with visual impairments that came along. She became aware of the virtual lack of literature available worldwide in the area of adapted sports and recreation for people with visual impairments or deafblindness during that time, and the idea for this manuscript began to grow in her mind. The publication of this book, along with that of Foundations of Rehabilitation Teaching *(AFB Press, 1996), is one of the two crowning achievements of her life. We are blessed to have been able to work with her on this project and to have helped her make her dream a reality.*

—L. J. L. and P. E. P.

Contents

Foreword, *Louis M. Tutt* vii

Preface: Views from Two Athletes, *James Mastro and Jennifer Armbruster* ix

Acknowledgments xiii

Introduction xv

PART 1 Visual Impairment, Deafblindness, and Physical Activity

1 The Impact of Visual Impairment and Deafblindness on Learning and Development 3

2 Visual Impairment and Deafblindness: An Overview 27

3 Providing Physical Education to Students with Visual Impairments or Deafblindness 52

PART 2 Modifications and Adaptations for Teaching Physical Activities

4 Modifying Instruction to Meet Students' Needs 91

5 Principles of Adapting Games, Sports, and Related Activities 135

PART 3 Teaching Physical Skills throughout the Lifespan

6 Early Childhood Development: Movement and Play in Early Childhood *Tanni L. Anthony* 159

7 Elementary Education Programming 187

8 Physical Education and Sports Activities in Middle School, High School, and Adulthood 227

9 Organized Sports for Children and Adults with Visual Impairments: Goalball and Beep Baseball 266

10 Recreational Activities and Their Adaptations: Toward a Positive Quality of Life 286

11 Fitness: A Lifelong Pursuit 312

12 Sports and Related Organizations of Special Interest 338

References 345
Appendix: Camp Abilities Activity Assessment 363
Resources 375
Index 387
About the Authors 395

Foreword

Physical education teachers, adapted physical education teachers, and activity leaders in the trenches are always on the lookout for new, appropriate, and appealing games and activities for their students. When it comes to working with individuals who are visually impaired or deafblind, however, most of them confront what may seem like a greater challenge: how to include these students in physical activities and adapt activities so that they may participate fully along with others. In *Physical Education and Sports for People with Visual Impairments and Deafblindness: Foundations of Instruction,* Lauren Lieberman, Paul Ponchillia, and Susan Ponchillia contribute compelling resources for these efforts and for these professionals, as well as for recreational therapists, physical therapists, teachers of students with visual impairments or deafblindness, and anyone concerned with the full inclusion of children and adults who are visually impaired in athletics and the other essential activities of life.

Capitalizing on their wide-ranging experiences in teaching and reaching students of all ages with blindness, visual impairments, and deafblindness, the authors have created a definitive guide on fitness, sports, and recreation activities for children, youths, and adults. There is some information on physical activity for all ages in this excellent book, which is divided for readers' ease of understanding, with Part 1 speaking to Visual Impairment, Deafblindness, and Physical Activity, Part 2 addressing Modifications and Adaptations for Teaching Physical Activities, and Part 3 focusing on Teaching Physical Skills throughout the Lifespan.

As readers explore the range of topics encompassed in this book, they will experience how Lieberman, Ponchillia, and Ponchillia carefully and clearly present methods, techniques, and tips to assist teachers, leaders, and coaches in working more effectively with their students, clients, and athletes. Experienced professionals as well as those seeking information on an often-neglected topic will find this book a bona fide resource on proven activities, methods, and approaches. For novices and seasoned practitioners alike, this book provides a wealth of information on what to do, how to do it, when to do it, and why.

The authors are aware, however, that learning is accomplished most effectively in environments providing enjoyment, pleasure, and fun. We should all therefore focus on the learner and learning and untapped potential and opportunities. Congratulations to the authors—my physical education colleagues and friends—especially as we remember Susan, on an outstanding professional job that will benefit persons with blindness, visual impairment, and deafblindness throughout their lifespan.

Louis M. Tutt
Executive Director
Association for Education and Rehabilitation
of the Blind and Visually Impaired
Alexandria, VA

Preface: Views from Two Athletes

JAMES MASTRO

It seems that every generation has to be reminded that children and adults with visual impairments or deafblindness have the right to as normal a life as possible. When individuals are not permitted to join in society's activities, they are being deprived of achieving their fullest potential. It is amazing that in the 21st century, with the many forms of information, resources, and organizations that exist, how many people still do not know about sports and recreation activities that have been adapted to meet the needs of individuals with visual impairment or deafblindness.

The past two decades have seen the growth of organizations whose reason for existence is to develop sports specifically designed for individuals with visual impairment. Sports such as beep baseball, goalball, beep kickball, audio darts, and showdown have given these populations a previously unavailable opportunity to participate in recreation or competition. Yet many individuals with visual impairments or deafblindness do not realize that they are able to participate successfully in games, sports, and recreation. School districts usually provide adapted physical education, and community park and recreation programs may have modified activities. However, parents, educators, and recreation specialists often do not have the confidence or knowledge to help these individuals participate in games, sports, and recreation and may even have some fears about interacting with members of these groups or doubt their capabilities. In addition, physical educators, administrators, and coaches can be overwhelmed by the complexity of adapting activities for people with visual impairments. Visual impairment and deafblindness are low-incidence disabilities, making it difficult to obtain the resources to develop physical education, recreation, and sport programs. Denied the right to discover their own capabilities, many individuals with visual impairments and deafblindness are likely to adopt a sedentary lifestyle that can overshadow their health.

This book has been written to help people who work with children, youths, or adults with visual impairments or deafblindness obtain the knowledge and confidence they need to include them in every kind of physical activity program. Lauren Lieberman, Paul Ponchillia, and Susan Ponchillia, who have had many years of experience working with these populations, describe practical, effective methods for physical educators, recreation specialists, teachers of students who are visually impaired, parents, and administrators of programs designed to mainstream individuals with these low-incident disabilities to teach physical fitness, modifications of games and rules, fundamental sports skills, and motor performance.

While participating in physical activity, individuals with visual impairments and deafblindness are introduced to the benefits of games, sports, and recreation. They become aware of the physical demands and skills needed in different activities so they may become proficient in their preferred games and sports. They discover their own abilities and the feelings of self-actualization they can have when participating in activities that have been modified to meet their unique needs. By giving activity providers ideas for modifying games, sports, and recreation to meet those needs, the authors of this book are giving individuals with visual impairments and deafblindness the opportunity to improve their quality of life.

Individuals with visual impairments and deafblindness have the right to enjoy the benefits of games, sports, and recreation that may help them take their place in society. They must be allowed to join the rest of the world and march to the same drummer. This must start as early in life as possible.

Although much has been gained in recent years, more needs to be done to make existing programs accessible to individuals with visual impairments and deafblindness. With this excellent publication in hand, specialists in games, sports, and recreation, along with parents and professionals in visual impairment, can use their creativity and initiative to make these programs work for everyone.

James Mastro, Ph.D.
Seven-time Paralympian in four sports and three-time gold medalist
Professor of Physical and Professional Education
Bemidji State University
Bemidji, Minnesota

JENNIFER ARMBRUSTER

As an individual who is totally blind, I know the importance of being active and the role that physical activity, sports, and recreation has played in my life. It taught me responsibility, hard work, time management, and teamwork. It also taught me to set goals, to achieve them, and to try everything to find what works for me and what I enjoy. Regardless of whether you exercise for general fitness or are a highly competitive athlete, the benefits are great. The social aspects of recreation with family and peers, the physical benefits of being in shape—both in terms of cardiovascular health and overall strength—as well as the lessons learned by playing sports are invaluable.

I was fortunate, when I lost my vision starting right before my freshman year in high school, to have a wonderful and supportive family that was always involved in sports and recreation, so when I lost my vision nothing really changed for me at home. We still went out and shot baskets and tried batting practice as well, trying to find what worked and what didn't work so well.

I also had a supportive school atmosphere. My coach at the time was wonderful and so were my teammates. I went through my high school career and college after going totally blind my senior year of high school with the trial and error system. My friends and I were creative and did what we needed to do for me to play in a flag football intramural league and to compete on my high school track and field team. There is not always one way to modify a sport or activity, as each person is different, but I love the creative process of figuring it out.

The process of coming up with solutions so that I could participate in sports as a competitive athlete was a positive one for me, but this is not always the case for children or adults with visual impairments or deafblindness who don't have the advantages that I did. Way too often the process is blocked by fear and the lack of creativity and education. *Physical Education and Sports for People with Visual Impairments and Deafblindness: Foundations of Instruction* will help to break down those barriers, inspire ideas and solutions, and get individuals who are blind, visually impaired, or deafblind off the sidelines and onto the field of play!

Jennifer Armbruster
Five-time Paralympian and Captain, 2012
U.S. Women's Goalball Team
Inclusive Recreation and Community Services
Coordinator
Portland State University
Portland, Oregon

Acknowledgments

I would like to thank Paul and Susan Ponchillia for their partnership in this incredible book journey. I have learned a tremendous amount working with them over the years. Paul, thank you for your dedication and commitment through extremely hard times. Your perseverance and courage are a testament to your incredible commitment to the field. Our field is so fortunate to have a professional like you who has changed the way people see children with visual impairments.

I thank all of the children I have worked with at Perkins School for the Blind, in schools throughout the country, and at Camp Abilities throughout the world. You are the best teachers anyone could have, and I have learned so much from you.

A huge thank you goes to Natalie Hilzen and Ellen Bilofsky from AFB Press for their tenacity, professionalism, and cheerleading through this book project. You were there through each step, and you truly made it happen.

Thank you to the College at Brockport, especially President John Halstead, Provost Anne Huot, Dean Frank Short of the School of Health and Human Performance, and Susan Petersen, Chair of the Kinesiology, Sport Studies and Physical Education Department, for embracing programming for individuals with visual impairments throughout the years, helping us train the future leaders about how to teach children with visual impairments and deafblindness, and supporting research in this important area.

Many thanks to my wonderful and encouraging family Stan (Pop), Ann, Pat, Marc, Diane, and Eric. Thank you to my amazing partner Dr. Katrina Arndt. Your unwavering support, positive attitude, and open mind have helped me through the exciting and the hard times of this project. I could not have done it without you!

—Lauren J. Lieberman

I would like to acknowledge the important roles that so many people played in the development and creation of this manuscript. First I must thank those who filled me with the love of sports in early childhood, my parents, Paul A. and Jean Ponchillia, and the first person I remember calling coach, Herb Gavin, my Saturday morning YMCA "gym teacher." Also, many thanks to those who have helped me learn the things I have written in this book. Among them are the hundreds of young athletes who dared to challenge themselves by attending one of the Western Michigan University (WMU) Sports Education Camps across the country and who taught me so much. Thanks to special friends, Collette Bauman, Nancy Boucher, Susan Bradley, Tom Coyne, Leanne Ford, Scott Ford, Jean Friedel, Patrick Gafney, Kevin Kimbrough, John McMahon, Mark Sinclair, and Hal Wolf, whose dedication to children, tireless efforts, and continuous advocacy have moved so many students with visual impairments "from the sidelines to the goal line." Thanks, too, to the literally thousands of volunteers, the lucky ones who interact directly with the young athletes at the Sports Camps, for they are truly the camps' heart. In addition, thanks to Mark Lucas and the United States Association of Blind Athletes and to Michigan Ski for Light for helping me get back to an active life of sports and recreation following my own vision loss and for teaching me all the great things they know about blind sports.

Thanks also to those at WMU who helped me so much professionally and who also provided the clerical and library research assistance required for this project. In particular, thanks to Dr. John Dunn, President of the university, Dean Early Washington, and Associate Dean for Research Richard Long, both of the College of Health and Human Services, and Dr. James Leja, Chairperson of the Department of Blindness and Low Vision Studies for providing the people-centered research environment that exists at WMU and that ultimately led to the writing of this manuscript.

Many thanks to those who helped directly with the research, compilation, and writing of the manuscript. I give tremendous thanks to Dr. Lauren Lieberman for her pioneering work in leading the field of adaptive physical education into the realm of serving students with visual impairments and deafblindness. Since I have known her, I have viewed her as the one person who could and would broaden the focus of that profession and consequently be responsible for vastly improving physical education services for visually impaired children in public schools. I believe that the completion of this book will take her one more giant step toward that goal. I also want to thank her for her high level of energy and unceasingly positive attitude during this project, which kept me from bailing out when I was facing some difficult times.

I offer much appreciation to my wife Jimmy Sue for proofreading, checking references, putting up with my occasional ill moods, and her continuous encouragement. Thanks also to my friend and sports photographer, Chuck Comer, not only for his great work, but for saying, "Yes, sure" so many times during this project.

Next, a million thanks go to Natalie Hilzen, editor in chief at AFB Press, for her gargantuan effort to bring this book to press, for her well-timed phone calls of encouragement, and for that most uncommon ability of hers to transform my face from a slack-jawed frown into a big happy smile. Perhaps the most deserved thanks go to Ellen Bilofsky, editor extraordinaire, whose suggestions, guidance, encouragement, dogged persistence, and fine editing have led to the quality readers will enjoy in this book.

—Paul E. Ponchillia

Introduction

In deciding to write a book about physical activity and people with visual impairments or deafblindness, our primary motivation was to share our experiences as educators and active sportspeople in working with individuals with visual impairments and deafblindness of all ages. Time and again, we have witnessed how the opportunity to participate in physical activity, such as a sport or recreational pastime, can have a life-altering effect on a child who has been blind since birth or an adult who recently lost most of his or her vision, ranging from improved health and physical ability, to increased self-confidence, opportunities for friendship, and even the discovery of a lifetime passion for a sport. Having also witnessed firsthand how often physical activity is lacking in the lives of individuals with visual impairments or deafblindness and how difficult it can sometimes be for them to get access to the physical education, sports, or leisure activities that others take for granted, our objective in this book is to provide teachers, rehabilitation and other professionals, and parents with information and tools that will assist them in increasing the physical skills of their students, children, and clients and their access to such activities.

This text, then, is intended primarily as a hands-on instruction manual demonstrating with specific examples and illustrations how individuals of any ability with visual impairments or deafblindness can participate and be included in the widest possible range of activities. Although the book has been written primarily for physical educators, adapted physical educators, recreation therapists, teachers of children with visual impairments, orientation and mobility specialists, vision rehabilitation therapists, and occupational therapists, its content will also assist parents, state project directors of programs for children who are deafblind, classroom teachers, coordinators of after-school and community fitness and recreation programs, and anyone who might work directly with individuals who are visually impaired or deafblind.

RESEARCH AND EXPERIENCE

We have based much of the content of this book on the literature and research in the areas of visual impairment, sports, and recreation; however, as authors we also draw heavily on our combined experiences in university personnel preparation instruction and operation of specialized short-term sports camps that have served more than 4,000 students with visual impairments or deafblindness since 1988; on more than 50 combined years of managing adult adaptive sports and recreation programs at the local, state, national, and international level; and on an immeasurable number of direct teaching, coaching, and participation experiences in sports and recreation activities designed specifically for individuals with visual impairments or deafblindness. We have also played a significant role in the development of the sport of goalball for athletes with visual impairments in the United States. In addition, we have all taught university-level courses in adapting sports and recreational activities for children with visual impairments or deafblindness in our respective professional teacher preparation programs.

Lauren Lieberman founded and directs Camp Abilities in Brockport, New York, the first of a network of similar camps around the country. Susan and Paul Ponchillia founded and directed the Michigan Sports Education Camp for Students with Visual Impairments from which was developed the National Sports Education Camps Project, a cooperative program in over 11 states, developed by Western Michigan University and the U.S. Association of Blind Athletes (USABA) with funding from the U S. Department of Education (Ponchillia, Armbruster & Wiebold, 2005). These sports camps are primarily designed to introduce children from 8 to 19 years of age to basic physical, health promotion, and fitness skills. The activities taught at these camps have included aerobic exercise, archery, beep baseball, bowling, canoeing and kayaking, goalball, gymnastics, horseback riding, ice skating, judo, kick boxing, power lifting, rock climbing, roller blading, rowing, showdown, swimming, tandem cycling, track and field, and wrestling. Campers also participate in interactive sessions on topics such as healthy eating, exercise, sports adaptations, and self-advocacy. Depending on the campers' ages, individual camps range from a few days up to one week in duration, and campers participate directly in educational programming from approximately 20 to 32 hours.

The camps also serve as hands-on experiential educational laboratories and practicum and internship sites for students in personnel preparation programs in blindness and low vision studies, adapted physical education, and other academic programs, such as at the College at Brockport, State University of New York; Western Michigan University; and other colleges and universities across the country. In addition, the camps have served as sites for research that has led to best practices in teaching techniques, camp programming, and inclusion of physical skills in local school curricula (Goodwin, Lieberman, Johnston & Leo, 2011; Ponchillia, 1995; Ponchillia, Armbruster & Wiebold, 2005; Scheib, & Ponchillia, 1999). This research, as well as our own observations, has demonstrated the success of the targeted methods used at these camps and presented in this book in adapting activities and teaching sports and fitness skills.

It is equally important, however, for students to have access to this type of instruction throughout the year, not just during the two weeks of camp, and for youngsters and adults to have access to the same variety of sports, recreation, and fitness activities in their communities as their sighted neighbors. Indeed, research comparing the athletic success of adults with visual impairments who received physical education in school as children to that of visually impaired adults who received none supports the crucial importance of such access (Ponchillia, Strause & Ponchillia, 2002). Sixty-nine percent of the group that had received physical education in school played on sports teams in school or college, while only 20 percent of the group who reported being left out of their physical education classes as children did so. Similarly, 75 percent of those who played on school or college sports teams later participated in races, marathons, and other events open to the general public, while only 40 percent of the group that never played in school competed against sighted athletes in public events. By making available the instructional techniques and methods of adapting activities for people with visual impairments and deafblindness in this book, we hope that even more such achievements might be expected, and on a broader scale.

SCOPE OF THIS BOOK

The structure of this book is designed to build on basic information about working with individuals with visual impairment and deafblindness, physical education, and instructional principles and then delve into a more detailed presentation of instruction for various age groups and types of activities. This organizational plan allows teachers and other professionals with different backgrounds to find more easily the information they need when working with a particular student or adult learner.

Part 1, Visual Impairment, Deafblindness, and Physical Activity, begins by discussing the importance of physical activity to all people and particularly to those with visual impairments and deafblindness as well as the factors affecting individuals with visual impairments or deafblindness that influence their potential for learning. These early chapters focus on concepts and definitions related to visual impairment and deafblindness and information necessary for understanding the needs of children and adults with visual impairment and deafblindness, as well as the principles of physical education and the special education system in the United States. The following chapters in Part 2, Modifications and Adaptations for Teaching Physical Activities, introduce the methodologies that have been developed to overcome the instructional barriers faced by teachers of learners with limited or no vision and the methods of adapting various activities.

In Part 3, Teaching Physical Skills throughout the Lifespan, Chapter 6 first presents the skills and activities of early childhood, from infancy through preschool and the importance of early development for later physical skills. Chapter 7 demonstrates how to include students with visual impairments or deafblindness in the physical education curriculum of elementary school and how to teach basic skills when they cannot be learned visually. Following this, Chapter 8 discusses the changing physical education curriculum in junior high and high school and then presents detailed descriptions of how youths and adults with visual impairments or deafblindness participate in virtually every competitive sport. Two sports created specifically for individuals with visual impairment, goalball and beep baseball, are covered in Chapter 9. Treatment of recreation and fitness activities follows in Chapters 10 and 11, respectively, and national and international umbrella sports organizations and associations that involve people who have visual impairments or deafblindness in sports and sponsor competitions for athletes who are visually impaired are described in Chapter 12. Organizations that sponsor specific sports are listed in the Resources section at the back of the book, along with other sources of information and products.

The heart of this book is the presentation in sequence from birth to adulthood of the skills that individuals with visual impairments and deafblindness need to participate in physical activities and how to teach them, along with the adaptations for specific activities and sports that might be engaged in at any age. The aim is to cover the needs of everyone who falls under the definitions of visual impairment or deafblindness as well as to demonstrate the possibility of participating in physical activities throughout the lifespan.

Role Models

The sequence of skills presented in this book is offered in part as a blueprint to follow for parents who are told at some time in their child's life, "Your child will never see normally" or "Your child cannot hear." If parents, teachers, and others advocate for that child to receive the kinds of services and instruction described in this book, their hopes of rearing a healthy and skilled youngster—or even an Olympic athlete—might be fulfilled.

There is a good deal of evidence to demonstrate that determined athletes with visual impairments have had great success, even reaching the level of Olympic competition. A few are well known to the general public, such as Erik Weihenmayer, the first person with total blindness to reach the summit of Mount Everest, who is also a high school wrestling champion, acrobatic skydiver, long distance biker, marathon runner, and skier; and Marla Runyan, track and field athlete and marathon runner, who is the first legally blind athlete to compete in the Olympics as well as a gold medalist in the Paralympics. But many others, though less well known, have reached success as well, such as those highlighted as role models in Part 3 of this book. Those who have succeeded are highly determined, wonderfully skilled, and likely had good support during their early childhood, elementary school, and high school years, such as James Mastro and Jennifer Armbruster, two notably successful individuals with visual impairments who have grown and prospered through their love for sports and who offer their own perspectives in the Preface. Perhaps their stories will provide the impetus to a parent, spouse, friend, or loved one to motivate an athlete to greatness:

- *James (Jim) Mastro, an outstanding all-around athlete who has received special recognition in wrestling, judo, track and field, beep baseball, and goalball, lost all of his vision at 18 years of age while a senior in high school. Like many who lose vision as young adults, he was devastated. A local newspaper quoted him as saying, "At first, I thought participating in sports was all over for me. I thought people who are blind are helpless. I thought I would have to sell pencils on a street corner. But in college, I went out for wrestling. My senior year, I was the conference champion."*

  After rediscovering sports, Jim's life has been filled with a rapid blur of successes. From 1972 to 1976, he was ranked nationally as a wrestler. And in 1976, Mastro was the first blind person to become an alternate to the U.S. Olympic Greco-Roman wrestling team. He was also named to the National Beep Baseball All Tournament team four times, was the tournament's most valuable player in 1978, and was named to the National Beep Baseball Hall of Fame in 1996. Judo became Mastro's primary sport after wrestling was dropped from the Paralympic program before the 1996 games. He has won medals in the U.S. Judo Championships Master's Division, the International Blind Sports Federation (IBSA) World Judo Championships, and the IBSA Pan-American Games. Mastro competed in seven Paralympics, becoming the first Para-

lympic athlete ever to earn medals in four different sports, earning 10 medals while competing in wrestling, judo, track and field, and goalball, as well as 17 international medals in other competitions. In 1995, Mastro was named Blind Athlete of the Year by the U.S. Olympic Committee. He received a nomination to the U.S. Olympic Committee Hall of Fame in 2008.

Jim has been equally successful in his working life. A professor of professional education and physical education at Bemidji State University, in Minnesota, Mastro has also been a pioneer in education as the first student with a visual impairment to receive a Ph.D. in physical education in the United States and is a prolific author and speaker on adapted and developmental physical education.

■

■ *Jennifer Armbruster has dedicated her adult life to playing goalball and to the athletic development of young people with visual impairments. She, like Jim, is dedicated to two of her life's passions: goalball and sports education. The U.S. Paralympic website reports her to be one of the top five women goalball players in the world and she is certainly the most well-known player in the U.S. Optic neuritis began to take her vision at age 13 and resulted in total blindness by age 17, ending a highly promising future in basketball. Like Mastro, she credits sports as the major factor in overcoming the effects of the onset of blindness.*

Jen's goalball career started near the top and has zoomed skyward since then. In her first national tournament, she led her team to the silver medal at the 1990 USABA National Championship. Jen and her USA teammates have won gold at the British Invitational, the Pan American Games, the Malmo Ladies Intercup (Sweden), the IBSA World Championships, and the 2008 Paralympics. She has been most valuable player more than 10 times at the USABA nationals and leading scorer of every major international goalball event held. Watching Jen propel her missile-like 5 foot 8 inch, 145-pound frame around a goalball court is to see athleticism at its finest. Her "ear-hand" coordination and her sense of place on the court are incredible. Like all outstanding athletes, Armbruster works hard to keep prepared for goalball action, spending an average of 3 hours a day in training.

Armbruster has been just as successful professionally. Her first job was project director of the National Sports Education Camps Project, which established 22 sports camps for students with visual impairments across the United States. Armbruster is now the Inclusive Recreation and Community Services Coordinator at Portland State University, responsible for creating inclusive activity programs on campus. The mother of a young son, she has become a national authority on adapted sports for children with visual impairments.

■

Both these outstanding athletes and role models had similar backgrounds. They had vision until they were teenagers and participated in sports to a great extent before losing their sight. As a consequence, their early childhood development was completed while they could see, and their sports skills were developed with the aid of vision up through their early teens. Their challenge was adjusting to the vision loss they faced as teenagers, and this adjustment was facilitated by their participation in sports—in the case of Jennifer Armbruster, goalball, and wrestling for Jim Mastro.

However, other successful athletes from every background imaginable are worthy of the label of role model. Many of them are highlighted in the chapters in Part 3 of this book, but others, omitted for lack of space, could just as easily have been singled out: *Asya Miller,* who overcame Stargardt's disease to win more than 50 medals in power lifting, goalball, and track and field, holds several world records in power lifting, and helps lead the USA women's goalball team to international gold with her powerful throws; *Ed McInnis,* who lost his vision to diabetes as a young adult, but who fights diabetic complications by staying physically fit by working out every day in his home gym; *Heather Vercoe,* a young athlete with low vision who won award after award for her great grades and hard work in earning her degree in recreation therapy; and many others. These, too, are role models of success for children, youths, or adults with visual impairments

VICTORY THROUGH SELF-DETERMINATION

In using this book, readers should keep in mind that the definition of the word *victory* does not relate only to outperforming others in competition. In fact, many of the athletes just mentioned or featured in this book gained their true victory in another way. Victory may be measured by the degree to which we have attained control of our choices, a degree of performance at the highest level our bodies are capable of, and comfortable and meaningful relationships with our teammates and friends (also known as autonomy, competence, and relatedness; see the discussion of self-determination theory in Chapter 3.). While few may have the inborn athletic ability and early support of a Jim Mastro or Jen Armbruster, teachers, parents, coaches, and advocates can help youngsters with visual impairments or deafblindness to become just as motivated by helping them achieve self-determination. A child or adult who feels the inner power provided by achieving autonomy, competence, and relatedness is also a great athlete. It is hoped that teachers, parents, and advocates will use this book to help the individuals they know with visual impairments or deafblindness to attain that level of victory.

In addition to support, the key to achieving self-determination through becoming physically active as a person with visual impairment or deafblindness is *access,* the freedom to participate in physical activities and sports across the lifespan. The most critical time to pursue access is during early childhood, when physical skills are being developed. People who do not have access to learning physical skills as youngsters can learn them later in life, but learning as an adult is rarely as effective as learning as a child. However, access refers not only to one's ability to participate in events or classes offered in a school or a community, but also to *knowledge*—in this case, knowledge of the adaptations required for a child who is blind or deafblind to learn to throw, hop, or skip or to gain the ability to play games with other students in an inclusive setting. It is to that end that we offer the contents of this book. We sincerely hope that the knowledge that lies between its covers will serve to provide teachers the tools needed to educate the bodies and minds of children with visual impairments or deafblindness, so that they can become the role models of the future.

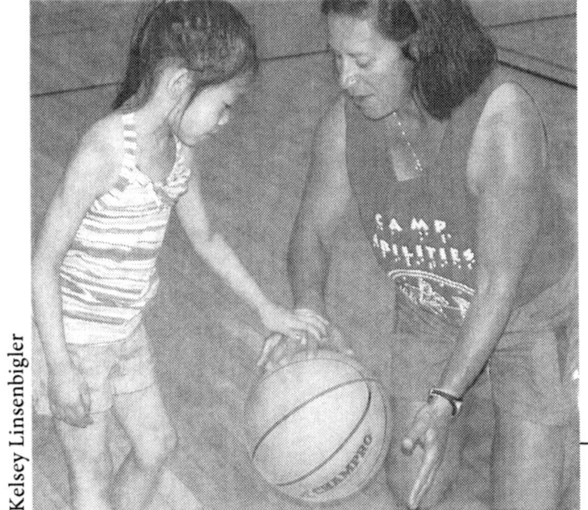

Kelsey Linsenbigler

PART 1
Visual Impairment, Deafblindness, and Physical Activity

The Impact of Visual Impairment and Deafblindness on Learning and Development

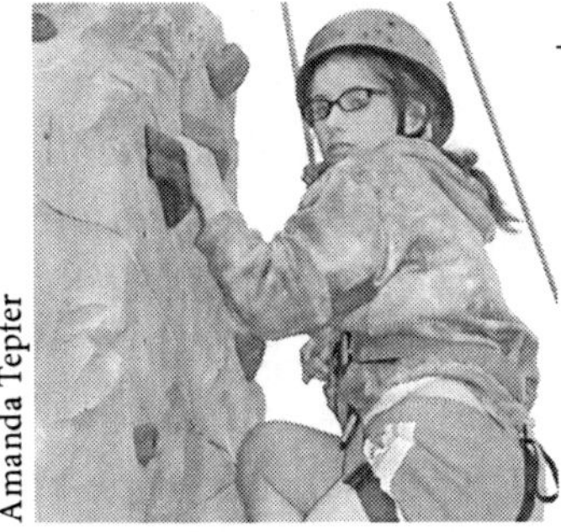

Amanda Tepfer

IN THIS CHAPTER

- **Why Physical Activity?**
- **Visual Impairment, Deafblindness, and Physical Activity**
- **Other Barriers to Physical Activity**
- **Consequences of Limited Physical Education**
- **Overcoming Barriers**

When Christopher was 13 years old, he didn't fit in well with his classmates. His total blindness wasn't the problem, though. Most of his middle school classmates could accept that he couldn't see. However, they didn't understand his constant cursing, unfriendly manner, eye poking, and repetitive rocking back and forth while standing or sitting.

Christopher resisted participating in physical education class, having convinced his mother to write him an excuse to get out of it, even though his teachers, including the teacher of students with visual impairments, physical education instructor, and adapted physical educator, tried their best to get him involved in physical education class. He needed it; his posture was stoop-shouldered and bent forward, his basic physical skills were poorly developed, and he was some 40 pounds overweight. During the winter of that school year, his teacher of students with visual impairments received a notice about an annual sports summer camp that was to be held for students with visual impairments. She and the adapted physical educator began to work on convincing Christopher and his parents that sports activities might be good for him.

Christopher mustered the courage to attend the camp, where he was introduced to basic track and field, swim racing, gymnastics, tandem cycling, wrestling, and goalball, a competitive sport for individuals with visual impairments. His behavior when he arrived at the camp continued to be disruptive. However, during the camp's wrestling competition, Christopher showed a spark of competitive drive. In a match with a much larger opponent, he simply refused to be pinned. His surprising display of spirit led the staff to encourage him to try out for his middle school wrestling team.

During the next school year, Christopher's life was turned around by his wrestling experiences. He resolutely lost 40 pounds (and even more later) to meet the weight classification in which he wrestled; his profanity and asocial behaviors were reduced to an insignificant level; and he even became somewhat popular among his classmates at school. He continued to wrestle throughout high school.

▀

Takisha, a Harvard Law School student who had graduated near the top of her class at a high school for the performing arts, was an outstanding sprinter on the high school track team and was among the most popular students in her class. She dressed well, looked terrific, and had her professional sights set on a law partnership. The casual observer might ask how a girl who was born with extremely low vision ever developed such great skills, self-confidence, and motivation.

In part she got them from her mother, who encouraged her to pursue her dreams, and from her innate intellect and skills. However, Takisha had also received weekly visits when she was 3 through 5 years of age from Ms. Welty, an orientation and mobility specialist, who helped her overcome poor walking posture caused by fear of colliding with objects around her. She also received services in middle school from Mr. Davis, an adapted physical education teacher, who noticed her athletic potential. He worked with her and the track coach to help her learn the adaptive running skills that eventually led to her outstanding track performance. When Takisha moved from middle school to high school, the level of competition she faced in city high school track leagues overwhelmed her. But the high school track coach, Ms. Wiley, along with Mr. Davis, spent extra hours with her each night at practice, working with her to develop her sprinting style to a level that gave her the confidence to continue and to succeed. All these "victories," obtained with the help of professionals, were as responsible for her self-confidence as were her innate skills. ▀

How is it that Christopher and Takisha, who were both born with visual impairments and grew up in the same city, had such different experiences when it came to participating in physical activity? Many factors influence an individual's abilities, personality, and involvement in the activities of life. In the case of individuals with visual impairments—those who are blind or have severe vision loss (low vision) and who may have additional sensory or other impairments—the impact of vision loss may be profound. Often, visual impairments can interfere directly with an individual's ability to gather the information required to learn necessary concepts and physical skills. However, as the stories of Christopher and Takisha as well as others presented in this chapter demonstrate, a number of other factors affect a person's involvement in physical activities and sports. Additional barriers related to social attitudes and institutionalized bias, as well as receipt or lack of services, may preclude exposure to physical education, sports, and physical activity and the resulting development of the skills necessary for individuals with visual impairments and additional disabilities to be physically active (Lieberman, Houston-Wilson, & Kozub, 2002; Lieberman & MacVicar, 2003; Lieberman, Robinson, & Rollheiser, 2006; Stuart, Lieberman, & Hand, 2006).

WHY PHYSICAL ACTIVITY?

Physical activity can be defined as "movement of the human body that results in the expenditure of energy at a level above the resting metabolic rate" (Anshel et al., 1991, p. 113). Physical activity is important to the health and well-being of every individual. For all of us, including individuals with visual impairments, physical activity not only provides the benefits of increased physical stamina and fitness but also improves self-esteem, perception of one's own competence, one's sense of autonomy, and relationship skills (described in detail in Chapter 3).

These benefits are enjoyed most fully when an individual has the ability to participate in physical activities and sports across the lifespan. However, the most critical time to pursue access to physical activity may be during early childhood, when physical and other important skills are being developed. People who do not have access to learning physical skills as youngsters can learn them later in life, but learning as an adult may not be as effective as learning as a child. Because of their contribution to overall health and fitness, skills in this area need to be encouraged from the start of a child's life. Moreover, as explained further in Chapter 3, for students with visual impairments, participation in physical education is an important component of the expanded core curriculum—the additional areas of education needed by students who are visually impaired that are essential to their well-being and independence (Sapp & Hatlen, 2010). By providing a student with increased physical strength and skill and the opportunities for social and group interaction, a well-rounded, individualized program of physical education can support a child in pursuit of each of the areas of this essential curriculum, which also includes compensatory or access skills, career education, independent living skills, orientation and mobility skills and concepts, social interaction skills, self-determination skills, use of assistive technology, and sensory efficiency skills.

As already noted, the barriers to participation in physical education and activities encountered by individuals with visual impairments can be numerous and diverse. Some stem directly from visual impairment or additional disabilities; some relate to the often prejudicial attitudes of other human beings; some to children's fears, lack of knowledge of options, or their reluctance to try new things; some to families' fears or misunderstanding of the importance of physical fitness; others from a frequent lack of training about students with sensory disabilities in university physical education teacher preparation programs or to deficiencies in and constraints on public school systems and the services they provide. However, as also demonstrated in the vignettes of Christopher and Takisha, appropriate support from professionals, including instruction in concepts and skills necessary for physical activity, can enable individuals not only to overcome these barriers but also to excel athletically.

This book, therefore, is intended to be an essential sourcebook on the teaching of children and adults with visual impairments and deafblindness the skills that will enable them to participate in physical education, recreation, sports, and lifelong health and fitness activities. The emphasis is on methods for encouraging and providing physical activities to individuals throughout the lifespan. Although individuals with visual impairments frequently have additional physical, sensory, intellectual, and cognitive disabilities, this book is focused on those with whom the authors have the greatest experience: children and adults with visual impairments and deafblindness—that is, who have vision loss or both vision and hearing loss. It is to be hoped that in the future, the provision of physical education and activities to students with additional disabling conditions will be addressed.

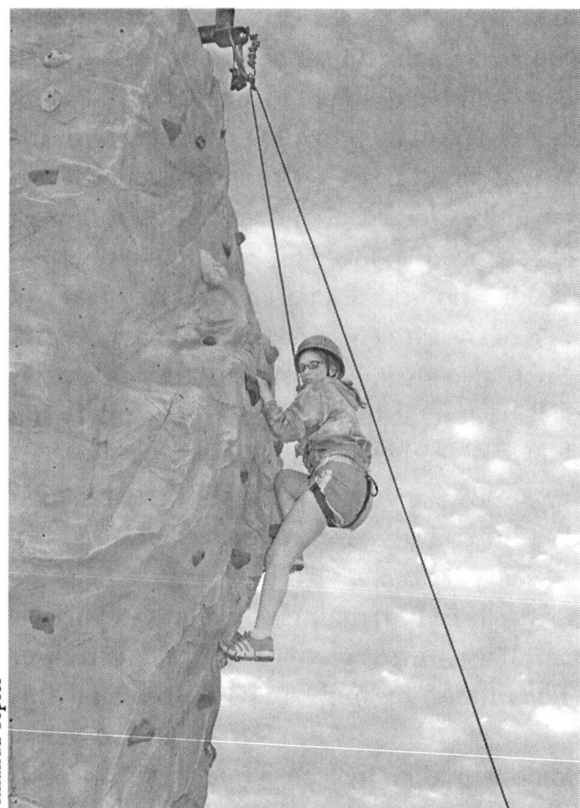
Amanda Tepfer

Rock climbing. Children and adults with visual impairments or deafblindness can participate in almost any physical activity, given the right instruction and adaptations, and have the potential to excel athletically.

VISUAL IMPAIRMENT, DEAFBLINDNESS, AND PHYSICAL ACTIVITY

Visual impairment or deafblindness does not in itself cause poor physical skills or lack of fitness. In a variety of ways, however, a visual or auditory disability can create obstacles to participating in physical activity. For example, the inability to see movement can affect the development of physical skills. Impediments to physical activity for individuals with visual impairments or deafblindness may vary depending on when in the person's life the vision or dual sensory loss developed, as well as the family, social, and organizational environments in which they find themselves. This chapter examines a variety of factors that may have an impact on the individual.

Factors Related to Early Vision Loss

The effects of severe or total vision loss on early childhood development may vary greatly from child to child, and are discussed in Chapter 6. In general, however, the early onset of a severe visual impairment or blindness can interfere to some extent with every area of human development: the affective domain (emotional, social, and personality development), the cognitive domain (an individual's body of knowledge as well as conceptual knowledge of such constructs as objects and space), and the motor domain (physical and movement skills) (Fazzi & Klein, 2002; Ferrell, 2000, 2011; Houwen, Hartman, & Visscher, 2009; Houwen, Visscher, Hartman, & Lemmink, 2007; Houwen, Visscher, Lemmink, & Hartman, 2008; Lowenfeld, 1973; Scholl, 1986; Strickling & Pogrund, 2002).

Vision is the primary sense through which individuals typically receive the majority of their input from and information about the surrounding environment. The quality and quantity of information obtained by many children with visual impairments during early development may be reduced because it is entirely or mostly gathered through the somewhat limited sensory modalities of audition and touch (Fazzi & Klein, 2002; Lowenfeld, 1973). (Although touch will be discussed in detail in Chapter 2, it should be noted that use of the word *touch* here refers not only to the sense of touch through which one's hands and fingers are used to identify objects but also to a more complex form of sensory feedback from the body's muscles, ligaments, and tendons, known as *kinesthetic touch* [Carello and Turvey, 2000; Heller, 2000; Millar, 2000], which also assists in learning certain physical skills.) Therefore, deliberate instruction in motor skills and spatial concepts may be required to overcome these limits.

Motor Skill Development

The need for a child with a visual impairment to learn complex movements, such as throwing or jumping, without the benefit of visual observation seems especially problematic because of the role that incidental learning plays in development of concepts and skills related to physical activity. *Incidental learning* is that which takes place automatically, perhaps unconsciously, through observation of persons and activities within the surrounding environment (Zabelski, 2007). Most young would-be athletes watch their heroes carefully and try to emulate the details of their throwing, running, or swimming styles; children with visual impairments do not have that advantage. They often cannot get even a rough idea of the motions used in throwing, running, or swimming, let alone the particulars of a style, solely through observation—whether visual or through listening or touching (Pogrund and Fazzi, 2002; Ponchillia, 2008). Physical skills can be taught to such children and, if they receive preschool services from a teacher of students with visual impairments who has been educated in the development of early physical skills, the difficulties caused by the barrier to incidental learning can be somewhat alleviated (Pogrund & Fazzi, 2002). Techniques for teaching physical skills to young children are described in Chapter 6.

Concept Development

Although this book is concerned primarily with motor skills, the early development of the affective and cognitive domains also indirectly relates to physical skills such as movement. Poor development of certain cognitive concepts can result in poor movement skills, even for children who have a high level of motor skill development (Fazzi & Klein, 2002; Ferrell, 2000; Houwen, Hartman, & Visscher, 2009; Houwen, Visscher, Hartman, & Lemmink, 2007; Houwen, Visscher, Lemmink, & Hartman, 2008; Lowenfeld, 1973; Scholl, 1986; Strickling & Pogrund, 2002). Concepts of objects and physical space, for example, are aspects of the cognitive domain that affect an individual's ability to move and interact with objects. As a result, children with visual impairments who have outstanding physical skills may still not move as well as expected within a given environment, because they lack understanding of particular related cognitive or affective concepts. Instruction in such concepts from a teacher of students with visual impairments or an orientation and mobility specialist, starting in a child's earliest days, is therefore crucial.

Object Permanence

The concept of object permanence—the understanding that objects continue to exist even when they cannot be seen, heard, or touched (Piaget, 1981, and discussed further in Chapter 6)—can have a dramatic effect on movement skills, as illustrated by the examples of Mykala and Tyrone:

■ *Mykala, a typically sighted toddler, has learned that objects such as her fuzzy teddy bear exist. She squeals with delight when her bear is handed to her or when she randomly encounters it. Thus, Mykala has reached a level of cognitive development known as object recognition (Ginsberg & Opper, 1969), in which she understands that objects exist separately from herself and can recognize them. Mykala's mother always places her bear in a group of stuffed animals near her door, and Mykala has come to understand that the bear is there, even if she can't see it from where she is in the room. She has thus demonstrated that she has also reached the developmental level of object permanence (Ginsberg & Opper, 1969), knowing that objects continue to exist even when she can't directly perceive them. If she wants her bear but does not see it, she automatically begins to move toward the place where the bear is always kept and expected to be. This pattern of wanting the bear and then moving to get it provides a good deal of purposeful movement within her room.*

■

Tyrone, a child of similar age and physical ability, has extremely limited vision. Tyrone understands the concept of object recognition; he too smiles with glee when he has his fuzzy bear. However, he does not yet understand the concept of object permanence, as he gives no indication that he is aware of his bear's existence when he is not holding it. Consequently, Tyrone has no tendency to move around his room looking for his bear or his other toys when they are located anywhere outside the limited range of his vision or his touch. Tyrone's mother has expressed concern about Tyrone's "lethargy" to the occupational therapist, because she assumes his lack of movement is due to a physical problem. In fact, however, Tyrone's inactivity results from a conceptual difficulty, not a physical one. ■

Some studies (Bigelow, 1992) indicate that a lack of understanding of the concept of object permanence may be a relatively common source of delayed movement in children with severe visual impairment, since without awareness of objects' existence they are not motivated to move to retrieve them. Bigelow suggested that giving objects an auditory presence—for example, by equipping Tyrone's bear with a sound beacon—might help children such as Tyrone establish the concept of object permanence more readily, because they could monitor an object's comings and goings into, through, and out of their immediate environment.

Spatial Concepts

Considering that delayed development of a relatively simple cognitive concept such as object permanence can have such a significant effect on movement skills, imagine the severity of the limitations that might result from conceptual difficulties in more complex concepts related to space. If toddlers with severe visual impairments are to develop into physically active children, they need to come to understand space through a sequence starting with body concepts and extending to the spatial concepts required to move freely within environments ranging from a modern traffic intersection to a soccer field. The steps in this learning sequence are the following:

1. Body concepts
2. Self-to-object concepts
3. Object-to-object concepts
4. Map concepts, or cognitive mapping (Guth, Rieser, & Ashmead, 2010)

Very young children first learn about their bodies, such as the names of their body parts and the body's planes (that is, left and right and front and back). In general, a visual impairment tends to interfere little with the development of such body concepts. Learning then moves away from a focus on the self and centers on the relationship of the self to objects in the environment, and then on the still more complex concept of how any two or more objects relate to one another in space. Object-to-object concept development is especially difficult if a severe visual impairment is present, because when objects are out of tactile or visual range a child has no sensory input available to monitor the location of objects and how they relate to one another (unless the objects happen to emit a sound). The last and most complex step in the developmental sequence of learning about space—map concepts, also called cognitive mapping—is to understand the relationship of all the parts of a complex environment in order to move through space effectively, whether that environment is a city block, the intersection of two streets, or a sports complex.

Understanding how a variety of unseen objects relate to one another—for example, the relationship of a volleyball net to boundary lines on a gym floor as well as to the door to the locker room and the bleachers along the wall—is a complex task requiring that all the possible objects in a given environment be held in a single conceptual framework, without sensory feedback from all the objects. It is relatively common to encounter gaps in the conceptual knowledge of individuals who experienced blindness or severe visual impairment at or shortly following birth. Ponchillia and Ponchillia (1996) described the case of an individual who demonstrated sound self-to-object concepts but who lacked understanding of object-to-object concepts. When starting from her apartment door, she could locate her couch or her favorite chair, but when sitting in the chair, she did not know the location of the couch, unless she first returned to the apartment door. She clearly understood the location of each object, but she could not conceptualize how they related to one another in space.

Movement and Sports Concepts

More complex concepts relating to movement through space and sports activity, including concepts of space awareness and effort, are usually learned during physical education classes starting when children reach elementary school. Because students with visual impairments or deafblindness often do not receive physical education instruction, as discussed in more detail later in this chapter, they frequently do not have a good grasp of these concepts, and this can hamper their ability to learn more complex physical skills. Professionals working with children or adults who are visually impaired or deafblind need to be aware that they may require additional instruction in these concepts before they can participate successfully in many physical activities.

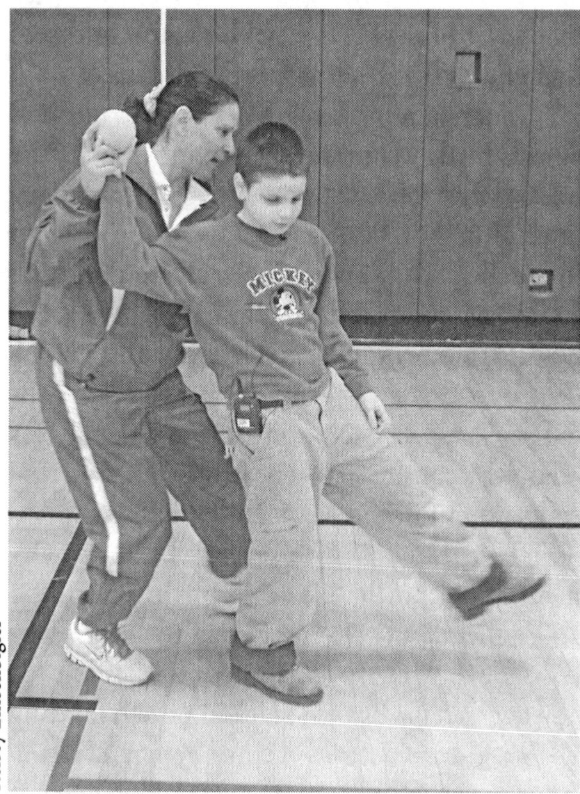

Kelsey Linsenbigler

Teaching an overhand throw to a student using physical guidance. With appropriate instruction, students can master such basic motor skills that they may have not learned through observation and imitation.

Space Awareness Concepts. *Space awareness* relates specifically to movement or so-called locomotor skills that are taught in the physical education curriculum and are the basis for concepts needed for sports and other physical activities. Some writers (Graham, Holt/Hale, & Parker, 2009) theorized that space awareness is prerequisite to learning locomotor skills. They subdivided space awareness into five categories (see Sidebar 1.1):

- location
- direction
- level
- pathway
- extension

Location refers to the individual's place in space. Its components are self-space, which includes a range of skills, from a knowledge of one's body parts to that space reached without moving from a given starting point, and *general space,* which refers to all the space away from self-space that is reachable by locomotion, such as the remainder of a room or playground in which an activity is taking place. Location space is similar to the spatial concepts described in the previous section.

The remaining four categories of space awareness define the relationship of the child's body to the space. *Direction* involves all the possible dimensional movements of a person or his

SIDEBAR 1.1

Categories of Space Awareness

- Location: One's place in space
  - Self-space: Space including body parts and the space that can be reached without leaving one's starting point
  - General space: Space in the room or area that can be reached by locomotion
- Direction: The dimensional possibility into which the body or its parts move or aim to move, expressed in relation to the self rather than the room
  - Forward-backward (generally learned first)
  - Left-right (more complex and cognitively difficult than forward-backward)
  - Clockwise-counterclockwise (also learned after forward-backward)
- Level: Height of space relevant to a standing student
  - Low level: Space below the knees
  - Medium level: Space between knees and shoulders
  - High level: Space above the shoulders
- Pathway: An imaginary design that the body or its parts or a ball or other objects create on the floor when moving through space
  - Straight
  - Curved
  - Zigzag
- Extension: Relative space between body and body parts, such as distance of arms and legs from body
  - Near extension
  - Far extension

Source: Based on G. Graham, S. A. Holt/Hale, and M. A. Parker, *Children Moving: A Reflective Approach to Teaching Physical Education* 8th ed. (New York: McGraw Hill, 2009).

or her limbs, such up and down, forward and backward, right and left, clockwise and counter-clockwise. *Level* describes the areas of a person in a standing position, with *low level* being the space below the knees, *medium level* the space between the knees and the shoulders, and *high level* the space above the shoulders. The concept of *pathway* refers to patterns or trajectories of the child's movement or that of a thrown or struck object, such as a zigzag pattern walked across the gym floor, the arc of a basketball shot, and the horizontal arc of a pitcher's curveball. Finally, the concept of *extension* refers to the size of movements of the body or its parts in space, for example, small versus large arm circles or tucked versus open forward rotating dives.

Skills in self-space are typically taught to children first (Graham, Holt/Hale, & Parker, 2009). Then learning proceeds through complex combinations of body movements through generalized space, with varying directions, levels, pathways, and extensions.

Effort Concepts. The concept of *effort* is also fundamental to the physical education curriculum. Graham and colleagues (2001, 2007) describe three aspects of the concept of effort: *time,* the rate at which a movement is accomplished (fast or slow); *force,* the degree of strength with which a movement is done; and *flow,* the degree of control one exhibits over the course of a movement. (Running wildly down a hill is considered *free flow* and running down the same hill with a beanbag on top of the head is *bound flow.*)

If Bigelow's (1992) contention is correct that the lack of the relatively simple concept of object permanence inhibits the movement of children with early-onset visual impairments, one can only imagine what missing all or part of these complex concepts that form the basis for the physical education curriculum would have on a child with a visual impairment.

Although at present there appears to be no research or literature to tell us, the authors' experiences at their sports camps (described in the section on Consequences of Limited Physical Education) point to severe limitations created by this lack of instruction. Chapter 9 contains an example of how appropriate, targeted instruction in a sports setting can serve to remediate such limitations.

Factors Related to Early-Onset Deafness

If early-onset visual impairment can have a wide-ranging effect on individuals, influencing such critical aspects of development as the learning of concepts, language, and motor skills, the early onset of a severe hearing impairment or deafness also has developmental effects (Axelrod, 2004). Skills vary widely among people with deafblindness; in general, the interplay among the age of onset, degree of sensory loss, and stability of each loss are the primary factors in the extent to which deafblindness may affect a child's development (Huebner, Prickett, Welch, & Joffee, 1995). Forms of deafblindness may be thought to fall into four broad categories that may assist teachers and other professionals in understanding a child's or adult's needs and identifying helpful instructional modifications:

1. Born with congenital deafness but later develops acquired visual impairment. The most well-known example is Usher syndrome, which is also the leading cause of deafblindness in the United States. It combines congenital deafness with acquired retinitis pigmentosa, a group of inherited eye conditions that cause deterioration of the retina (National Eye Institute and the National Institute on Deafness and Other Communication Disorders, n.d.).
2. Born with both hearing and vision impairments. CHARGE syndrome, a complex genetic disorder resulting in holes in one or both eyes, narrowed or blocked nasal passages, cranial nerve problems, hearing impairment, and other abnormalities that are present at birth, is a frequent cause.
3. Born with a visual impairment but later acquires deafness.
4. Acquires both hearing and vision loss later in life after hearing, speech, and visual abilities have been developed.

Individuals whose deafblindness falls within the first two categories differ from those in the second two because congenital deafness or severe hearing impairments have common consequences, particularly to language development (Axelrod, 2004). For example, those with early-onset deafness are likely to have learned sign language as a communication method, while those who became hard of hearing later in life may use both speech and written communication for expressive communication.

Those with early hearing impairments commonly face similar barriers as those with early-onset visual impairments, but they may also experience significant difficulties in communication and interpersonal interactions because of their hearing loss (Axelrod, 2004). Consequently, their interaction with their caregivers and teachers may be affected, resulting in further difficulties in the areas of connection and attachment, feelings of security, interpersonal relationships, learning, and communication

(Axelrod, 2004). Communication with students who are deafblind is discussed in Chapter 4.

The development of communication skills includes the learning of turn-taking during parent-infant interactions, in which the infant acts, is reacted to, and in turn responds. This early pattern of statement and response is the model for later communication. A visual impairment can interfere with easy back-and-forth sharing, and deafness can interfere with it significantly as the child's parents or caregivers may have difficulty recognizing the child's communication signals, which may differ from those of typical infants, and, conversely, the diminished sensory input received by the child affects his or her ability to recognize parental signals. Since harmonious interaction between caregiver and child may affect the development of brain structures and functions that regulate emotions, learning, and psychosocial development, children with limited ability to receive and interpret sensory information may demonstrate strong emotions and unusual social behaviors that may pose barriers to learning (Axelrod, 2004).

Factors Related to Acquired Vision or Hearing Loss

Osmund, a 15-year-old high school freshman, has mild cerebral palsy, which affects the strength in his left leg. However, his determination allowed him to become an outstanding soccer goalie on both his high school varsity and local club teams. He is also popular at school, president of the freshman class, and active in school plays. In addition, he has been on the honor roll through middle school and his first semester in high school.

One day when he was reading a book, the bill of his cap accidentally slipped down and covered his left eye. To his amazement, he couldn't see the print with his right eye. The family optometrist referred him to a retinal ophthalmologist in a nearby city, who diagnosed the problem as Leber's hereditary optic neuropathy. The ophthalmologist told his mother and father that the disease would likely take all of Osmund's central vision in the affected eye and that it might also affect the left eye in the future, possibly even within a few weeks or months.

At first, Osmund took the news surprisingly well and even told his friends and classmates about his condition. He also spent hours on the Internet looking for cures. After months of fruitless visits to specialists and holistic medicine practitioners around the country, he became withdrawn and extremely unhappy. Although he continues to attend his classes, he is not completing his homework, is doing poorly on exams, has resigned from student government, and has pulled away from all of his friends.

His teachers and the school counselors became concerned, and even though he was not yet legally blind, the counselor asked if he would like to receive lessons from the school district's teacher of students with visual impairments. Osmund responded, "She can't help me get my vision back, can she? Of course she can't, and I can't do anything without it. I'm going to flunk my classes or maybe even just drop out of school! I just can't do anything without my vision! What am I going to do?"

James, a 28-year-old man in a rehabilitation program, has lost all but 2 degrees of central vision in his right eye as a result of acute glaucoma. He was an avid bowler with a 182 average in his weekly bowling league before the onset of his vision loss. He initially refused the recreation therapist's invitation to go on the rehabilitation center's Tuesday night bowling outing, but after two weeks at the center, he finally agreed to go with the others.

The recreation therapist accompanied James to the bowling alley the first time. She ascertained that he was able to see the step up onto the lane itself, the arrows and dots on the surface of the lane, and the ball return mechanism, and he could safely get on and off of the lane. However, he could not see the pins.

James was excited to start bowling, but after four frames, he had a score of 5 and finished the first game at 43. He was reluctant to bowl again, but after much encouragement from the recreation therapist, he bowled a second and third game with scores of 64 and 78. On the way back to the rehabilitation center, James told the therapist that he didn't want to bowl any more, because it was just too depressing. He said, "How would you like it if you once bowled 180 and the best you could do now was not even 80?" The therapist expressed an understanding of his frustration but also explained that it was common to start below 100 and that it really wasn't fair to him to compare his old scores to the new ones. She encouraged James to think of bowling as a competition with himself for now and that if he kept improving, he might want to join the local bowling league. In time, James did return, achieved an average of 118, and joined a local league for blind bowlers and another one consisting of sighted bowlers. ■

The barriers to participation in physical activity are significantly different for individuals who have experienced permanent and significant change, such as loss of vision, hearing, or both, after having use of these senses for a number of years than they are for children who have congenital visual impairments or deafblindness. These individuals have already learned spatial concepts and motor skills as a sighted and hearing individual, and may even be accomplished athletes. Although they may require the same kinds of adaptations and modifications to the activities in order to perform them, some of the barriers that prevent individuals such as Osmund from participating in sports and other physical activities may have more to do with their reactions and lack of adjustment to their vision loss. Therefore, it is crucial that teachers and other people who work with these individuals understand the process of adjusting to an acquired visual impairment so that they can help them overcome their resistance to physical activity, as the recreation therapist was able to do with James. Knowing the common behaviors associated with adjustment enables teachers to utilize techniques that foster learning and promote growth.

Reaction and Adjustment to Loss

For many individuals, typical responses to a major loss, such as the loss of vision or hearing or both, the death of a loved one, or the breakup of a marriage, may include a rapid and significant decrease in self-image or self-worth that can leave the person feeling as if he or she has little value or worth (Livneh, 1991; Tuttle, 1984). Adjustment to such loss is not considered to be a choice; rather, it is a process of recovering the former level of self-image (Livneh, 1991). Theorists and clinical researchers working in the area of adjustment to disability hold that psychological defense mechanisms are used in the process of adjustment to move people through a set of progressive stages that can culminate in adaptation to the loss (Livneh, 1991; Tuttle, 1984). Because psychological defense mechanisms have an unconscious aspect that generally exhibits itself in some degree of irrational thought and counterproductive behaviors, instructors cannot use simple problem-solving techniques to foster growth; rather, they need to understand how the psychological defense mechanisms function in the adjustment process before they can adequately help foster positive adaptation to loss.

A psychological defense mechanism can be defined as an unconscious distortion of reality that reduces painful feeling and conflict through the use of automatic and habitual responses (Clark, 1991). Simply put, it is an unconscious psychological reaction to an unacceptable reality—in this case, the loss of sight, hearing, or both. Common defense mechanisms include the following:

- *denial,* characterized by ignoring the problem at hand and exemplified by a statement, such as, "Well yes, I can't see anything now, but I'll be okay after my upcoming surgery."
- *withdrawal,* characterized by decreasing one's need for and involvement in social interaction with others and exemplified by a statement, such as, "I don't want to hang around with all my old friends; I just want to stay here and listen to my iPod."
- *regression,* characterized by returning in one's mind to a safer time or place and exemplified by a statement such as, "I'm giving up on all this modern music. I just got a bunch of '70s downloads, got my old '70s haircut and a bunch of my old college clothes out of the attic. I'll live in the past, a place that treated me right." (Clark, 1991)

Tuttle (1984) suggested that children with congenital impairments experience similar reactions to loss as do adults, beginning at the moment they first become aware of their visual limitations, which commonly occurs during play with sighted children.

The Unified Model of Adjustment

A unified stage model of adjustment to loss was developed by Livneh (1991), following an exhaustive analysis of the models of adjustment proposed in the literature. Livneh's unified model posited five stages of adjustment—initial reaction, defense mobilization, initial realization, retaliation, and reintegration (described in Sidebar 1.2)—and was based on the following set of assumptions, among others:

- The onset of a traumatic event has a sudden, unexpected, and massively extensive effect on a person's life
- Adjustment is dynamic, and adaptation is the desired outcome of the process.
- Normal adaptation to loss involves a sequence of psychosocial development stages.
- The initiation and progression of the stages of adjustment to disability occur more or less automatically.

SIDEBAR 1.2

The Stages of Livneh's Unified Model of Adjustment

Stage I: Initial Reaction

In the initial reaction stage, the person generally responds to the loss with a shock-like state that begins with numbness of thought and action and ends with frenetic actions and anxieties. The anxieties related to vision loss can be realistic ones about future job prospects, transportation difficulties, and child-rearing challenges, or they can be irrational fears, such as a terror of falling into an abyss while walking or being abandoned by loved ones because of the impairment. Rehabilitation and education professionals may not often see individuals experiencing this early stage.

Stage II: Defense Mobilization

Defense mobilization entails the first use of psychological defense mechanisms, typically including denial, often exhibited with irrational statements about how the individual's sight will soon be restored, even if there is no medical possibility of this restoration. The strong sense of conviction in such beliefs often creates a feeling of comfort and safety.

This might be called the "I don't need" stage, because many people may reject offers of services during this time, based on the "fact" that they will soon have their sight back. An effective way for teachers and rehabilitation professionals to respond to "I don't need" statements is to offer services just to meet the individual's immediate needs while waiting for the hoped-for improvement. Confronting an individual in denial by trying to convince him or her that "your sight isn't coming back" can result in loss of rapport with the person and should be avoided until a relationship of trust is established (Clark, 1991).

Stage III: Initial Realization

Initial realization occurs when denial finally breaks down and an individual becomes aware that the loss is permanent and irreversible. This stage is characterized by depression, withdrawal, and unhappiness. Anger, though felt, may be held inside. The authors call this the "I can't" stage, because during this time individuals commonly feel they are helpless and often believe they will never be functional again. Ironically, even though this stage brings sadness, the teacher or rehabilitation professional should be encouraged to see the movement from the false comfort of denial to the unhappiness of this stage, because this movement represents progress in adjustment.

Stage IV: Retaliation

During the retaliation stage the inner anger held during the initial realization is let out. This stage is characterized by outward anger, blaming others, and the use of strongly aggressive defense mechanisms. The authors term this the "I won't" stage, and it can be identified by the individual's refusal to participate in adapted instruction or programming and a general belligerence in attitude. Here again, these behaviors may likely signify growth and may be welcomed in spite of their negative aspects.

Stage V: Reintegration

The fifth and final stage, reintegration, is characterized by cooperation, willingness to participate in instruction or rehabilitation activities, creative thinking about how to overcome the limitations of the disability, and plans for the future. The defense mechanisms used during this stage are in general mild, and the thought process exhibited is rational and sound. This is called the "I will" stage.

Source: Based on H. Livneh, "A Unified Approach to Existing Models of Adaptation to Disability: A Model of Adaptation," in R. P. Marinelli and A. E. Dell Orto (Eds.), *The Psychological and Social Impact of Disability,* 3d ed. (New York: Springer, 1991), pp. 111–138.

- Success in making the transition through the different psychosocial stages of adaptation produces increased psychosocial growth and maturity.
- Although most people experience most of the stages, not all people will exhibit all of them.
- The process of adaptation does not necessarily consist of discrete and categorically exclusive stages, and the stages may fluctuate, blend, or overlap.
- Most stages may and do fluctuate in their length as a result of individual differences and may extend from hours or days to months or years.
- Not all individuals who become disabled reach the theoretical end point of the adaptation process, the so-called final adjustment; many will be "stuck" at a certain phase along the adaptation continuum.

Knowing about the irrational nature of thought during the early stages of adjustment and that stages have recognizable characteristics has practical value to instructors. For example, knowing that psychological defense mechanisms can cause people to act out angrily or make highly critical statements helps teachers understand that both are natural consequences of the healing process and enables them to avoid internalizing the anger or the statements.

Being able to identify an individual's stage of adjustment to vision or hearing loss gives an instructor or other helper a way of monitoring growth along the adjustment continuum through change in an individual's behaviors, even when the behaviors on the surface do not appear indicative of growth. Although a detailed treatment of the stages of adjustment to loss is beyond the scope of this book, practitioners will have little trouble spotting when most people move from the defense mobilization or "I don't need" stage to the initial realization or "I can't" stage, or the important and dramatic change to the "I will" stage of reintegration. (For more information about identifying stages of adjustment, see Livneh [1991].)

The psychological defenses employed in the early stages of loss of vision or hearing can become obstacles to learning methods of resuming physical activities. The behavior of Osmund, introduced at the beginning of this section, reflects the depths of the "I can't" stage of the unified model. Osmund believes that his successful sports competition days are gone and has withdrawn to avoid having to face the challenges. Professionals working with individuals like Osmund need to make every effort to get them reinvolved and help them move from feeling that their impairment is an "unacceptable reality" to viewing it as something that they can accept. When Osmund learns that he can cope with his vision loss, just as he has with his cerebral palsy, he will move on to an "I will" stage. Without a teacher's intervention, however, he might linger in the "I can't" or "I won't" stages. As teachers and rehabilitation professionals support and encourage Osmund to become involved in his life and activities again, he may be unhappy at first, but as his feelings that he is confronted with an unacceptable reality vanish, his negative behaviors should diminish as well. He will begin the healthy process of coping, eventually coming to view his visual impairment simply as one of his attributes.

There has been some debate over when in the process of adjustment educational or rehabilitation services should be initiated. Early writers, including Carroll (1961), felt that rehabilitation services should be withheld until people are "ready" for services; that is, they must have reached Stage 3, the Initial Realization stage, and have "accepted" their impairment. However, Dodds (2006), Tuttle (1984), and the authors feel that services should be initiated as quickly as possible, regardless of level of adjustment. Although convincing people who are in early stages of adjustment to accept services is sometimes difficult, under most circumstances, the sooner they get started on the road to gaining adaptive skills, the sooner they lose the belief that a visual or hearing impairment is an unacceptable reality, which in turn eliminates the need for psychological defense mechanisms and promotes adjustment. As adaptive skills are learned, such as alternative methods of reading and writing, getting around independently, or playing soccer, it becomes clear that coping with reality is quite possible in spite of any degree of vision loss.

The encouragement provided by instructors is also key to helping someone regain his or her former level of physical activity. The vignette of James at the beginning of this section shows how professional intervention is often needed during the reintroduction of former recreation or sports activities and how important well-timed encouragement from a professional can be in helping individuals with acquired visual impairments or deafblindness become motivated to participate in physical activities.

OTHER BARRIERS TO PHYSICAL ACTIVITY

Attitudinal Factors

Antwan, a 30-year-old man who lost most of his vision as a result of long-term diabetes, had excelled in basketball as a youngster. Until his sight loss, he worked out on a regular basis to maintain a trim, muscular physique and took great pride in his physical appearance. After becoming totally blind, Antwan entered a 10-week residential rehabilitation program to learn alternative ways of dealing with everyday tasks of reading and writing, caring for personal and household needs, and traveling in his environment. He studied adaptive techniques for reading and writing, personal management, and recreation with the help of a vision rehabilitation therapist and training in the use of a long cane from an orientation and mobility specialist.

After completing his rehabilitation program, he moved to a new community where he had obtained a job managing a vending machine operation. The first thing he did for himself after the move was to look up a reputable health club so he could resume his workout regimen. He purchased a membership over the Internet and showed up for the first time on a weeknight after work. To his great surprise, the owner stopped him after he had taken a first few steps in the door and said, "I'm sorry, but I'm afraid you can't work out here. This place is filled with big machines and is far too dangerous for someone who's blind! You'll break a leg or something and I'll be facing a big lawsuit!" Antwan responded, "But I used to work out all the time at a gym back home." "Well, that wasn't here, and it's not going to be here," the owner replied.

Antwan, not having the confidence in himself or his skills to argue, gave up and left. To meet his goal of working out regularly but avoid the barrier he had encountered at the health club, he took out a loan and bought some inexpensive equipment for his apartment.

Maria had lost most of her vision by age 35 from a hereditary disease that left her with only a small pinpoint of sight in the center of her visual field and that caused her to be totally blind at night. She had grown up training horses and riding them in jumping competitions, but when her vision worsened significantly, she gave up riding and training. She entered a rehabilitation program at that time, which, in addition to the usual skills training, offered a comprehensive therapeutic recreation program.

While at the rehabilitation facility where she was learning the methods that helped her to read and write, travel independently, and take care of her personal and home care needs and to adjust to her vision loss, Maria regained her old confidence in working with horses through the agency's equestrian recreation program. With the help of the occupational therapist, she worked out adaptations that gave her the ability and confidence to return to her old training and riding roles.

Maria went back to her home community following her rehabilitation program, where she worked in a travel agency booking tours. She also applied for a position as a part-time instructor at a therapeutic horseback-riding program. The owner of the stable turned her application down, saying: "I'm sorry, but I just don't know how you could possibly do the job with such limited vision." Fortunately for Maria, her experience during rehabilitation taught her how to advocate for herself, and she explained in detail just how she would manage to do the required job duties. The owner was convinced to try her out, and Maria landed the job.

Additional access barriers to participation in physical activities can result from commonly held prejudicial attitudes about the capabilities of individuals who are blind or visually impaired. For example, it is well known that some people believe that individuals with disabilities are dependent on others or are not generally competent (Smart, 2009). Since such attitudes are represented in all segments of the population, it is reasonable to expect that they would be present in people in positions of authority, such as school administrators, fitness facility owners, coaches, and physical educators who have influence over students' and adults' activities. Such individuals who have negative attitudes about individuals with visual impairments might consciously or subconsciously limit access to school physical education programs, fitness centers, sports teams, and the like.

Faced with such negative attitudes, even skilled athletes such as Antwan may not be able to surmount the barrier to access. Whereas Maria's horseback riding lessons during rehabilitation gave her the confidence to challenge the director of the training facility, Antwan's rehabilitation services were not as comprehensive, and he was not comfortable enough with his skills to challenge the fitness center manager's rebuff. Antwan was also not made aware of sports and recreational resources outside the rehabilitation system. If he had been, perhaps he might have gotten involved in a local goalball, bowling, skiing, or tandem cycling club, or some other specialized program sponsored by an organization such as the United States Association of Blind Athletes (see Chapters 7 and 11).

For children, attitudinal barriers to inclusion in regular physical fitness activities are typically invisible, stemming from uninformed attitudes about the potential and abilities of children with visual impairments (Stuart, Lieberman, & Hand, 2006). In addition, a child's lack of skill, which can negatively affect his or her confidence and willingness to attempt an unfamiliar athletic activity, can in turn create a vicious cycle of never participating, and therefore never learning the necessary skills, and therefore continuing not to participate (Ponchillia, 1995). Families and teachers can play a significant role in this dynamic. Winnick (1985) reported that the negative attitudes and behaviors of a physical education teacher often affect a student's willingness to participate. The value placed by families on physical activity also appears to affect children's motivation to participate (Jacobs & Eccles, 1992; Lieberman, Haibach, & Schedlin, 2012; Stuart, 2003; Stuart, Lieberman, & Hand, 2006).

The Medical Model of Disability

One of the major sources of prejudicial attitudes is the way society has viewed disability in the past (Smart, 2009). For example, the traditional perspective or model through which disability has often been regarded is the so-called medical model (Smart, 2009), according to which any of a number of human conditions, ranging from disability to pregnancy to menopause, is seen as an illness to be treated. In this model, which is based on the traditional physician-patient relationship, people with a disability are seen as having a disorder or something wrong that needs to be corrected in order to render them functional. Thus, given Maria's extremely limited vision, which makes it difficult for her to see the boundaries of the horseback riding arena under its existing lighting conditions, the medical approach would focus on what Maria's disability has prevented her from doing—that is, seeing the arena. According to the medical model, since her eye condition cannot be corrected medically and she cannot view the arena under existing conditions, she cannot ride horses safely there. Since the medical model has been so pervasive in the thinking of the past, there is a tendency to generalize its application from the medical condition of lack of vision to the functional issue of competence (Smart, 2009). This negative belief can also spread to the person with the disability and become self-limiting (Smart 2009).

Environmental and Functional Models of Disability

More recently, the medical model of disability is being replaced by the environmental and functional models. The environmental model holds that barriers to the participation in society of people with disabilities generally result from limitations in the design of the environment rather than from the biological impairment. According to this model, the limitations of an individual such as Maria are caused by poor design, such as the poor visibility of the environment.

The functional model, the third paradigm through which disabilities may be viewed, holds that Maria's limitation stems from a lack of skills training or lack of access to equipment or a methodology that would enable her to navigate the arena. In this view, Maria could improve her ability to ride safely and efficiently through the arena either by receiving adequate adaptive skills training or by using an engineering solution, such as an electronic navigation device to monitor the boundary and other parameters of the arena. Today, many professionals think of disabilities in the context of the environmental and functional models. The chapters in this book that cover activity modifications are based on the environmental and functional models.

Lack of Professional Training

Lack of knowledge on the part of professionals about the abilities of individuals with visual impairments can also cause barriers to access. For example, physical educators may not have adequate training about how to teach adaptive physical skills, since university teacher preparation training programs in that field usually include little specific content regarding blindness or deafblindness (Lieberman et al., 2002). Likewise, an examination of personnel preparation program curricula in special education and visual impairment indicates a general lack of coursework in adapted physical education.

School-Related Barriers

Other barriers to students' participation in physical education in school relate to the nature of the education system in our society. The large size of many public school classes affects the ability of classroom teachers to attend to individual students with or without special needs, and resulting time constraints can also limit a child's access to responsive instruction. This is especially true for those who cannot keep up with the pace of the main body of the class (Goldfine, 1993; Trippe, 1996). Other aspects of students' visual impairments or deafblindness may also prevent students from benefiting from their physical education classes: they may not be able to see or hear demonstrations of activities and motor behaviors, they may lack the physical ability or cognitive concepts to participate in class, or they may have developed a negative attitude about their ability to participate in physical activities.

Another school-related barrier to students' participation and involvement is the difficulty of finding time for physical education classes in the usually overcrowded schedules of students who receive special services (Conroy, 2012). Often, the choice is to pull children out of a physical education class to participate in orientation and mobility instruction or to receive some other specialized service (Lieberman et al., 2002). The next section focuses on the effects that the lack of physical education provided in most school systems for students with visual impairments or deafblindness has on the students throughout their lives.

CONSEQUENCES OF LIMITED PHYSICAL EDUCATION

Takisha, introduced at the beginning of this chapter, represents a good example of how early intervention and physical skills instruction can affect a child born with a significant visual impairment, whereas Christopher during his pre-wrestling days is an example of what can happen when children do not receive instruction in physical skills. Takisha is fit and has solid physical and social skills; Christopher was overweight and had poor social and physical skills before he became involved in team sports. Much of Christopher's difficulty was attitudinal; that is, it related in part to his level of affective development, which acted as a barrier to involvement in sports activities. Christopher's increased involvement in sports resulted from a change in attitude brought on by a learning experience outside the usual education curriculum.

The consequences of restricted access to physical education can cause limitations for children in a variety of areas, including:

- concepts of movement and space
- physical skills
- health and fitness

As discussed earlier, some conceptual limitations and physical and motor difficulties may stem from the visual impairment itself. For example, early childhood developmental barriers caused by Christopher's having to learn object-to-object concepts with little or no visual feedback may have limited his ability to create mental images of increasingly complex environments. For example, he might be able to move from the door of the gym to equipment such as a pommel horse or parallel bars, but not to move directly from the pommel horse to the parallel bars without going back to the door first. In such cases, an individual might be able to visualize the route to each object, but not be able to create an image of the entire scene and locate items in relation to one another. The conceptual ability to hold an image in the mind's eye of something as complex as a high school track and field facility, with all of its various competition areas, vending stands, entrance gates, and other features and be able to move from one place to another is an extremely complicated task for students such as Christopher. As a consequence, such students may be able to move independently from one part of the facility to another, but it should be no surprise if they require assistance in some aspects of this task.

Concepts of Movement and Space

Lack of access to physical education classes can have significant consequences for concept development in children (Ponchillia, 2008). Although the effect of limited understanding among children with visual impairments of the concepts described earlier of space awareness and effort is virtually unreported in the literature, based on the observations of the authors at their summer sports camps, young participants with visual impairments seemed to have particular difficulty with space concepts of direction and extension and effort concepts of time and force. Often, these children exhibit somewhat similar behaviors. For example, when they are introduced to goalball, a sport in which a bell-filled ball is rolled across a volleyball court–sized area in an attempt to force it through three defensive players, children who are totally blind appear to know exactly where the audible ball is as it rolls across the gym floor. However, when playing defense, they commonly do not extend their arms to the degree necessary to reach the ball as it passes them. Instead of lying on their sides and extending knees, hips, shoulders, elbows, wrists, and fingers in a burst of speed to block the goalball, most stay fixed in their position on their hands and knees. Some make a reaching gesture with one hand toward the ball, but too frequently the effort is significantly limited in force, timing, and speed. Also, these children often throw the ball with little velocity, have difficulty lining up parallel along the raised lines of the goalball court, are not able to take steps with their throws, cannot transfer their weight from one foot to the other during a throw, and seldom extend their

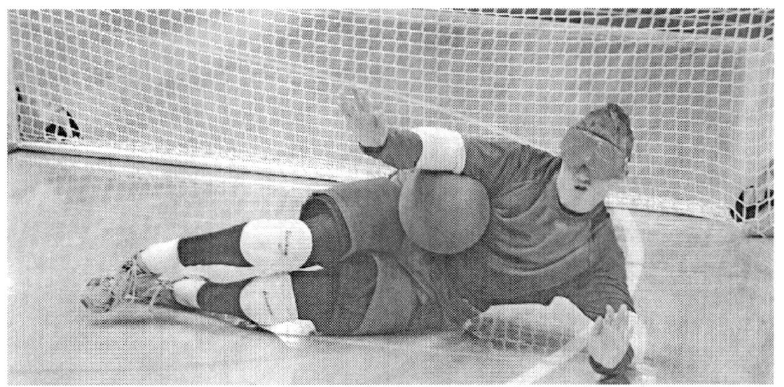

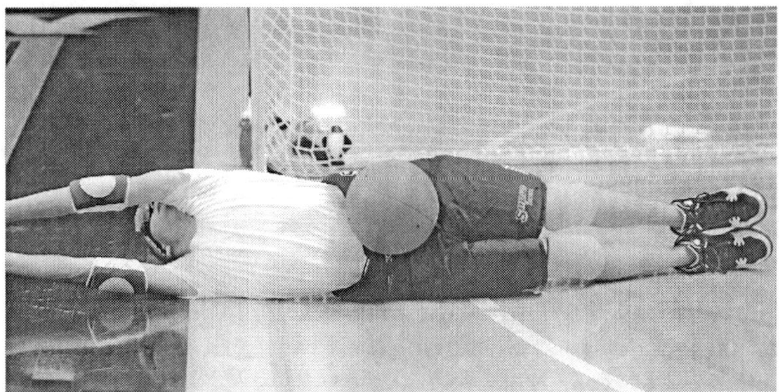

Chuck Comer

When attempting to block a moving goalball, young students with visual impairments frequently remain on hands and knees and reach tentatively toward the ball (top) instead of lying on their sides and extending knees, hips, shoulders, elbows, wrists, and fingers fully (bottom).

arms and legs fully in correct goalball blocking form.

Physical Skills

A number of observers have noted that the physical abilities of many children who have early-onset visual impairments differ somewhat from those of their classmates with unimpaired vision (Cratty, 1971; Fazzi & Klein, 2002; Ferrell, 2000, 2011; Fraiberg, 1968, 1977). The physical skills and body mechanics observable in many children who attend sports camps and who have had a visual impairment since early in their life often reflect developmental lags and an apparent lack of instruction in physical education. Many children appear to have a limited repertoire of skills. For example, in a typical group of 10- to 12-year-old campers who are asked, "Do you know how to throw a softball overhand?" most will answer "Yes." However, when asked to demonstrate the overhand throw, fewer than half can actually execute it (Ponchillia, Armbruster, & Wiebold, 2005). In addition, only a few—usually those whose families have either

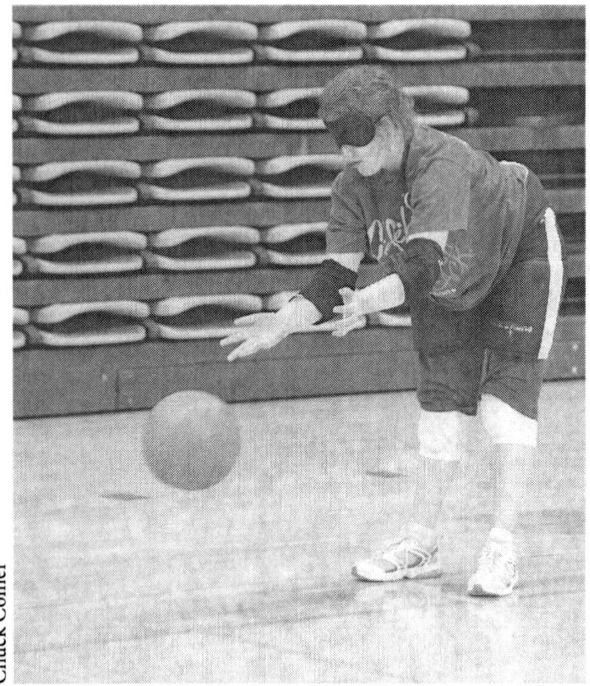

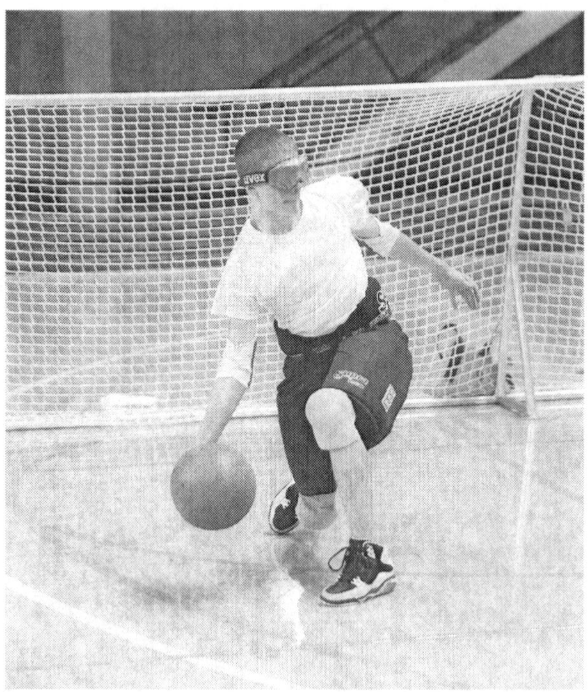

Chuck Comer

Students with visual impairments often throw the goalball with little velocity while standing in one place (left), instead of taking a step and transferring their weight from one foot to the other during a throw (right).

taught them athletics or arranged for special lessons—will be able to perform certain fundamental sports skills, such as the basic standing ready position, a hop or skip, a standing long jump, the down wrestling position, or a basketball hook shot.

Another noticeable limitation among those with early-onset impairments is the somewhat delayed mechanics seen in basic skills, such as throwing, jumping, kicking, and the like (Lieberman, 2011). That is, in contrast to the smooth, quick movements of an athlete such as a professional baseball pitcher, which are generally accomplished in one fluid motion, individuals with early or severe visual impairments often throw with a motion in which each part is distinguishable and the transition from one part to the next appears mechanical. Also, in some cases, children with early-onset visual impairments sometimes add extra movements to a skill such as the throwing motion, in order to reproduce sounds heard while listening to the performance of role models. For instance, one goalball player, attempting to make a typical underhand throw, first jumped in the air and brought his feet down on the floor with a big bang, presumably to emulate a sound he heard an outstanding thrower make when he took his running approach before releasing a hard goalball throw.

Health and Fitness

Being physically fit has clear benefits for good health. Sedentary lifestyles are related to risk factors for diseases associated with lack of exercise, such as obesity, hypertension, diabetes mellitus, coronary artery disease, and osteoporosis, as well as to reduced life expectancy (Kenney, Bryant, Humphrey, Mahler, Froelicher, Miller, & York, 1995; Corbin, Welk, Lindsey, & Corbin, 2004). According to Buell (1982), the tendency of children with visual impairments to be more sedentary than their sighted counterparts and the fact that they are often left out of physical education activities place such students at higher risk for disease. (See Chapter 11 for discussion of fitness activities for people with visual impairments or deafblindness.)

Children with visual impairments overall exhibit lower levels of fitness than their typically sighted peers (Blessing, McCrimmon, Stovall, & Williford, 1993; Buell, 1973; Hopkins, Gaeta, Thomas, & Hill, 1987; Jankowski & Evans, 1981; Kobberling, Jankowski, & Leger, 1991; Lieberman, Byrne, Mattern, Watt, & Fernández-Vivó, 2010; Lieberman & McHugh, 2001; Meek & Maguire, 1996; Shindo, Kumagai, & Tanaka, 1987; Short & Winnick, 1986; Sundberg, 1982; Winnick & Short, 1985). Skaggs and Hopper (1996) estimated that 36 percent of students with visual impairments in the United States are overweight because they lack physical activity. Lieberman and McHugh (2001) reported that only 20 percent of their study population of 46 children with visual impairments were able to pass four tests on the Fitnessgram (an assessment in which students are evaluated in areas of health-related fitness and compared to objective standards that indicate a level of fitness necessary for health; see www.cooperinstitute.org/fitnessgram and www.fitnessgram.net) compared with 70 percent of their sighted classmates who performed at the same level. Jankowski and Evans (1981) found that the physical education of children with visual impairments was insufficient to maintain normal levels of body composition, strength, and aerobic capacity.

In addition, there may be inconsistency among schools in providing children with visual impairments adequate levels of exercise. Data collected from 321 sports camp athletes in 12 states from 2001 through 2003 indicate that opportunity to participate in specialized programs, such as goalball or beep baseball, is still limited in local schools (Ponchillia, Armbruster, & Wiebold, 2005). Another indicator of lack of programming for students with visual impairment or deafblindness in local schools was demonstrated by the fact that slightly more than two-thirds "never" or only "sometimes" "play games with other athletes with visual impairments" (Ponchillia, Armbruster, & Wiebold, 2005).

OVERCOMING BARRIERS

Individuals with visual impairments respond positively to specific training programs such as regular adapted physical education classes or sessions of vigorous endurance activity several times per week; in a number of studies, the study groups reached fitness levels comparable to those of the general population (Blessing, McCrimmon, Stovall, & Williford, 1993; Lee, Ward, & Shephard, 1985; Lieberman, Stuart, Hand, & Robinson, 2006; Ponchillia, Powell, Felski, & Nicklawski, 1992; Williams, Armstrong, Eves, & Faulkner, 1996). These same literature and experience factors also tell us that children and adults with blindness, deafblindness, or visual impairments can learn physical skills readily (Ponchillia, Armbruster, & Wiebold, 2005). Many individuals with visual impairments have outstanding athletic potential, and when those individuals are given full access to coaches and specific programs, they can become world-class competitors. However, as indicated throughout this chapter, both studies and experiences with children who are served at summer sports camps have repeatedly demonstrated that access to quality physical education services continues to be a serious problem.

Consequently, the remainder of this text presents approaches designed to overcome the barriers to participation in physical education, sports, and other physical activities described in this chapter. The approaches taken include techniques to improve the quality of inclusive education and a novel short-term specialized training developed at the nationwide network of summer sports camps operated by the authors. The text will provide information on the following:

- appropriate interventions during early childhood, elementary school, middle school, high school, and beyond
- the modifications to teaching style and the adaptations required to make physical activities accessible in inclusive educational and recreational settings
- specialized adaptive equipment
- techniques for motivating children and adults with visual impairments or deafblindness to engage in self-advocacy to overcome the barriers that prevent them from living active, healthy lifestyles

The text offers an approach that includes active involvement of all those within a given community to overcome the present disadvantages faced by individuals with visual impairments and deafblindness.

CONCLUSION

Visual impairments and deafblindness do not directly cause poor physical skills or fitness. Rather, the lack of ability to perceive movement visually can affect the normal development of physical skills. This coupled with the reduced opportunities to learn to perform sports and fitness activities that may result from psychosocial barriers can lead to below-average physical abilities for an individual. Those who do not have typical or usual opportunities to be involved in sports and physical education may not advocate for themselves, and family members and teachers who do not know adaptive techniques may unintentionally exacerbate the situation. However, effective interventions can remove barriers, increase skills, heighten a desire for physical activity, and improve fitness and the individual's self-concept. The following chapters explore these themes in detail and provide a model for overcoming barriers to learning and access, particularly by utilizing the power of a team composed of educators, teachers, athletes with sensory impairments, families, and individuals with visual impairments or deafblindness themselves.

Visual Impairment and Deafblindness

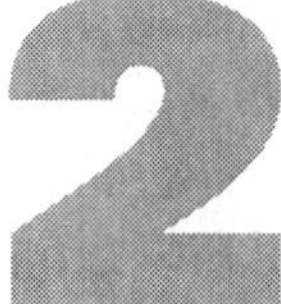

AN OVERVIEW

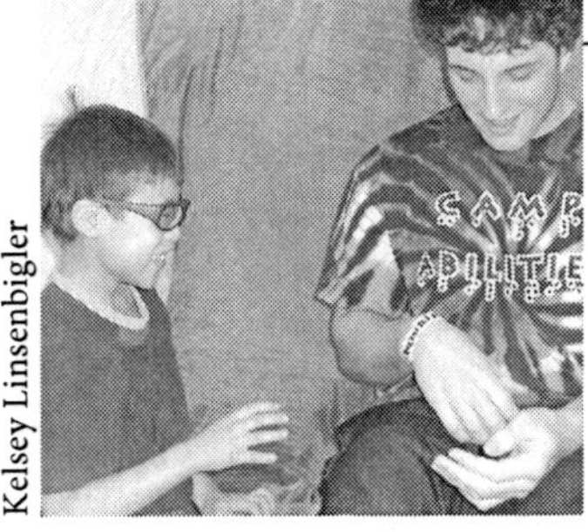

Kelsey Linsenbigler

IN THIS CHAPTER

- **Terminology**
- **Classification Systems**
- **Demographics of Visual Impairment and Deafblindness**
- **Causes of Visual Impairments**
- **Causes of Deafblindness**
- **Methods of Compensating for Vision Loss**
- **Professionals who Teach Individuals with Visual Impairment or Deafblindness**

William is a 15-year-old high school freshman who has Usher syndrome, a condition associated with the dual sensory loss of both vision and hearing. Neither he nor his parents knew of this diagnosis until he reached his early teens. Aware of William's severe deafness when he was only an infant, William's parents knew he could hear their voices only if they stood directly in front of him and spoke clearly and loudly. Because his hearing was so limited, William learned American Sign Language

(ASL) as a young child and now communicates through a combination of ASL and lip reading.

Although William's vision had deteriorated for several years, the decrease was slow and gradual and did not affect him significantly until he was 12 years old. Only when his night blindness became severe enough for him to note the differences between his and others' abilities to see in dim light did William become aware of his vision loss. He and his parents reacted strongly to the subsequent diagnosis of Usher syndrome. His peripheral field loss has progressed significantly, leaving him with only 6 degrees of central vision in his left eye and 4 degrees in his right, resulting in a kind of tunnel vision. William describes his vision as similar to looking at the world through a paper towel tube.

In William's high school physical education class, an aide assists William, primarily by interpreting the teacher's instructions using ASL. William and his aide also work closely with the teacher of students who are visually impaired, who provides adaptive equipment and consultation on how to adapt activities tailored to William's visual abilities. William performs well at activities such as running and jumping that do not require rapid visual tracking of balls or other moving objects. Before he became aware of his visual diagnosis, he was a competitive swimmer on a local club team.

■

Devonte is a 12-year-old sixth grader whose visual impairment is caused by albinism. He is included in his school's physical education classes, where he demonstrates good physical skills. Devonte performs well in most activities, even some of the ball sports, if the ball has good contrast with its surroundings.

When he entered middle school, he tried hard to impress his new physical education instructor. He did very well during the running lessons that were covered early in the school year, which caused the instructor to think of Devonte as a good natural athlete who did not need a lot of attention during class. When the class began its unit on outdoor soccer, however, the instructor was extremely surprised to find that Devonte's entire attitude changed. He reacted angrily and refused to participate. It seemed as though even the weather affected his mood, but not as might be expected. Devonte seemed to hate going out on the nicest, brightest, sunny days. ■

As discussed in Chapter 1, it often takes the intervention of families and professionals—physical education teachers, coaches, and rehabilitation and recreation personnel—to help people with visual impairments or deafblindness learn the concepts and skills they need to become physically active and participate in physical education, sports, and recreation. However, some professionals may not have previously worked with individuals who are visually impaired or deafblind. In such cases, it can be difficult to know how to provide instruction or give feedback to someone who may not be able to see the instructor's movements and may not be able to hear them well, either. This chapter contains information about the nature of visual impairment and deafblindness that will be helpful in working effectively with individuals with sensory impairments. Modifying instruction to meet the needs of students who are visually impaired or deafblind is discussed in detail in Chapter 4.

TERMINOLOGY

Visual Impairment

Visual impairment is considered a "low-incidence" disability because, as detailed later in this chapter, the number of people who are visually impaired is small relative to the overall population. However, the types and degrees of vision loss are numerous and wide ranging, and the population of individuals with visual impairment is diverse (Corn & Lusk, 2010). As explained later in this chapter, there are many causes of visual impairment, and individuals with the same visual diagnosis may in fact see quite differently (Spungin, 2002); indeed, it is said that no two people see the same. As a result, the term *visual impairment* encompasses a wide range of visual disabilities, from total blindness through severe and moderate impairment, and a number of other terms exist to refer to types of vision loss.

The terminology used to describe various aspects of vision or hearing loss is frequently misused in everyday language, making it essential to define the meaning of specific terms before delving into the instructional methodologies presented later in this book. The terms used to describe visual impairment have changed over the years, and some have fallen out of use. In recent years, visual impairment has been viewed and defined functionally, that is, from the perspective of how a vision loss may affect the individual's ability to use his or her vision and perform daily tasks. It has been generally recognized that a functional point of view provides a more accurate understanding and more concrete description of a person's actual abilities than do terms based on the arbitrary numeric boundaries and measurements that are derived from the vision charts used in an optometrist's office (Barraga, 1976; Corn & Lusk, 2010; Koenig & Holbrook, 2000; Ponchillia & Ponchillia, 1996; Scholl, 1986). Sidebar 2.1 presents definitions of terms with which it is important to be familiar.

SIDEBAR 2.1

Definitions of Common Terms Related to Blindness, Deafblindness, and Visual Impairment

Term	Definition
Acquired	Not present at birth; also known as adventitious.
Blindness	Lack of functional vision.
Congenital	Developing at or soon after birth.
Deafblindness	Concomitant hearing and visual impairments, the combination of which causes such severe communication and other developmental and educational needs that the individual cannot be accommodated in special education programs solely for children with deafness or children with blindness.
Functional	Related to use; useful.
Functional vision	A degree of vision sufficient to be of use in performing a given task.
Legal blindness	A visual acuity of 20/200 or less in the better eye after standard correction, or a visual field of 20 degrees or less in the better eye.
Low vision	A degree of vision that is functional but limited enough to interfere with the ability to perform everyday activities and that cannot be corrected with standard eyeglasses or contact lenses.

SIDEBAR 2.1 *(continued)*

Term	Definition
Visual acuity	The ability to discern form visually; the sharpness or clearness of vision.
Visual disability	A limitation in functional ability resulting from visual impairment.
Visual field	The area that is visible without shifting the gaze.
Visual impairment	Any degree of vision loss, including total blindness, that affects an individual's ability to perform the tasks of daily life.

Sources: I. L. Bailey and A. Hall, *Visual Impairment: An Overview* (New York: American Foundation for the Blind, 1990); K. M. Huebner, J. G. Prickett, T. R. Welch, and E. Joffee (Eds.), *Hand in Hand: Essentials of Communication and Mobility for Your Students Who Are Deafblind,* Vol. 2 (New York: AFB Press, 1995); and National Consortium on Deafblindness, Glossary, retrieved 7/3/12 from www.dblink.org/lib/topics/feddef.htm.

The definitions of important terms such as *blind, low vision,* and *visually impaired* should be noted, as they are sometimes used in different ways. (The implications of terminology and how it is used to describe or classify individuals with disabilities are described later in this chapter.) An individual who is blind has no functional (usable) vision; someone with low vision has some functional vision, but it cannot be corrected to normal by using standard lenses or eyeglasses (Bailey & Hall, 1990; Huebner, Prickett, Welch, & Joffee, 1995). A person who is visually impaired has vision limited enough to cause difficulty conducting everyday tasks; the term generally encompasses those who are blind as well as those with low vision. A few terms that were once in common use, such as *partially sighted,* once used to refer to those with low vision, have become more or less outdated and are no longer used. In addition, the term *handicapped* has been largely replaced by *disabled* in today's society.

A visual impairment present at or soon after birth is known as a *congenital* or *early-onset* visual impairment. If the impairment had its onset after early childhood, when visual memory had already been established, it is known as an *acquired* or sometimes an *adventitious* impairment (Smart, 2009).

Deafblindness

The majority of individuals with visual impairments have some usable vision. Many, however, may have an additional disability, such as a hearing loss. The term *deafblindness* is used to refer to any degree of vision loss and hearing loss combined, and does not necessarily refer to a total absence of vision and hearing. However, the effects of deafblindness may be multidimensional, meaning that when the senses of vision and hearing are both impaired, the interplay of these sensory losses can be cumulative and complex (Huebner, Prickett, Welch, & Joffee, 1995).

It should be noted that although the term *deafblind* is used in this text, there is some debate about what term should designate the dual sensory impairment (Marschark, Spencer, & Nathan, 2010). Lagati (1995; Gallagher, n.d.) suggested the use of *deafblind* as opposed to the hyphenated deaf-blind because the condition is singular and cumulative in scope, the resulting disabilities representing more than the sum of the consequences of deafness and blindness, and therefore deserves to be represented by its own unique term. Alternative terms that have been proposed include *deaf-blind, dual sensory impaired, auditorily and visually challenged,* and *person with deaf-blindness* (Gallagher, n.d.; Marschark, Spencer, & Nathan, 2010).

The term *person with deafblindness* is an example of using so-called person-first language, or employing phraseology in which references to persons are literally placed first, before references to disability. Person-first language will be discussed in more detail in the following section. In this text, we will use the term *person with deafblindness* or *person who is deafblind* where practical.

The Influence of Terminology and Language

Although using specific terminology is essential for effective communication among professionals, the language used to describe groups of people can negatively influence others' perceptions of the group and result in prejudice (Smart, 2009). Consequently, anyone working in or around a disability-related profession needs to be aware of the subtle influence of word usage on attitudes about disability and disabled people and their potential for affecting the self-images of the target group. Speech that is considered racist or sexist is a well-known and much-discussed example of objectionable, prejudicial language. The language used to describe disability has the same potential for negative consequences for the people it in effect defines (Smart, 2009). In order to make the terminology as respectful as possible, many organizations and personnel today use the form referred to earlier, "person-first language," such as "a person who is blind" or "a person with blindness," rather than "the blind" or "blind person" and "a child with diabetes," instead of "a diabetic" or "a diabetic child." This shift in word use and placement is intended to recognize that an individual is a person first, who happens to have a particular attribute, such as a disability (APA, 2003; Lieberman & Arndt, 2004; Smart, 2009; Zola, 1993).

It should be noted here that long-standing agencies and organizations of and for people with visual impairments or deafblindness were named well before person-first language came into popular use and, therefore, sometimes contain older terminology, such as *the blind,* for example, the American Foundation for the Blind and the American Printing House for the Blind. The lack of person-first language in such names is often accepted in deference to their age and historical significance.

In regard to the term *deafblind,* as opposed to *deaf-blind,* there is some disagreement among the community of persons with deaf-blindness about whether or not to use person-first language. For example, many people who are deaf consider themselves part of a distinct subculture of society that has its own language, customs, and perception of whether deafness is a disability or not and may not feel that a phrase such as "the deaf" or "deaf people" bears a negative connotation. In fact, some prefer capitalizing the *d,* as in "the Deaf," to indicate that it is a proper noun and that they take pride in identifying their group as its own entity (Smart, 2009). Although the issue of person-first language continues to be a matter of ongoing discussion, in the present discussion the term *deafblind* will be used.

CLASSIFICATION SYSTEMS

Nature and Implications of Classification Systems

Disabilities, including visual impairment, are often divided into categories or classes. Classification is frequently used to determine eligibility for services such as special education and rehabilitation. It is also used to establish fair competitive categories in sports competitions among people with disabilities. Therefore, to ensure that professionals and the people they serve fully understand what to expect from service providers or competitive event holders across the nation and the world, it is essential for these categories and terms to be highly standardized and widely used.

At the same time, professionals need to keep in mind that traditional classification systems, like the descriptive terminology they employ, may also have negative effects on the people they designate. In essence, it is important to understand that classifications describe individuals but do not define them and that categorization can lead to focusing on people's disabilities and limitations, rather than on their abilities and potential, which in turn can lead to stereotyping and prejudicial treatment.

The most common classification encountered in relation to visual impairment is that of legal blindness, which, as noted in Sidebar 2.1, is defined in terms of measurements of visual acuity and visual field as obtained in the office of an eye care specialist, namely, a visual acuity of 20/200 or less in the better eye after standard correction, or a visual field of 20 degrees or less in the better eye. (Visual acuity of 20/200 means that the individual can see at a standard distance of 20 feet the letters on the standard Snellen eye chart that a person with unimpaired vision can read at 200 feet.) This classification was originally created to determine eligibility for benefits such as Social Security and is still used as a criterion for many services today. However, people who may fall into this category often have usable vision and therefore are not blind, as the term might seem to imply. Moreover, as noted earlier, the measurements of visual acuity and visual field obtained in the eye care specialist's office do not necessarily represent how an individual can function visually in daily life, and some people with low vision do not fall into the category of legal blindness. The use of this category may have a negative psychological effect on some individuals who are then described as "blind" or may arbitrarily designate them as eligible or ineligible for services (Corn & Lusk, 2010), an example of how classifications need to be used with caution.

Categories of Disabilities

A common categorization of disabilities is by symptom or manifestation (Bradsher, 1997; Brown, 1991). Smart (2009) describes four broad symptomatic categories of disability, including physical, intellectual, cognitive, and psychiatric disabilities. According to this system, blindness, low vision, and deafblindness are physical disabilities, as are mobility impairments, neurological impairments, musculoskeletal conditions, other forms of sensory loss, and many health disorders. According to Smart (2009), examples of intellectual disabilities include cognitive disability, Down syndrome, and autism; learning disabilities and traumatic brain injury are examples of cognitive disorders; mental illness and chemical and substance abuse are examples of psychiatric disabilities. When dealing with classification schemes, however, it is important to remember that categorizing a condition such as blindness as a disability does not limit what a person with the condition can do physically.

Classifications for Sports Competition

The International Blind Sports Federation (IBSA) and the United States Association of Blind Athletes (USABA), the international and U.S. bodies governing blind sports, respectively, hold competitive events in various sports for people who are blind or deafblind (see Chapter 11 for descriptions of these organizations). The competitive visual categories used by IBSA and the USABA for events are based on amount of vision, thereby enabling athletes to compete against only those with similar degrees of vision. For example, those who have no functional vision generally do not compete against those with any degree of vision. The four IBSA and USABA visual classifications are described in more detail in Chapter 8.

DEMOGRAPHICS OF VISUAL IMPAIRMENT AND DEAFBLINDNESS

Information about the population of people who are visually impaired in the United States is offered here to give readers a perspective on the nature and size of the book's target population. As indicated earlier in this chapter, the number of people affected by visual impairment is relatively small in relation to the general population. As was also pointed out, terminology used to refer to visual impairment varies, and vision loss is described in many ways, some of them overlapping—for example, *visually impaired* versus *legally blind*. For these reasons, the prevalence, or rate of occurrence, of visual impairment in the United States cannot be expressed simply, because the definitions of visual impairment used within surveys as well as the survey methods vary significantly.

The broadest measure of the number of people with visual impairments is from census data: the National Health Interview Survey, conducted annually by interviewers of the U.S. Census Bureau for the Centers for Disease Control and Prevention's National Center for Health Statistics. In 2010, this survey found that 21.5 million adults in the United States reported that they either are blind or had trouble seeing even while wearing eyeglasses or contact lenses (Schiller, Lucas, Ward, & Peregoy, 2012). Of these, about 16.1 million, or 74.9 percent, were between the ages of 18 and 64, while 5.4 million, or about 25 percent, were age 65 or older. However, the percentage of a given age group that is visually impaired increases significantly as people age. Whereas only 6.2 percent of those from age 18 to 44 had a visual impairment, 11.6 percent of those from age 45 to 64, 12.2 percent of those from age 65 to 74, and 16.1 percent of those 75 years of age and older had a visual impairment. Moreover, when using a stricter criterion for vision loss, that of legal blindness, as many as two-thirds of the legally blind population are people aged 65 or older who lost vision as a result of age-related eye diseases (American Foundation for the Blind, 2012).

Earlier studies that have not been duplicated indicated that of those who reported meeting the criteria for legal blindness, approximately

80 percent reported having low vision, while the remaining 20 percent reported having no functional vision (Chiang, Bassi, & Javitt, 1992; National Center for Health Statistics, 2007).

On the other end of the age spectrum, as of January 2009, the number of children through age 18 who met the criteria for legal blindness totaled 59,341 (www.aph.org/about/ar2010.html).

With regard to individuals with deafblindness, an annual count conducted by the National Consortium on Deaf-Blindness (NCDB) reported a total of 9,320 children and youths with deafblindness as of December 2010 (NCDB, 2011). While current estimates of the number of adults with deafblindness are lacking, a 1993 estimate put the population at 35,000 to 40,000 (Turkington & Sussman, 2000; Watson & Taff-Watson, 1993). Thus the total population in the United States might be estimated at roughly 45,000 to 50,000 individuals who are deafblind. (For further information from NCDB on the issues involved in determining the demographics of the American deafblind population, see www.nationaldb.org/ISSelectedTopics.php?topicCatID=16.)

CAUSES OF VISUAL IMPAIRMENTS

While a detailed clinical discussion of the types and causes of visual impairment is beyond the scope of this book, this section outlines some of the most common vision problems and causes of vision loss and the functional limitations associated with them. It is important for professionals who work with people who are visually impaired to have a basic understanding of the salient characteristics that might be expected within this group as well as the implications of their students' or clients' conditions and how they might affect their capabilities. (For more detailed information, see Goldberg & Trattler, 2012; Riordan-Eva & Cunningham, 2011; Schwartz, 2010.) In addition, readers can locate current information about eye diseases, statistics, and simulations of how eye conditions affect vision through the website of the National Eye Institute, www.nei.nih.gov.

Each individual's visual abilities are affected by the type and cause of his or her visual impairment, and in varying degrees. Visual impairment can be caused by a congenital abnormality of the vision system that is present at or soon after birth, by an acquired disease of the eye or the brain, or by an injury. Although the effects of such conditions are varied and wide ranging, most eye disorders limit one's vision by decreasing the degree of visual acuity or the size of the visual field (Schwartz, 2010). The most common causes of visual impairments are discussed in the following sections.

Conditions Affecting Visual Acuity

Most conditions that affect visual acuity—that is, how clearly someone is able to see—affect the clarity of the cornea, the eye's outer protective layer through which light enters the eye, or more commonly, the eye's crystalline lens, which helps bring light rays to a focus on the retina, the eye's inner sensory layer found between the anterior and posterior chambers of the eye (Schwartz, 2010; see Figure 2.1). Cataracts, the most frequent cause of blindness

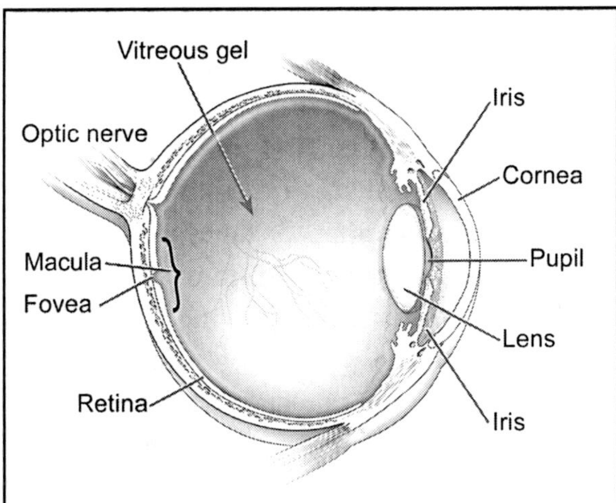

FIGURE 2.1 Cross Section of the Eye
Source: National Eye Institute.

worldwide, affect the clarity of the lens, resulting in a clouding of the entire visual field. In the presence of cataracts, as well as a number of other visual conditions, bright light or glare, light reflected from shiny surfaces, increases the difficulty of seeing.

Conditions Affecting Visual Field

There are three common forms of visual field loss: central, peripheral, and irregular losses. The most common central field loss is caused by *macular degeneration,* a condition usually found in people over 65 years of age and frequently referred to as *age-related macular degeneration* (AMD; Schwartz, 2010). The macula is the central portion of the retina and responsible for acuity or the eye's sharpest vision. Therefore, a central field loss is essentially a loss of acuity in the center of vision; peripheral or side vision is often unaffected. A similar condition that affects the central or macular vision of children is *Stargardt disease* (Schwartz, 2010).

In beginning stages of vision loss, a diffuse spot appears in the center of vision, which some persons describe as a blue dot. Over time, the occlusion generally becomes denser and more obtrusive. The functional result of such a loss is a severe limitation in reading and other near-vision tasks, while movement through the environment may sometimes not be affected greatly (Ponchillia & Ponchillia, 1996). Individuals with a central field loss can be helped to learn *eccentric viewing,* that is, focusing their gaze in such a way as to "look around" the blind spot, or *scotoma,* in the center of the eye, so that they view objects with their better peripheral vision. It is important to note that although large objects may be viewed with peripheral vision, people with central vision loss may "lose" objects such as targets or balls that appear in their central blind spot, making it difficult for them to play fast-moving games involving such objects.

Among the common causes of vision loss in the peripheral visual field are retinitis pigmentosa and glaucoma (Schwartz, 2010). Retinitis pigmentosa is an inherited disease that results in the progressive destruction of cells within the retina. *Glaucoma* is a condition in which there is damage to the optic nerve as a result of extreme pressure within the eye. Glaucoma, like retinitis pigmentosa, also occurs in children but is far more common in older people. In both conditions, the peripheral field is gradually reduced, resulting in a narrow tunnel of vision, sometimes to the point of total blindness. Although the outer boundaries of vision are lost, central acuity may be unaffected. In such cases, near-vision tasks can often be accomplished, but movement in unfamiliar surroundings is generally difficult, because it is hard to see what is underfoot or at one's elbow. In addition, because the peripheral portion of the retina is responsible for night vision, people with these conditions may be functionally blind after dark (Ponchillia & Ponchillia, 1996; Schwartz, 2010).

The loss of visual field in randomly placed, irregular patches is most frequently the result of *diabetic retinopathy*, a leading cause of blindness in North America (Schwartz, 2010). Diabetes causes circulatory problems that damage the tiny blood vessels in the retina, which not only affect the field of vision but also may cause extreme acuity problems as a consequence of intraocular bleeding, when blood components leak into the eye, blocking the course of light from cornea to retina.

Retinopathy of prematurity (ROP), a condition in which blood vessels grow uncontrollably on the retina of premature infants, thought to be due to exposure to high levels of oxygen in incubators, also causes randomly placed field loss in children (Schwartz, 2010). The practical problems imposed by intermittent field loss range from limitations in carrying out tasks that require near vision to difficulties with moving through unfamiliar environments, depending on the location of the retinal damage.

Cortical Visual Impairment

Terms referring to visual impairment caused by damage or injury to the brain include *cortical* or *cerebral visual impairment, neurological visual impairment,* and *brain injury–related visual impairment.* Cortical visual impairment (CVI), a common cause of visual impairment in children, results from damage or injury to the brain, rather than to the eye (Roman-Lantzy, 2007; Schwartz, 2010). Some of the highly variable consequences of this condition can be overall reduced vision, visual field reduction, impaired depth perception, difficulty perceiving movement, and photophobia, or sensitivity to light. Children with this condition may have trouble with reading and other near-vision tasks as well as moving through unfamiliar environments and other distance-vision tasks. They may show a preference for certain colors, be attracted to bright or moving objects, and stare at lights. The vision of children with this condition fluctuates a great deal, and they seem to have difficulty in interpreting the visual environment, especially when it is visually complex. The degree of difficulty a child experiences may vary considerably.

Photophobia

Photophobia, an extreme sensitivity to light, is associated with many causes of visual impairment. People who are photophobic, such as those with *albinism*, an inherited disorder of pigment development that affects the eyes,

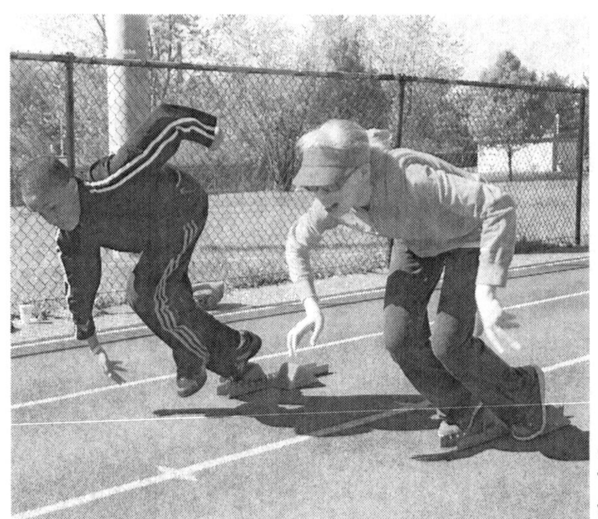
Chuck Comer

Simple adaptations such as wearing tinted lenses and a visor to minimize glare, like the sprinter on the right, can improve an individual's ability to participate in activities outdoors.

skin, hair, and brain, have extreme difficulty in direct sunlight or with situations in which glare is present. The change in attitude of Devonte, described at the beginning of this chapter, from cooperative and successful during indoor activities to angry and uncooperative during outdoor classes was related to his inability to see in the sunlight during outdoor physical education classes. Devonte's instructor could not understand Devonte's reaction and difficulty without some knowledge of the relationship of albinism to photophobia and its functional effects.

CAUSES OF DEAFBLINDNESS

Because deafblindness is relatively rare and because the specific disorders that cause it are numerous and yet affect few people, the leading causes are often presented as general categories. For example, the National Consortium on Deaf-blindness (www.nationaldb.org) lists the following as the leading causes:

- no determination of etiology
- hereditary syndromes or disorders
- complications of prematurity
- CHARGE syndrome

Consequently, the cause of deafblindness is often unknown or is the result of hereditary or nonhereditary prenatal factors. Complexes of physical, cognitive, and intellectual symptoms or conditions known as syndromes, such as Usher syndrome and CHARGE syndrome, are among the best-known causes.

CHARGE syndrome (formerly known as CHARGE association) affects specific areas of the body; its name derives from the first letter of the words describing its symptoms: *C*oloboma (eye defects), *H*eart defects, *A*tresia of the choanae (blocked nasal passages), *R*etardation of growth and development, *G*enital abnormalities, and *E*ar abnormalities and hearing loss (http://ghr.nlm.nih.gov/condition/charge-syndrome, 2011). The symptoms vary among those affected, but infants commonly have multiple life-threatening medical conditions. Diagnosis of CHARGE syndrome is complex, because symptoms vary widely. About half of the cases of CHARGE syndrome are genetic, either inherited or resulting from gene mutations, and occur in people with no family history of the condition.

The single syndrome known to cause the greatest number of cases of deafblindness is *Usher syndrome*, which commonly combines congenital deafness with acquired retinitis pigmentosa but also affects some individuals after early childhood (www.ushersyndrome.nih.gov). There are three types of Usher syndrome based on time of onset and the presence or absence of balance problems:

- *Type I:* Deafness from birth with severe balance problems from a young age; vision problems usually starting by age 10 and leading to blindness
- *Type II:* Moderate to severe hearing loss with normal balance; vision problems starting in the early teens and progressing more slowly than in Type I
- *Type III:* Born with normal hearing and balance, but developing vision problems and then hearing loss

Due to the variability of the causes of deafblindness, there is an equally wide range of skills among those defined as deafblind. In particular, the hearing and vision loss can be either congenital or acquired, and the severity of the sensory losses can range from little to total impairment. The age at which hearing and vision are lost can have a major impact on the skills and knowledge of individuals who are deafblind, particularly with regard to their awareness of their environment and ability to communicate with others. As a result, it is essential to conduct assessments of communication ability and skills early in any educational or rehabilitation program.

METHODS OF COMPENSATING FOR VISION LOSS

While vision loss may reduce or otherwise distort the visual information available to an individual, people with visual impairments or deafblindness use other methods to get information they need from the environment. The most common methods are enhancing the use of remaining vision and substituting touch and hearing for vision. Having a knowledge of how to manipulate environmental variables to increase visibility and how touch and hearing can be used as substitutes for vision can enable a teacher or coach to eliminate many of the limitations caused by a student's visual impairment and provides the basis for making physical activities accessible to individuals with visual impairments or deafblindness (see Chapter 5).

Enhancing Usable Vision: Environmental Modification

It is important to realize that the percentage of those with visual impairments who are totally blind is small, and similarly those with deafblindness are even more rarely totally deaf and blind. As a consequence, understanding the factors that enhance a person's remaining vision is extremely important to instructors of such individuals.

As noted in Chapter 1, vision that accompanies a visual impairment severe enough to interfere with the tasks of daily life that can be used for everyday activities is referred to as *low vision*. Children and adults who have low vision can learn to use their vision more effectively through the receipt of low vision services, a range of services involving assessment, prescription of special low vision devices such as magnifiers, and training in the use of these devices and other adaptive techniques (Wilkinson, 2010).

In addition, certain basic principles can be applied to modify the individual's environment to enhance his or her use of vision and the *visibility* of objects in the environment, that is, how easily they can be seen (Duffy, 2002; Sticken & Kapperman, 2010). For example, a game or activity can be made accessible to many people with low vision simply by adding a few strips of contrasting colored tape to a goal or ball, getting a larger and more visible ball, or adding artificial light to a play area (Ponchillia, 1995). Instructors and other professionals knowledgeable about the variables that improve visibility will have the ability to manipulate the environment to maximize its accessibility for their students and clients. (See Chapter 5 for more information on how to adapt sports and games.) Important variables to consider when modifying the environment to optimize the use of someone's remaining vision are illumination, contrast, and size (Ponchillia & Ponchillia, 1996; Sticken & Kapperman, 2010).

Illumination

Illumination, the amount of light reflected from the surface of a viewed object into the eye, is a critical factor in visibility. In general, as the degree of illumination is increased, so is visibility, up to the point at which the light may become overwhelming and difficult to look at for the viewer, and then it is considered to be *glare*.

Assessing the amount of lighting or illumination in an area where a game or activity is to be held is one of an instructor's first tasks when working with a student with visual impairment or deafblindness. Gymnasiums often have good lighting, but other activity rooms, such as those used for gymnastics, may not. If illumination is lacking in the gymnastics room, the simple addition of lights focused on equipment like the vaulting horse may be all that is required to make vaulting possible for a child with low vision. Rheostats (dimmer switches) are typically preferable features for lights, because they can be adjusted according to the needs of the individual.

Some factors relating to increased illumination need particular attention, such as the possibility of glare and the presence if any of a learner's oversensitivity to light (Zimmerman, Zebehazy, & Moon, 2010). If reflected light strikes the eye at an angle or is bright enough to cause the eye to close or blink, then glare is evident. Glare of this kind can interfere with the performance of visual tasks. It can be controlled by adjusting the angle of the light source or by placing the object to be viewed on a less shiny and less reflective surface and instead using a surface that is more absorptive (Zimmerman, Zebehazy, & Moon, 2010). For example, the glare from a glass basketball backboard can be controlled by temporarily covering it with paper or cloth. An outdoor activity can be set up so the sun is behind rather than in front of a student who has low vision.

As mentioned previously, many eye conditions result in oversensitivity to light, or photophobia. In such cases, too much light can be detrimental because it can decrease visual efficiency. Sunglasses, which act as light filters, or tinted prescription eyeglasses can be used to control light in circumstances such as these. The impact of overhead lights in classrooms and gymnasiums that might interfere with a photophobic child's vision or bright sunlight outside during sports or recreational activities can be controlled by using visors, caps with bills, or sunwear with side shields. Shades or blinds can be drawn in glare-filled rooms to decrease glare and sunlight effectively as well. Devonte, who was described at the beginning of this chapter, might have been more willing to participate in outdoor physical education classes if he had been wearing socially acceptable sunglasses and a cap that helped reduce and filter ambient light.

Contrast

The degree of color difference between an object and the surface against which it is being viewed is termed *contrast*. Heightening contrast can make objects more visible for many people with low vision (Smith & Geruschat, 2010; Sticken & Kapperman, 2010). The effective use of contrast can be illustrated when a dark-colored plate is placed against a white tablecloth. A practical and important way of increasing accessibility to physical activities and to teaching and learning environments is by increasing the contrast between the major components of the activity. Whereas increasing lighting often requires large floor lamps or even architectural modifications, alterations of contrast can be accomplished simply by adding contrasting color tape to objects or areas, changing the color of equipment, moving equipment from one place to another to make use of a contrasting background, or placing something contrasting, such as a carpet, under a piece of equipment (Ponchillia, 1995).

Examples of contrast modification include using a different-colored ball that shows up better against a playing surface; placing strips of gymnasium tape across the ends of a balance beam; placing dark tumbling mats under a light-colored weight bench so it is easy to spot; or placing a few strips of bright orange tape on a volleyball. These are simple and inexpensive methods of increasing visibility, and they do not negatively affect others who have normal vision who may be involved in the same sport or venue. Filters of certain colors, especially yellow filters, which tend to change blues, grays, and purples to black, can also enhance contrast. Thus, the use of sunwear can increase the contrast between objects being viewed. Color and contrast modifications such as these also make it easier for people to read print. Placing a yellow acetate sheet over reading material tends to make print, especially faint or colored print, appear blacker and more legible.

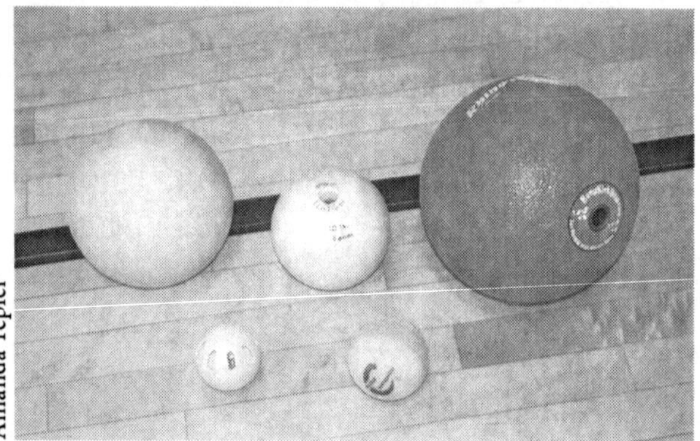

Amanda Tepfer

Using a larger ball or one in a color that contrasts with the gym floor or other background can improve the ball's visibility.

Size

Degree of visibility is also affected by the size of an object to be viewed. Perception of size can be manipulated by increasing the actual size of the object to be viewed, by bringing the object closer to the eye, or by creating a larger image of the object through magnification (Zimmerman, Zebehazy, & Moon, 2010). Using a larger ball in a particular activity or game may be all that is needed to make the game accessible to people with low vision. For example, using a colorful volleyball instead of a softball or using an exercise ball or beach ball instead of a volleyball may provide the means to include a person with low vision in a baseball or volleyball game.

Another way to increase perceived size is by bringing the object closer to the eye, which enlarges its image on the retina. This phenomenon is known as *relative-distance magnification*. When the distance from eye to object is decreased by one-half, the size of the image on the retina doubles (Zimmerman, Zebehazy, & Moon, 2010). Although it may not be possible to apply this principle while participating in an activity, it may be helpful when introducing a person with low vision to a new type of equipment; he or she may need to get closer to examine an object or area. However, bringing objects closer is not necessarily effective for everyone who has a visual impairment. For someone with severely limited visual fields, bringing an object closer may increase the size of its image on the retina so much that the individual can see only a portion of the entire image with his or her remaining area of vision. For this reason, the optimal distance for presenting visual information needs to be determined for every individual.

The apparent size of objects can also be increased by the use of *optical low vision devices,* such as magnifiers, telescopes, and other devices (Zimmerman, Zebehazy, & Moon, 2010). For people with appropriate training, a low vision device can be used for such activities as spotting the flag on a golf green or looking at a game scoreboard.

Touch as a Substitute for Vision

Touch is commonly used as a substitute for vision by many people with visual impairments. Teachers specializing in work with students who are visually impaired typically help their students learn to obtain as much information as possible through the use of touch and their other senses. However, the word *touch* encompasses a range of sensory experiences, as well as meanings that may be misunderstood (Millar, 2000). Several terms have been used in relation to the sense of touch, including *tactile, tactual, haptic, dynamic* (Heller, 2000), and *kinesthetic* (Millar, 2000).

"Tactile" and "tactual" are used broadly to refer to touch and are commonly used interchangeably. The following definitions of other terms, as used by Heller (2000), are used throughout this text:

- *Passive touch* describes the experience of contact without active movement on the individual's part.
- *Haptic touch* relates to active touch; feeling an object in order to perceive it.
- *Dynamic touch* refers to touch experienced through an implement or device.

According to this schema, when people are touched by someone or something else, they experience passive touch; when they perform an act such as reading braille or identifying an object by picking it up or stepping on it, they are using haptic touch; and when striking a baseball with a bat or swinging a long cane, they are experiencing dynamic touch.

In addition, *kinesthetic touch* can be described as a sensory dimension that monitors the environment through movement of muscles and joints (Millar, 2000). In addition to monitoring sensory feedback, kinesthetic touch also has a motor function, which can assist in learning certain physical skills (Carello and Turvey, 2000). Specifically, learning occurs when the human brain monitors the environment through the body's use of muscles and joints and the movements themselves are simultaneously memorized by the individual. This phenomenon is sometimes called *kinesthetic learning* or *muscle memory,* and provides the theoretical basis for teaching physical skills, such as jumping and throwing, through repetition (Fazzi & Klein, 2002). Kinesthetic learning occurs through a combination of repetition of the mental imagery of performing the skill and the involvement of the muscles, joints, tendons, and ligaments during the actual performance of the skill (Romiszowski, 1999).

In light of this broad and multifaceted conceptualization of touch, when adapting a physical activity for a person with a visual impairment, it is important to think of touch not just as an experience of the hands and fingers, but one of the body, mind, hands, joints, and limbs, in which even the sticks, rackets, and other equipment used in physical activities play a role. Consequently, the tactile adaptations made to physical activities or to instructional settings can involve all these aspects of touch. For example, when marking the boundaries of a game, several tactile approaches are possible:

- The feet can be used to monitor boundaries (haptic touch) if the out-of-bounds lines are made tactile by placing cords individually under the centers of strips of 2-inch vinyl gymnasium tape.
- Muscle memory can be used by having players run repetitive drills within the playing area until their bodies learn its parameters (kinesthetic touch).
- A long cane can be used by the individual to explore the boundaries of the playing area delineated by a wall or another object (dynamic touch) before playing a game.

(See Chapter 5 for a more complete explanation of adapting boundaries.)

It is known that many people with visual impairments are highly skilled at using touch, although there is considerable variation in this ability, both to accomplish tasks required in daily life and for more complex endeavors such as producing fine sculptures or performing athletic feats (Katz, 1989; Ponchillia, 2008; Revesz, 1950, pp. 218–222, 226). This kind of tactile ability was formerly assumed to be a function of increased experience in using the sense of touch. More recent research has offered strong evidence of the presence of a phenomenon known as *cross-modal brain reorganization* or *brain plasticity* that provides the mechanism by which many people with blindness are able to use touch effectively to interpret objects and even understand the space around them (Cohen, Celnik, Pascual-Leone, Corwell, Falz, Dambrosia & Honda, 1997; Merabet, Pitskel, Amedi & Pascual-Leone, 2008; Sathian & Lacey, 2008). Brain scan technology has shown that the loss of vision can trigger a reorganization of neural pathways within the brain so that touch sensations are sent to sites in the occipital cortex that are generally used for vision. Thus, in many instances, the brain images of someone who is blind that are produced by touch become virtually equivalent to the images once produced in the visual cortex through vision (Sadato et al., 1996; Merabet et al., 2008). Consequently, the source of the neural input to the brain—that is, vision or touch—appears to be less relevant than the part of the brain in which the neural transmission is deciphered. In short, researchers in the area of brain plasticity have demonstrated that the brain image produced in the occipital cortex of a person who is blind viewing an object through touch is—with the exception of its color—virtually identical to the image that would have resulted from observing it with vision.

In the experience of one of the authors, after 30 years of stone sculpting following an acquired vision loss, images available through touch appear to be visual in nature and remain stored in that form as long as three decades. This conclusion is reinforced by the fact that the images of objects viewed before and after the onset of vision loss are so identical in memory that it is impossible to determine just by their appearances whether they were "seen" by his eyes or hands.

The outstanding haptic abilities of many athletes with visual impairments, blindness, or deafblindness (Ponchillia, 2008) is well represented by the athletes playing the fast-moving sport of goalball, a six-person game played blindfolded on an indoor court marked with raised boundary and orientation lines, whose objective is to score a goal by throwing a hollow, basketball-sized ball containing bells through the opposing players and into their net (see Chapter 10 for a detailed description). It is apparent when observing goalball games at the authors' sports camps and at other goalball events that in spite of the constant movement required of goalball players during a game, most of those with experience have an almost uncanny ability to use nonvisual sensory input to keep track of their place on the court and monitor the locations of their teammates, their opponents, the opposing goal line, and the ball as they implement the strategy of the game. Experienced players report that while they are playing, they see fleeting visual images of the boundary and other court lines, their teammates, the opposing defensive players, and the opposing thrower. (It should be clear that orientation to the court and the other players is also a function of many factors besides touch, including the players' ability to conceptualize space, communication among teammates, practicing with teammates, sophistication of players' sports concepts, repetition through drills, and hearing, as discussed in the next section.)

Although brain plasticity may play a major role in the tactile ability of a person who is blind, the quality and efficiency of that person's tactile experience are also important (Ponchillia, 2008). For example, given the opportunity to touch a sculpture to see what they can discover, many museum patrons will just use the tips of one or two fingers to stab lightly at random parts of the piece (Ponchillia, 2008). Using this fingertip method of investigation is akin to viewing an object backward through a telescope, decreasing the field of vision and briefly disclosing only small parts of the object

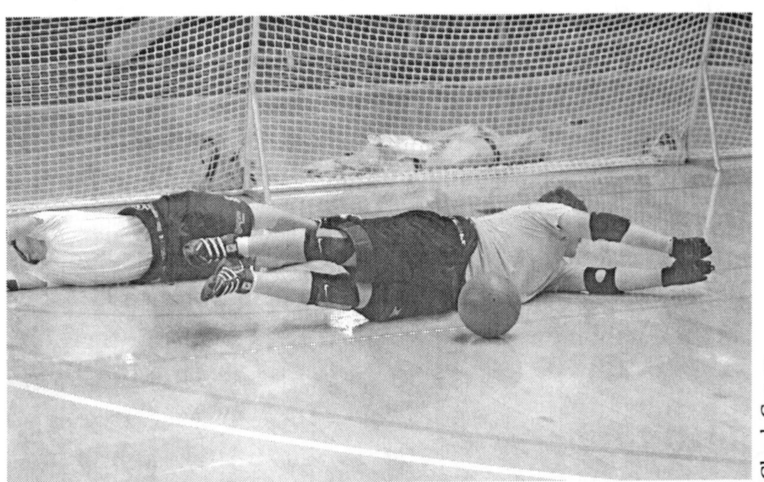
Chuck Comer

Practicing a movement over and over, such as this drill in goalball blocking technique, makes use of the sensory and kinesthetic components of touch to fix the correct movement in memory.

with each touch. However, scanning the object with the entire surface area of the palms and fingers may instead yield an image of the whole object (Ponchillia, 2008). In addition, efficiently recognizing objects, form, details, textures, and other characteristics of an object requires active scanning or moving the hands (Carello & Turvey, 2000).

Understanding the equivalency of touch and vision in many cases—knowing that students with blindness or deafblindness may be expected to "see" sports equipment with their hands the way others do with their vision—means that describing new equipment, such as high jump standards, baseball gloves, kayak paddles, and the like (discussed in Chapter 4) may not be as difficult as an instructor may have expected. Also, given that there are efficient and inefficient methods of using the hands to "look at" objects, students' tactile skills should be assessed and training offered if necessary. Further, understanding that touch has sensory and motor components that involve the "memory" of muscles and joints of the body helps teachers plan lessons that capitalize on training techniques such as repetition to instill the boundaries of a soccer field in a student's memory or to attain an outstanding soccer kick. Finally, knowing that there are athletes who are totally blind and are successful because of their well-developed senses of haptic and dynamic touch helps instructors understand the potential for others with visual impairments or deafblindness.

Hearing as a Substitute for Vision

Hearing, or audition, is another sensory modality that can be used as a substitute for vision and provides people with visual impairments information that is supplemental to that available through touch. Although, as just described, touch can provide extremely accurate information for the recognition of objects and yields kinesthetic feedback that helps people learn physical skills and understand spatial concepts, touch is nevertheless limited in what it can yield to the user, because information can typically be obtained only within the area immediately adjacent to one's body or within arms' reach. Hearing significantly increases that effective sensory range.

There is a great deal of variation, as is true of touch, among people who are visually impaired in their ability to interpret and use hearing as a substitute for vision in their activities. There are people who are blind who have what might be considered extraordinary skills. For example, a higher percentage of musicians who are blind than are sighted have absolute pitch and can identify pure tones as specific musical notes, while others with longstanding blindness can use sound echoes from buildings and other structures to accurately describe their environmental configurations (Emerson & Ashmead, 2008). More commonly, people with visual impairments in general are able to use hearing to gather environmental information that helps them deal with everyday situations, such as listening to traffic sounds to know when to cross streets, paying attention to a teacher's voice to know where to face while listening, or using the bubbling sounds from water jets to locate a nearby hot tub.

Some of the variability in use of auditory skills is thought to be a function of the human brain's ability to reorganize its pathways following the onset of blindness (Merabet et al., 2008). The phenomenon of brain plasticity or cross-modal brain reorganization may apply equally to the sense of audition as to touch and provides a plausible reason for the development of extraordinary auditory abilities in some people who are blind. People with total blindness have been shown to process auditory input in the occipital cortices of their brains, increasing their ability to recognize sounds and use hearing to substitute for vision (Merabet et al., 2008). Teachers who are aware of this potential can encourage students to make use of their sense of hearing and can use this knowledge to create adaptations that make physical activities accessible. As with tactile skills, listening skills can be learned and taught (Barclay, 2011) and environments modified to support auditory skills.

Perception of sound depends in part on the quality of a sound signal, which is affected by environmental factors, such as interference from ambient noise, the sound-reflecting nature or degree of echo produced by the wall or floor coverings in a room, or the clarity of the sound signal. For example, a sound beacon placed in a gymnasium to help someone find a basketball hoop may be impossible to hear over the din of the other students in class; a teacher's voice may not be understood because it is echoing loudly off the hyper-reflective surface of ceramic tile in the swimming pool area; or the frequency of the sound source may be so high that it is impossible to locate with hearing. Under proper conditions, however, people with adequate binaural hearing are generally extremely effective at pinpointing the location of a sound source (Lawson & Wiener, 2010). Therefore, sound-emitting devices can be used to provide access to an activity such as soccer by indicating the location of the ball or the goal or by delineating the boundaries of the playing field (Ponchillia, 1995). Other examples of using auditory cues to make physical activities more accessible include placing a beeping device at the back edge of a basketball hoop, inserting bells into a soccer ball, or placing a CD player with music at the opposite corner of a mat as a sound beacon for a gymnastics diagonal floor routine.

As substitutes for vision, audition and touch are not necessarily separate entities. The interplay of the senses is complicated. The ability of a goalball player who is blind or blindfolded to use his or her haptic sense to maintain orientation on the court, discussed in the previous section—a task that involves a player's continual repositioning and reorientation throughout a 24-minute game—requires an extremely complex interaction of both hearing and touch. Players establish their place on the court by using the raised lines on the floor; once they move away from the starting position, they maintain their place on the court by listening to and interpreting the movements and voices of the other players and by following the feedback signals sent to their brains from their muscles.

Auditory Adaptations

Three important factors to consider when designing auditory adaptations for physical activities or games are the following:

- frequency or pitch of the sound being produced as the beacon
- construction materials used in the walls, floors, and ceilings of the facility being modified
- ambient sound or noise present during the activity

Sound beacons producing acoustic signals of extremely high frequency are not useful, because such sound waves tend to bounce off all surfaces, making them impossible to localize

(Lawson & Wiener, 2010). By the same token, if the walls of the facility in which the activity is being held are made of tile or other extremely hard substances, a similar problem occurs. Sound beacons are seldom used in indoor aquatics areas for this reason, and they are difficult to use in some gymnasiums as well. Types of sound beacons will be discussed in Chapter 5, but one simple solution is using a portable radio emitting a human voice. Because voices are made up of multifrequency sounds, they may be good beacons in general and are certainly superior to single-tone beepers in aquatics and gymnasium areas.

The skill of *sound localization,* or determining the source of a particular sound, is based on the binaural hearing system of human beings. Recognizing that a sound is coming from one direction or another is possible because the sound waves strike the closer ear a split second before they do the other, and the brain is capable of distinguishing that difference (Lawson & Wiener, 2010). It is sometimes difficult for people who have hearing losses to use sound beacons for orientation, with or without hearing aids, because this binaural ability can be impaired. Some digital and software-controlled hearing aids are designed to replace many of the ears' abilities, so they might be exceptions to this generalization.

At first glance, it might appear that sound beacons would not be effective for people with deafblindness. Assessment of each individual is key. Since deafblindness is defined as having virtually any degree of hearing loss along with a visual impairment, some individuals who are deafblind will be able to locate a sound source and use an auditory adaptation to access many games, and others will be able to hear the sound source without being able to localize it. In either case, certain adaptations would be unnecessary for these individuals, such as replacing the starter's pistol by tapping a sprinter who is deafblind at the time of the pistol shot.

Cochlear Implants

A cochlear implant is an electronic device designed to enhance hearing in people who are profoundly or totally deaf due to certain inner ear anomalies (www.umm.edu/otolaryngology/cochlear.htm). The device is composed of two parts, an internal receiver and electrode array that is surgically implanted under the skin and an external processor/microphone component housed in an earpiece. Cochlear implants are not hearing aids, since they do not simply amplify or clarify sound signals; nor do they reproduce voices and other sounds as they are heard by people without hearing impairments. Rather, users experience improvement in perceiving environmental sounds and receive the sensation of sound when conversing with others. The implant's user needs to interpret the sounds and learn to recognize rhythms and patterns of speech and use these perceptions to enhance lip reading (www.umm.edu/otolaryngology/cochlear.htm). With experience, most users can eventually learn to carry on everyday conversation and some even to talk on the telephone. The best candidates for cochlear implantation are very young children or adults with recent hearing losses. It should be noted that using cochlear implants has been controversial among some members of the deaf community with long-standing deafness. The controversy centers on these individuals' belief that people with deafness constitute a culture and that their difference is a point of pride.

Cochlear implants generally do not provide sufficient binaural hearing and sound localization to permit the use of sound beacons for orientation. However, sound can be heard, so whistles and the like can be used to signal the beginning and end of playing periods, races, and so forth.

PROFESSIONALS WHO TEACH INDIVIDUALS WITH VISUAL IMPAIRMENTS OR DEAFBLINDNESS

Children and adults with visual impairments may be taught physical activity skills by a wide variety of professionals in an education setting, a rehabilitation setting, or a transitional situation between education and rehabilitation. The descriptions of these professionals provided in this section are intended to introduce members of the book's potential audience to one another and to provide an overview of the services each member provides.

Personnel in Educational Settings

The majority of children with visual impairments or deafblindness receive services, including physical education training, in their local schools with their sighted classmates (Ponchillia, Strause, & Ponchillia, 2002). In many cases, given the low-incidence nature of these conditions, as noted earlier in this chapter, a child who attends his or her local school may be the only student there with a sensory impairment.

Some states provide educational services to students with visual impairments or deafblindness in state residential schools. In those settings, students commonly live and learn at the residential school during the school week, receiving instruction from teachers who have many students with visual impairments and several with deafblindness. In addition, such residential schools play important roles in the provision of blindness-specific educational services during the summer or on weekends, as resources to students and teachers throughout the state, and provide professional development for teachers.

In the United States, the education of students with disabilities, including visual impairments or deafblindness, is governed by federal law known as the Individuals with Disabilities Education Act (IDEA). A key provision of this law is that in a school system, all students with a disability who have been determined to be eligible for special education service must have created for them an Individualized Education Program (IEP), which identifies their educational goals and the services required to attain them. The services are predicated on an initial eligibility determination and are based on an assessment of the student's abilities and needs (see Chapter 3). Professionals who provide the services identified as necessary to help the student in reaching those goals are included on the student's IEP team, which is responsible for the writing and maintenance of the plan.

As mentioned in the vignettes in Chapter 1 of Christopher and Takisha, who were both in school, an adapted physical education teacher, teacher of children with visual impairments, and orientation and mobility (O&M) specialist were involved in their programs. Teaching assistants referred to as paraeducators (or sometimes as aides, teacher assistants, support teachers, or paraprofessionals) may also be involved with students as noncertified staff members working under the direction of certified personnel to support student learning, such as the "aide" described in the case of William earlier in this chapter. The teacher of students with visual impairments and the certified O&M instructor typically work within the school district's special education service program, but the adapted physical education teacher frequently does not. Instead, this teacher is usually a service provider within the physical education department of the school or school district and is not always part of the special education service system. The following sections describe these personnel in more detail. The responsibilities of professionals when working with students with deafblindness are discussed in more detail in Chapter 4.

Teacher of Students with Visual Impairments

The primary member of teams that serve children with visual impairments in this country are teachers of students with visual impairments, who are sometimes referred to as vision teachers, teachers of the visually impaired, or teacher consultants. Although the titles used are often a matter of geographical or other custom, the term *teacher consultant* is usually applied to a teacher who provides consultation during the majority of his or her work time and who consequently does direct teaching less than 50 percent of the time (Lewis & Allman, 2000). The teacher of students with visual impairments is an expert in the needs of students and the principles of instructing students who are visually impaired and prepares adaptations required to instruct students in reading, writing, math, and other academic subjects, as well as physical education. The teacher of students with visual impairments is also commonly responsible for teaching daily living, personal care, and social skills, among other components of the expanded core curriculum, described in Chapter 3.

Orientation and Mobility Specialist

An O&M specialist providing services in an educational setting teaches students techniques for safe and independent travel. Depending on the student's age and needs, O&M specialists also teach movement skills to children who are not yet walking, mobility skills prior to a child's use of a long cane, travel with the long cane, orientation to school and other environments, and concepts of space. This specialist often works with the teacher of students with visual impairments, with the occupational therapist on early childhood development, and with the adapted physical education instructor on physical skill development.

Adapted Physical Education Instructor

The adapted physical education instructor is a physical educator with special training in adapting the physical education curriculum to the needs of students with disabilities. Although they do not work in every school district, in general, adapted physical education instructors work either alone or jointly with the general physical education teacher to meet the physical education goals indicated on a student's IEP. The services provided by these teachers include designing students' physical education program; assessment of individuals and environments; student placement; teaching, counseling, and coaching; evaluation of services; coordination of resources; consulting with other teachers; and student advocacy (Block, 2007; Lieberman & Houston-Wilson, 2009; Sherrill, 2004). Adapted physical education teachers are considered direct service providers under IDEA (rather than a related service provider), because adapted physical education is a federally mandated component of special education services (U.S.C.A. 1402 [25]). This means that physical education needs to be provided to the student with a disability as part of the child's special education service plan (Sherrill, 2004).

Paraeducator

Paraeducators, also known as paraprofessionals, teacher's assistants, teacher's aides, educational aides, or just aides, are staff members who provide a range of support services to students under a teacher's supervision. They are generally provided for students with disabilities who need individual assistance in the classroom. In many cases, students with visual impairments or deafblindness will need the support of the paraeducator in physical education class (Conroy, 2012; Lieberman, Haibach, & Schedlin, 2012). The paraeducator works alongside the physical education teacher to ensure that the students with visual impairment or deafblindness are receiving the intended benefit from the physical education class, regardless of whether physical education is provided in an inclusive setting with nondisabled students, in a modified setting, or in a separate class. Paraeducators working in this situation should be trained in working with children with visual impairments or deafblindness as well as in physical education (Lieberman & Conroy, in press).

Interpreter and Intervener

Interpreters are professionals who translate communications for individuals who are hard of hearing and use sign language to communicate. Interveners may work with students with deafblindness to give them visual information in addition to interpreting for them. The roles of these professionals are discussed in Chapter 4.

Occupational Therapist

Occupational therapists have received training in human growth and development with specific emphasis on the effects of illness and injury on activities of daily living. They work with people who have physical, emotional, mental, and developmental disabilities. Occupational therapists work in the educational system with physical educators on the development of early physical skills, and with teachers of students with visual impairments or O&M specialists as consultants to provide assistance with children who have additional physical or other disabilities.

Personnel in Rehabilitation Settings

The rehabilitation system generally serves adults or older children who are making the transition from their education programs into rehabilitation training or vocational programs, rather than young children, and was primarily designed to help people with acquired disabilities resume work (Ponchillia & Ponchillia, 1996). Therefore, rehabilitation settings represent a model that differs considerably from that found within the education system. This system is a federal-state cooperative program through which the federal government provides the states the majority of the funds needed for them to offer direct rehabilitation services to people with visual impairments or deafblindness (Ponchillia & Ponchillia, 1996).

After eligibility is established and an Individualized Plan for Employment (IPE) is written, the state provides services known as personal adjustment training to people such as Antwan and Maria, the two adults described in Chapter 1, who are in need of adaptive skills, followed by vocational evaluation and training. Personal adjustment training is the portion of rehabilitation in which instructors teach individuals the adaptations that enable them to continue to perform the tasks of everyday life and to make them ready for vocational services. Although both Antwan and Maria received their services in a residential rehabilitation center, other recipients of personal adjustment training services might receive them in their homes, rather than in center-based settings. Antwan and Maria each worked with a vision rehabilitation therapist, an O&M specialist, and an occupational therapist. The roles of the O&M specialist and occupational therapist in rehabilitation settings are similar to the roles they play in the school setting, but they address skills at an adult level, depending on the needs of their clients. The vision rehabilitation therapist is described in the following section.

Vision Rehabilitation Therapist

A vision rehabilitation therapist (formerly known as a rehabilitation teacher) is a teacher who provides instructional services in communication skills, such as braille reading and writing, electronic listening and recording devices, handwriting, adaptive computing, reading with low vision devices, and adapted mathematics; home management skills, such as food preparation, home care, and home repair; personal management skills, such as personal hygiene, personal appearance, and medication management; leisure time and recreation skills, such as indoor and outdoor recreation, arts and crafts, games, and physical activities; and orientation and movement skills, such as walking with a human guide, indoor orientation and mobility, and room familiarization (Ponchillia & Ponchillia, 1996).

In Maria's case, center-based vision rehabilitation therapists taught her how to use braille, operate a talking computer, prepare meals, care for her apartment, and organize her new job. An O&M specialist who works with adults taught travel skills, use of a long cane, use of distance low vision devices (telescopes), orientation skills, and use of public transportation to both Antwan and Maria through the rehabilitation center. The occupational therapist at the rehabilitation center primarily taught arts and crafts activities, but also worked directly with Maria on adaptations to enable her to continue her equestrian hobby. The inclusion of weight machines in Antwan's program would surely have better prepared him to advocate for himself in the situation he faced at the health club.

The major differences in approaches between education and rehabilitation services are reflected in the vignettes in Chapter 1. Antwan and Maria, both past school age, had received physical education instruction in elementary and secondary school, in college, and in nonacademic training programs for adults. As a consequence, they were equipped with specific physical skills well before the onset of their visual impairments. The vision loss had no real effect on their physical abilities, only on their confidence to participate and on the degree of access they had to places where they could practice their skills as individuals with visual impairments. They received services as part of rehabilitation programs, which were designed to teach them adaptations to the activities in order to enable them to use the skills they knew. For example, Maria knew how to ride a horse before receiving rehabilitation services, so she needed help in figuring out how horseback riding could be adapted to her level of vision, not learning how to ride.

■

The professionals just described, along with the parents, friends, and community volunteers, are potential players on the team working to promote the acquisition of physical education and sports skills and activity access for adults and children with visual impairments or deafblindness. Not only these professionals but also highly skilled volunteers, such as athletes with disabilities; students in university teacher preparation programs in adapted physical education, visual impairment, or deafblindness; professional coaches; and many others play significant roles in this endeavor. Such volunteers staff the many physical education, sports, and recreation summer camps and other programs offered annually across the country that provide supplemental educational services.

CONCLUSION

Understanding the nature of visual impairment and deafblindness enables professionals who are working with children or adults to better understand their needs and their abilities. Applying this knowledge to modify methods of instruction in physical skills and activities and adapting activities, games, and sports for the participation of people with visual impairments are described in Chapters 4 and 5. First, however, Chapter 3 provides an overview of physical education in the school system and its importance for children with visual impairments or deafblindness.

3 Providing Physical Education to Students with Visual Impairments or Deafblindness

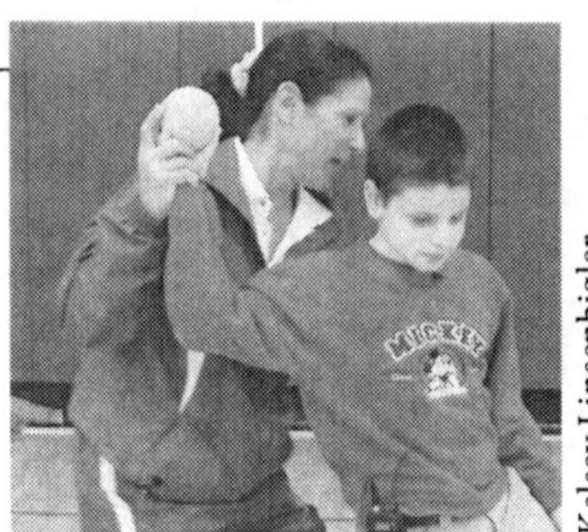
Kelsey Linsenbigler

IN THIS CHAPTER

- **What Is Physical Education?**
- **The Value of Physical Education for Children with Visual Impairments or Deafblindness**
- **Physical Education and the Law**
- **Assessment**
- **Planning a Physical Education Program**
- **Transition Services and Physical Education**

Viva is a 9-year-old girl who has been blind from birth. She is just beginning fourth grade at her local elementary school. Her physical education teacher does not know how to provide accommodations that would allow her to participate in activities that involve balls. She participates in fitness units and kicks and throws balls with her para-educator on the side. She has played games at home with her older brother and knows how to kick and throw, and walk and swim.

When she attended a summer sports camp for children with visual impairments, at the suggestion of her teacher of students with visual impairments, the director asked her what experiences she had in sports or physical activities. She answered that she cannot "do sports in PE" because she is blind. The games move too fast and they are "not safe" for her. Her physical education teacher believed this to be true; the teacher's university professional preparation courses had not prepared her to include children like Viva in physical education classes. Unfortunately, because Viva has had the same teacher for four years, Viva has begun to believe this to be true as well.

Situations such as that described in Viva's scenario, in which children with visual impairments languish on the sidelines while their classmates participate in sports and other activities in physical education class, are all too common. Chapter 1 described many of the various reasons why people with visual impairment or deafblindness frequently do not develop skills in physical activities. This chapter focuses on physical education in the schools, and a common reason why students who are visually impaired do not participate actively in physical education is the lack of preparation that their teachers have for including them in their classes.

Physical education teachers typically feel that they do not have the appropriate professional preparation to include children with visual impairments in regular physical education activities (Conroy, 2012; Lieberman, Houston-Wilson, & Kozub, 2002). Parents of children who have visual impairments and who are included in their neighborhood schools confirm that their children's physical education teachers often appear not to know how to teach their child, and some of their children are aware of this as well (Perkins, Bailey, Columna, & Lieberman, 2012; Stuart, Lieberman, & Hand, 2006).

Although some professionals may not have worked with a student with a visual impairment or deafblindness before, it is important to remember that the student with a visual impairment or deafblindness is a student like any other who may have certain individual needs. Detailed information on working comfortably with students with disabilities is provided in the following chapter. In general, helpful ways of preparing for instruction with a student who is visually impaired include reading the student's past records and familiarizing oneself with any conditions the student may have; contacting the teacher of students with visual impairments ahead of time to discuss the student's needs and begin thinking about any necessary adaptations or modifications; and if possible, talking to family members to obtain more information about the student.

Physical education is an important part of the general education program for all students at every age and grade level, providing a range of benefits, from health and fitness to lessons in socialization, teamwork, competition, and cooperation that can have lifelong benefits. It is no less beneficial for students with visual impairments or deafblindness; indeed, physical education can have additional advantages for this group of students who may have fewer opportunities in the community than other students to experience those benefits. A position statement written for the Council for Exceptional Children's Division of Visual Impairment (see Sidebar 3.1) emphasizes that physical education is a core subject area that every student, including those with visual impairments and deafblindness, needs to experience. Yet students like Viva are missing out on these benefits every day and receiving the message that they are not considered as able as their sighted classmates.

SIDEBAR 3.1

Physical Education for Children and Youths with Visual Impairments

Louis M. Tutt, Lauren Lieberman, and Bob Brasher

Physical activities, whether structured or recreational, are important in the lives of boys and girls, men and women. All people deserve formal and informal opportunities to fully develop physical skills and abilities. Children and youths who are visually impaired should have every opportunity to participate in physical activities with other children, including those who are sighted, and have specific physical activities adapted when necessary to meet their individual needs at various growth and developmental stages (Blessing, McCrimmin, Stovall, & Williford, 1993; Lieberman, Robinson, & Rollheiser, 2006; Stuart, Lieberman, & Hand, 2006).

Physical education is the development of motor skills and patterns through individual and group games, aquatics, dance, cooperative activities, and lifelong recreational activities (IDEA, 2004, PL 108-446). It contributes to the student's cognitive, affective, and psychomotor development. Adapted physical education is defined as physical education modified to meet the unique needs of students with disabilities (Lieberman & Houston-Wilson, 2009). Adapted physical education instruction can be delivered in a variety of placements, including those found in both public and special school settings. The entire multidisciplinary team makes such placement decisions, taking into consideration factors such as fitness level, motor skills development, ability to be in large groups, social needs, and safety (Columna, Davis, Lieberman, & Lytle, 2010). There is no separate curriculum for students with visual impairments (Lieberman, 2010). All students should learn the same units, with modifications when necessary, and students with visual impairments should typically receive an equal amount of instruction per week or more as their sighted classmates receive. Skilled peer tutors and paraeducators can be a resource to assist with games, fitness, or other activities when needed (Rusotti & Shaw, 2004; Wiskochil, Lieberman, Houston-Wilson, & Petersen, 2007). When students who are blind or visually impaired are in a class with sighted peers, the entire class should learn blind sports such as goalball, beep baseball, 5-a-side soccer, tandem biking, or running with no sight when possible. Such action provides disability awareness and gives sighted peers knowledge of the sports that students participate in who are blind or visually impaired (Foley, Tindall, Lieberman, & Kim, 2007).

Without physical education, students with visual impairments are at risk of not developing good locomotor skills necessary for fitness and wellness (Houwen, Hartman, & Visscher, 2009). Stereotypical barriers or fear of liability must not exclude students with visual impairments from participating in physical education activities.

Source: Position paper revised for review by the general membership, Division on Visual Impairments, Council for Exceptional Children, retrieved 2/28/12 from http://www.cecdvi.org/positionpapers.html.

Moreover, students with visual impairments who are not given appropriate guidance in how they can engage in physical activity throughout their life may be at risk of developing a predominantly passive lifestyle, without the pleasure or health benefits physical activities can bring (Lewis & Wolffe, 2006). This book aims to provide professionals with information and resources that enable them to include children who are visually impaired or deafblind in physical education and thereby help them experience the benefits of physical activity: positive self-esteem and a potentially active lifestyle.

Subsequent chapters offer detailed information about how physical educators can provide an appropriate program for students with visual impairments or deafblindness who include them in physical education classes with their sighted classmates. This chapter provides an overview of the purposes and content of physical education, its importance for students with visual impairments, the provisions of the law that mandate physical education for students with disabilities, and the relevant components of physical education for children with visual impairments or deafblindness.

WHAT IS PHYSICAL EDUCATION?

Physical education is the foundation of fitness, health, and participation in sports, as well as of a healthy lifestyle for all children and youths. Physical education programs offer the opportunity to provide physical activity to all children and to teach them the skills and knowledge needed to establish and sustain an active lifestyle (NASPE, 2011). Physical education is part of the educational curriculum from the early grades through high school and beyond. A good well-rounded, accessible physical education program provides the basis for physical activity, sport, and recreation for a lifetime and can lead to increased participation in social activities with others and improvements in social skills, as well as increased self-esteem.

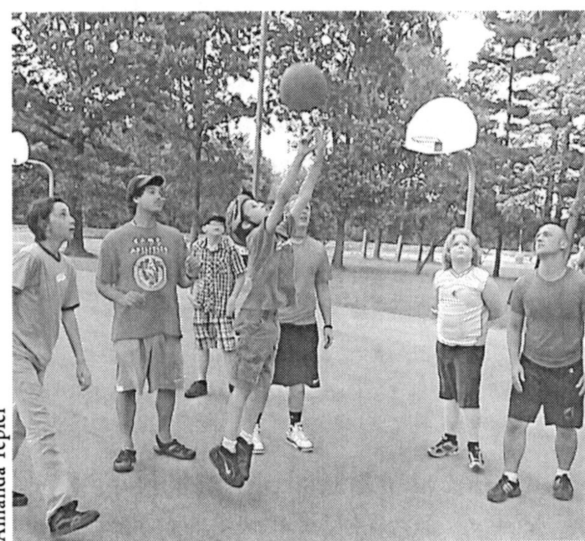

Amanda Tepfer

A well-rounded, physical education program with a variety of activities provides the basis for a lifetime of physical activity and opportunities for socializing with classmates.

As defined in the Individuals with Disabilities Education Act (IDEA), the federal law that regulates special education in the United States, physical education is the development of physical and motor fitness; fundamental motor skills and patterns; and skills in aquatics, dance, and individual and group games and sports (including intramural sports) (IDEA, Sec 300.39[b][2]). According to the National Association for Sport and Physical Education (NASPE, 2004, 2011), an organization whose mission is to enhance knowledge, improve professional practice, and increase support for high-quality physical education, sports, and physical activity programs, the content of physical education should include the following:

- instruction in a variety of motor skills that are designed to enhance the physical, mental, and social/emotional development of every child
- fitness education and assessment to help children understand and improve or maintain their physical well-being
- development of cognitive concepts about motor skill and fitness
- opportunities to improve emerging social and cooperative skills through physical activity and gain a multicultural perspective
- promotion of recommended amounts of physical activity now and throughout life

NASPE (2004) has also set forth national standards for physical education to provide the framework for a high-quality physical education program and as a structure around which states and local school districts can develop standards and curricula with realistic and achievable expectations for students' performance (see Sidebar 3.2). These standards apply to all children, including those with visual impairments. Although instruction for students with visual impairments may vary from that provided for their sighted classmates, the standards that students with visual impairments and their sighted classmates need to work toward are the same.

To fulfill the goals outlined in the NASPE standards, physical education programs focus on instructional units relating to different skills and based on students' developmental needs at each level. The following are typical physical education instructional units commonly used at each level (see Sidebar 3.3):

SIDEBAR 3.2

National Association for Sport and Physical Education Standards

The purpose of the National Standards document is to provide the framework for a quality physical education.

Standard 1

Demonstrates competency in motor skills and movement patterns needed to perform a variety of physical activities.

Standard 2

Demonstrates understanding of movement concepts, principles, strategies, and tactics as they apply to the learning and performance of physical activities.

Standard 3

Participates regularly in physical activity.

Standard 4

Achieves and maintains a health-enhancing level of physical fitness.

Standard 5

Exhibits responsible personal and social behavior that respects self and others in physical activity settings.

Standard 6

Values physical activity for health, enjoyment, challenge, self-expression, and/or social interaction.

Source: National Association for Sport and Physical Education, *Moving into the Future: National Standards for Physical Education,* 2d ed. (St. Louis: Mosby, 2004), retrieved 7/3/12 from http://www.aahperd.org/naspe/standards/nationalStandards/PEstandards.cfm.

SIDEBAR 3.3

Typical Physical Education Skills Taught at Different Levels

Skills Taught in Preschool Programs

- object control (such as throwing, catching, batting, and rolling)
- locomotor skills (such as running, hopping, skipping, and jumping)
- play
- orientation (teaching concepts such as *in, out, under,* and *through* by the use of obstacle courses and games and activities)

Skills Taught in Elementary School

- locomotor skills (such as running, hopping, skipping, and jumping)
- object control skills (such as throwing, catching, batting, and rolling)

SIDEBAR 3.3 *(continued)*

- "lead-up" games and sports-related skills (games with a small number of players on each side that develop foundational skills to prepare children for sports and recreational activities, such as relay races, tag games, and three-versus-three keep-away soccer games)
- physical fitness
- aquatics
- rhythm and dance

Skills Taught in Secondary School

- sports skills (such as soccer, basketball, ultimate Frisbee, and volleyball)
- physical fitness (such as running, biking, weight lifting, aerobics, and Pilates)
- aquatics (such as swimming, diving, water aerobics, water polo, and kayaking)
- lifetime activities (such as badminton, archery, bocce, and bowling)
- rhythm and dance
- adventure-based activities (such as hiking, rock climbing, kayaking, and mountain biking)

In order to teach these skills, physical education professionals not only need to have knowledge of the particular activities but also need a thorough grounding in physiological and biomechanical concepts, motor learning, and principles of development. They need to know effective instructional methods that are flexible and geared to students' developmental levels and individual needs, such as demonstrations and modeling, cues and prompting, and ways of providing feedback, all while maintaining a safe and secure environment. Physical educators also have the responsibility of developing and teaching a curriculum that meets the state and national standards for physical education for their grade.

In most cases, students with visual impairments or deafblindness will be included in the general education physical education class, so the general physical educator is the teacher, but he or she is not alone in working with a student who has special needs. A team of professionals can help and may be necessary in the process, and may include a teacher of students with visual impairments, an orientation and mobility (O&M) instructor, an adapted physical educator, and a paraeducator, as described in Chapter 2. (Additional sources of assistance are described in Sidebar 3.4.) The teacher may use peer tutors as well. In some cases, however, depending on the student's Individualized Education Program (IEP, introduced in Chapter 2 and discussed in detail later in this chapter) and based on his or her needs, a student with a visual impairment or deafblindness is placed in a separate class that will be taught by an adapted physical educator, general physical educator, or both, with the support of the paraeducator and a peer tutor. (See Chapter 2 for more information on the roles of these professionals.)

Physical education teachers who teach children with visual impairments or deafblindness need to ensure that they modify class activities so that these students have equal access to the curriculum and the opportunity to achieve the same standards as their classmates (as described in detail in Chapter 4 and throughout Part 3 of this book). The physical educator can turn to the teacher of students with visual impairments, the O&M instructor, or the adapted physical educator, if one is available, for more help with questions about how to modify the activities or instruction to include their students in the class activities. Sidebar 3.5 suggests some ways that these team members can collaborate.

SIDEBAR 3.4

Resources and Information on Working with Students Who Are Blind or Visually Impaired

When a physical educator or other professional needs assistance and support in knowing how to work with a student with a visual impairment or deafblindness, the primary resources to consult are the members of the student's educational team, such as a teacher of students with visual impairments, an O&M specialist, an adapted physical education instructor, or an intervener who works with students who are deafblind. The office of the director of special education for your school district may be able to provide additional resources.

Should further assistance be needed, however, most states have the following agencies, which are principal sources of assistance:

- the state's special school for students who are visually impaired
- the state department of education, and in particular the consultant from this state department who specializes in the education of students who are visually impaired, often referred to as "the state vision consultant"
- the state commission for persons who are visually impaired, or a unit focusing on people who are visually impaired within the state department of rehabilitation or vocational rehabilitation
- state departments or agencies that focus on education, training, employment, and rehabilitation issues for individuals who are visually impaired
- federally funded deaf-blind projects in each state that provide technical assistance to families and professionals

Specific contact information for each state's agencies is available from the American Foundation for the Blind (AFB) through its help-line number ([800] 232-5463 in the United States), or the AFB Directory of Services search feature on AFB's website at www.afb.org. Information about state deaf-blind projects is available from the National Consortium on Deaf-Blindness (www.nationaldb.org), a national technical assistance and information dissemination center for children and youths who are deafblind.

Finally, the organizations listed in the Resources section at the back of this book are important sources for additional information.

SIDEBAR 3.5

Collaboration between Teachers of Students with Visual Impairments and Physical Educators

Teachers of students with visual impairments and physical educators or adapted physical educators can work together to support their students who are visually impaired or deafblind by communicating frequently, exchanging information, and sharing their special expertise. Communication should be conducted face to face when possible but also through any effective, regular means, such as lesson plans, e-mails, texts, or phone calls.

Teachers of students with visual impairments can

- explain the student's visual impairment and any other disabilities and their implications for the student's physical performance
- share the IEP goals and objectives
- offer assistance with adaptations and accessible materials

SIDEBAR 3.5 *(continued)*

- describe equipment and other products designed for people with visual impairments and where it can be purchased
- explain instructional techniques for working with students with visual impairments or deafblindness
- explain the expanded core curriculum
- provide print and other instructional materials needed by a student in an alternate medium or format the student can access
- observe the student in the physical education class to see if additional support is needed
- suggest that students meet adults with visual impairments who are active physically who can serve as role models and suggest ways to identify such role models
- provide information on sports organizations for people with disabilities the student and family can be encouraged to join
- provide pre-teaching for the student or assist another professional in pre-teaching components of physical education lessons

The physical educator can

- share all physical education units for the year, including skills to be taught and length of the unit
- provide information about the class's physical education goals
- ask for support from the teacher of students with visual impairments or the adapted physical education instructor
- share the student's successes with the teacher and family and indicate how physical activity can be incorporated into the student's life at home
- communicate about the sports that the student excels in and encourage the student to train for after school sports or the United States Association for Blind Athletes programs (see Chapter 11)
- provide written instructions or other materials to be adapted for the student ahead of time

The adapted physical education instructor can

- become familiar with the student's IEP goals and the goals of the physical education class as a whole
- ask the teacher of students with visual impairments for information about working with students with visual impairments and deafblindness and suggestions for adaptations
- suggest adapted physical education equipment and products that may be useful for the student

Together the teacher of students with visual impairments, the physical educator, and the adapted physical education instructor can

- train the paraeducator
- train peer tutors
- train after-school coaches
- make sure that pre-teaching is taking place when necessary
- share information about summer sports camps and other events with the family

THE VALUE OF PHYSICAL EDUCATION FOR CHILDREN WITH VISUAL IMPAIRMENTS OR DEAFBLINDNESS

Physical education is part of the general education curriculum, and therefore it is mandatory for every student. In addition to its role as part of the curriculum in general education, physical education also provides the foundation for instruction in the area of recreation and leisure skills of the expanded core curriculum for students with visual impairments or blindness. The expanded core curriculum consists of the areas of specialized skills that students with visual impairments need to learn to be able to access the general core curriculum, succeed in their education, and become functioning, independent adults (Sapp & Hatlen, 2010), including the following:

- compensatory or functional academic skills, including communication modes
- O&M
- social interaction skills
- independent living skills
- recreation and leisure skills
- career education
- use of assistive technology
- sensory efficiency skills
- self-determination

Key components of many of these other areas of the expanded core curriculum are also infused into physical education classes. For example, in addition to specific physical skills that can be used in recreation and leisure activities, physical education also teaches social skills. According to Farrenkopf and McGregor (2000, p. 440), "students learn valuable social skills, including cooperation, competition, communication, turn taking, sportsmanship, and getting along with others in physical education classes. Physical education affords students with visual impairments the opportunity to interact with other students in a positive and socially appropriate manner." O&M, communication, and sensory efficiency skills are all utilized as well. Moreover, the sense of competence and self-determination that can be achieved through active participation in physical activities with classmates can contribute to greater independence and success in other areas.

It is a premise of this book that providing physical education for students with blindness or visual impairments in an inclusive environment with their classmates (in addition to being required by law under most circumstances, as discussed later in this chapter) will provide students with more opportunities for learning in the various areas of the expanded core curriculum. In an inclusive class, students with blindness or visual impairment will be more likely to be exposed to a greater variety of experiences (sports, physical activity, and recreation), interact with same-age classmates, gain independence within the sports arena, and learn about potential careers in sports than in a separate class. In addition, when individuals with disabilities are included side by side with their peers in everyday activities, they are more likely to be viewed as valued in society (Wolfensberger, 1972), which can have a positive effect on the students' self-esteem.

As part of both the general curriculum and the expanded core curriculum, physical education is a key area to study for students who are visually impaired for their health and well-being and for future success in life. Some of the research showing improvements in students' physical stamina and fitness, perceived competence, self-esteem, self-determination, and socialization as a result of physical education is summarized in the following sections.

Improvement in Physical Stamina and Fitness

The lack of participation in physical education by students with visual impairment and deafblindness that has already been noted may be related to the fact that both children and adults with visual impairments have been found to be less active and less physically fit when compared to others of the same age (Holbrook, Caputo, Perry, Fuller, & Morgan, 2009; Lieberman & McHugh, 2001). For example, although individuals with visual impairments tend to utilize more energy during activities of daily living than their school classmates (Buell, 1982), they also tend to have lower levels of physical activity and health-related fitness (Lieberman, Byrne, Mattern, Watt, & Fernández-Vivó, 2010; Skaggs & Hopper, 1996; Wyatt & Ng, 1997). But research has also shown that with appropriate programming, students with visual impairments can equal their sighted classmates in the area of fitness (Blessing, McCrimmon, Stovall, & Williford, 1993; Williams, Armstrong, Eves, & Faulkner, 1996). In addition, as discussed further in the next section, higher levels of physical activity and health-related fitness can improve students' perceptions of their abilities and competence and increase their self-esteem (Ponchillia, Strause, & Ponchillia, 2002).

Providing an appropriate amount (number of times per week) and quality (appropriate degree of participation) of physical education will increase the likelihood that students with visual impairments or deafblindness will enjoy sports and recreation in the future. It will also increase the likelihood that they will become physically active adults (NASPE, 2011).

Perceived Competence

The way a person thinks about himself or herself in a particular area or endeavor, such as physical activity or social interactions, is known as *perceived competence*. Children may have different perceptions of their competence in different areas. Positive perceived competence in athletics may lead to increased participation and success in this area. It has been suggested that negative perceptions of their own athletic competence among children and youths with visual impairments may reflect a lack of meaningful community and school-based opportunities for physical activity (Shapiro, Moffett, Lieberman, & Dummer, 2005). Children's feelings about their social competence also can be related to their involvement in physical activity as well as how well they perform; those who score high on measures of social competence tend to be more physically active and have better scores on selected measures of physical fitness (Page et al., 1992).

Physical activity provides more social opportunities and an additional avenue to having common bonds with peers (Farrenkopf & McGregor, 2000). With a proper physical education program that teaches each child at his or her developmental level, all children can learn and grow, and these successful experiences can, in turn, lead them to develop improved perceptions of their own competence and enhance their self-esteem (Farrenkopf & McGregor,

2000; Ponchillia, Strause, & Ponchillia, 2002; Schedlin, Lieberman, Houston-Wilson, & Cruz, 2012).

Self-Determination

Self-determination is the perception of the ability to possess control, power, and decision-making ability over one's life (Wehmeyer, Agran, & Hughes, 1998). A perception of self-determination—that is, the sense that a person has control over his or her own behavior and choices—is an important factor in becoming an independent and successful person. According to Sapp and Hatlan (2010),

> Self-determination refers to a person's right to decide freely and without undue influence how he or she wishes to live his or her life. To develop self-determination skills, children or adolescents who are visually impaired must be provided with the necessary knowledge and experience. They must learn which choices are available to them, have the skills necessary to take advantage of these choices, and be given opportunities to make age-appropriate choices for themselves.

Participating in activities such as physical education provides opportunities for choice in participation, social connections, and adaptations and modifications. However, children with visual impairments have been found to have low levels of self-determination when it comes to both physical education and friendships (Lieberman & Stuart, 2002; Perkins, Bailey, Columna, & Lieberman, 2012; Robinson & Lieberman, 2004). The provision of a well-rounded physical education program with a variety of sports, games, fitness, and lifetime recreation can increase the variety of opportunities and choices for children with visual impairments or deafblindness and lead to an increase in their sense of self-determination (Lieberman, Haibach, & Schedlin, 2012). Therefore, it is important for teachers to ask themselves whether a student with disabilities has the same choices and options as his or her same-age classmates.

Socialization

The ability to socialize and get along with others is a crucial skill for everyone, preventing social isolation and enabling everyone to succeed in future endeavors that require getting along with others, in both family life and work (Sacks & Wolffe, 2006). Yet, children with disabilities often experience negative attitudes and interactions from their classmates (Blinde & McCallister, 1998; Goodwin, 2001; Taub & Greer, 2000), which increase their feelings of loneliness and isolation (Taub & Greer, 2000). For example, it has been found that both children and youths with visual impairments have low and stable perceptions of social acceptance (Shapiro et al., 2005). Achieving satisfactory social situations becomes even more difficult for teenagers (Rosengren & Undemar, 2001). This might reflect a consistent experience of peer rejection and loneliness on the part of students with visual impairments throughout their school years. Because these students have often had such negative experiences with their classmates, their ability and opportunity to engage in community events and activities may be impeded. Participation in physical education and developing the constellation of skills involved can help counteract this effect.

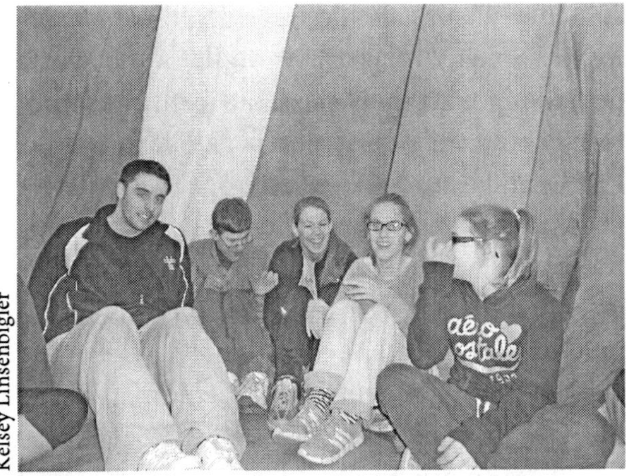
Kelsey Linsenbigler

Participation in physical education and activities, such as this parachute game, can help counteract common feelings of loneliness and isolation.

The Particular Value of Physical Education for Students with Deafblindness

For students with deafblindness, the need for learning in the psychomotor domain and for socialization is as great as or greater than that of their classmates with visual impairments or those with typical sight. Because it results in the diminution or absence of input from two primary sensory channels, deafblindness can be extremely isolating and can cut a child off from socializing and friendships with peers (Miles & Riggio, 1999). This isolation has many causes, but in essence because individuals with deafblindness frequently rely on interpreters or interveners (discussed in Chapter 2) and often can converse with only one person at a time, they commonly have a limited variety of experiences, and as a result have limited social development (Miles & Riggio, 1999).

Active participation in physical education provides the following benefits for students with deafblindness:

- clear concepts of common sports and activities
- a shared experience and knowledge they will have in common with classmates
- a clear idea of the students in their class as individuals
- an opportunity to be part of a team, which can provide them a sense of belonging and ownership
- opportunities for socialization
- improved language skills
- self-determination skills
- increased mobility, independence, and stamina
- increased understanding of the world

Being part of a physical activity program can also open doors for leadership opportunities (Lieberman, Arndt, & Grassick, 2010).

For individuals who are visually impaired or deafblind, physical education and recreation can reduce physical, social, and psychological isolation (Blinde and McClung, 1997; Smith, 2002). Inclusion of students in regular physical education classes has a positive effect on their socialization skills as well as on their choice to participate in sports (Lieberman, Houston-Wilson, & Kozub, 2002; Ponchillia, Strause, & Ponchillia, 2002). Moreover, the likelihood of students with visual impairments reaping the rewards of physical activity increases when they are included in regular educational environments (Ponchillia, Strause, & Ponchillia, 2002), with supports when necessary (Conroy, 2012; Lieberman, Haibach, & Schedlin, 2012). It has been found that the physical educator is one of the more influential variables for socialization within the physical education class (Suomi, Collier, & Brown, 2003). This key professional, the physical educator, can have an important role to play in improving the opportunities for students with visual impairments to socialize in addition to improving their physical abilities (Conroy, 2012; Lieberman, Haibach, & Schedlin, 2012).

PHYSICAL EDUCATION AND THE LAW

Just like any other part of the general education curriculum, physical education is mandated for students with disabilities, including those with visual impairments, by the Individuals with Disabilities Education Act (IDEA). It is important to be aware of how the provisions of the law apply to physical education with students who are visually impaired or deafblind.

Least Restrictive Environment

IDEA requires that students with disabilities receive their education in the least restrictive environment—that is, that they be educated with their sighted classmates in the regular classroom to the maximum extent possible. This means that students with visual impairments should be removed from the general education environment only when the nature or severity of the disability will not allow the student to benefit from the program, even with the use of supplemental aids or supports. Put simply, students with disabilities should be educated with their same-age classmates (a situation usually referred to as *inclusion*) unless it would not be beneficial to the student. Thus, students with visual impairments or deafblindness not only are required to have physical education classes to the same extent as all other students but also should be taking those classes in the same gymnasium or on the same sports field along with their classmates, unless something about their condition prohibits it.

Should a student's educational team determine that general physical education is not appropriate, the student may be placed in a smaller modified class, a segregated class, or a combination of placements, depending on where the student would benefit most (Columna, Davis, Lieberman, & Lytle, 2010). Any physical education class that is modified to meet a student's unique need is referred to as *adapted physical education.* Adapted physical education is the service the student receives, not the placement in which the student receives it (Lieberman & Houston-Wilson, 2009); that is, even when a student with a visual impairment is included in the general physical education class, he or she may still be receiving adapted physical education services.

Qualified Personnel

In addition to requiring physical education for all students with disabilities as a direct service, IDEA also stipulates that such education should be provided by qualified personnel. Although federal legislation does not clearly define *qualified personnel,* most states define it in the regulations governing physical education in that state. For example, in New York State, the term *qualified personnel* with regard to physical education is defined as anyone certified to teach physical education. Other states may allow classroom teachers to provide adapted physical education, while still others may require certification in adapted physical education. Regardless of state definitions, whoever provides physical education to students with visual impairments needs to be aware of appropriate adaptations and modifications to be able to ensure successful and safe physical education experiences.

Most teachers educated to be adapted physical education specialists work as consultants with general physical education teachers to ensure appropriate programming and instruction (see Chapter 2). In some instances, the adapted physical education specialist may work on a one-to-one basis with students either inside or outside of the regular physical education class, train a paraeducator to work with the students, or teach a separate segregated class. In any of these situations, the general physical education teacher should work with the adapted physical education teacher to create the best program for students with visual impairments or deafblindness (Hodge, Lieberman, & Murata, 2012).

The Individualized Education Program

Under IDEA, all students with disabilities must be provided with a written document known as the Individualized Education Program (IEP) that identifies their specific educational needs; develops a program to address those needs, with specific and measurable goals and objectives for each area of instruction; and determines the appropriate resources to achieve those goals. (For a sample of a typical IEP form, see Appendix 3A.)

Typically, upon notification that a student with a visual impairment will be entering a district, an IEP team is assembled to determine an appropriate plan for the student. IEP team members (often referred to as the *educational team*) usually include the families, the student (when appropriate), special education teachers, teachers of students with visual impairments, O&M instructors, school psychologists, general education teachers, the physical education teacher, and any other representatives deemed necessary by the district or the families. During IEP evaluations and discussions, the team makes decisions about what types of classes the student should be placed in, determines modification and adaptation strategies, and finalizes goals and objectives specific to each curricular area.

In general, IEPs describe a student's current level of performance, identify goals and objectives for the future, and list educational services to be provided to meet these goals (Short, 2011). (See Sidebar 3.6 for a list of all the components of an IEP.) Current law states that the IEP must be revised annually at an IEP meeting called to discuss the student's progress toward his or her goals and objectives. Because

SIDEBAR 3.6

Components of the Individualized Education Program (IEP)

Although formats differ among Individualized Educational Programs (IEPs) in different states or localities, the following basic components are essentially the same:

1. Present level of performance
2. Annual goals and short-term objectives
3. Supplementary aids and support services
4. Statement of participation in regular settings
5. Assessment modifications
6. Schedule of services
7. Transition services
8. Procedures for evaluation and parental reports

physical education is a direct service—meaning the curricular area is mandatory and required by law—goals and objectives for physical education, as well as necessary adaptations to equipment, rules, and instruction, should be included in the appropriate section of the IEP.

The IEP serves the following functions in each area of instruction, including physical education:

- It serves as a communication tool for the whole IEP team, including the student's family, and the school administration.
- It holds the teacher accountable for the student's learning.
- It is a commitment of school resources and services.
- It ensures assessment is occurring.

Assessment of the student's strengths and weaknesses is part of the process of creating the IEP. For physical education, a student's IEP goals are determined by psychomotor assessment to see which areas need improvement. (Methods of assessment for physical education are discussed in the next section.) The general physical education teacher, the adapted physical education teacher, or both can propose goals for the IEP team to approve. Some of the physical education IEP goals may be similar to the goals of a student's class, such as increasing cardiovascular fitness. Some may be different than the class goals, for example, "developing independence in turn taking." Either way, the goals should be infused into the physical education class and the student should not be pulled out if the student's placement is inclusion. The only time it is not necessary for a student with a visual impairment to have physical education goals and objectives in his or her IEP is if the student can easily participate in general physical education with no modifications or adaptations.

Sidebar 3.7 provides examples of the physical education goals and objectives for three students, one who is blind, one who has low vision, and one who is deafblind and also has physical disabilities, showing how the programs are individualized for each student's unique needs. Chapters 4 and 5 provide detailed information about how instruction may be modified and activities adapted for students who are visually impaired or deafblind.

The importance of being specific on the IEP about the supports and services that the team is recommending for a student can be illustrated by the scenario at the beginning of this chapter. Viva's paraeducator came to physical education class but did not help her participate in the class activities. If her IEP had stated that in order for Viva to be successfully included, her paraeducator had to assist her in physical education class, she would have been provided with that support because the school had made that commitment.

As already noted, a student for whom the IEP meeting is being held may attend the meeting, but whether the student does so depends on scheduling of the meeting and the student's maturity or interest. Whether the student attends the meeting or not, however, it is important not only to include physical education on the IEP, but to ensure the goals and objectives are shared and discussed with the student. Discussing the goals with students helps them to be aware of their strengths and weaknesses and can help motivate them to realize their goals and potential. Unfortunately, this does not always happen. For example, in one study (Lieberman, Robinson, & Rollheiser,

SIDEBAR 3.7

Examples of IEP Goals and Objectives for Physical Education

The following examples of goals and objectives illustrate how they may be tailored to the needs of individual students:

MARCO

Marco is blind and is 14 years old. He has a trained peer tutor who works with him one on one during his inclusive physical education class. He has a paraeducator in his classes who comes to physical education with him, but his peer tutor works with him most of the time.

Performance Area: Aquatics

Present Level of Performance

Marco can swim the crawl stroke with proper form with arm extension, flutter kick, and rhythmic breathing for one length of a 25-yard pool in 45 seconds with verbal support from his peer tutor.

Annual Goal

Marco will improve on his swimming skills.

Short-Term Objective/Benchmarks

Marco will swim the crawl stroke with proper form with arm extension, flutter kick, and rhythmic breathing for one length of a 25-yard pool in 35 seconds with verbal support from his peer tutor.

Assessment Method

Marco will be assessed with the aquatics skills checklist through qualitative methods (skill analysis) and quantitative methods (distance and times).

Schedule

Marco will be assessed on swimming at the beginning and end of his swimming unit, which lasts eight weeks.

Special Education Program or Services

Marco will have a paraeducator in all classes. He will use a one-to-one trained peer tutor for physical education.

Related Services

Marco receives services from the teacher of the visually impaired every day, and orientation and mobility two times a week.

Testing Accommodations

Marco will be taught the skills on his assessments both verbally and through tactile means. He will also be permitted two trials before the actual testing to ensure he knows what is expected of him.

Participation with Students without Disabilities

Marco will be included with his same-age sighted classmates 100 percent of the time. He will be provided a trained peer tutor for each class, and his paraeducator will accompany him to physical education.

Transition Services

Marco is currently learning how to use a public pool, fitness facilities, a bowling alley, and an ice skating rink. He will also be going hiking and camping in a local park in May. Marco is also learning how to play modified Wii bowling and Wii tennis games.

Transportation

Marco is learning how to take public transportation to his community-based recreation facilities with his O&M instructor.

BEN

Ben is 16 and has Stargardt disease, which affects his central vision. He is independent in his physical education class. He enjoys his physical education class and is on his school's cross-country team.

Performance Area: Fitness

Present Level of Performance

Ben can perform 52 bent-knee curl-ups with proper form independently (47 is standard for his age).

(Continued on next page)

SIDEBAR 3.7 *(continued)*

Annual Goal

Ben will improve his abdominal strength.

Short-Term Objective/Benchmarks

Ben will perform 60 curl-ups with proper form independently.

Assessment Method

Ben will be assessed with his general physical education class.

Schedule

Ben will be assessed when his class is assessed on health-related physical fitness and units in the curriculum.

Special Education Program or Services

Ben does not need any special services at this time.

Related Services

Ben has a teacher of the visually impaired once a week for reading services.

Testing Accommodations

Ben does not need any accommodations to his testing.

Participation with Students without Disabilities

Ben will be included 100 percent of the time.

Transition Services

Ben is currently on his cross-country team in high school. Ben will learn with his class how to use a public pool facility, a community fitness center, and the local bowling alley. Ben will be going with his school on a camping trip to the state park and will participate in hiking and fishing. Ben participates in an after-school exergame club and plays the Wii and other active video games.

NADIA

Nadia is a student who is 8 years old, deaf, and visually impaired and has cerebral palsy. She uses a wheelchair but can walk with a walker and has a one-to-one paraeducator for all classes. She communicates with a combination of signs, gestures, and tactile symbols. She uses a tactile schedule each day and a tactile communication system that is in 4"×4" on the wall at head height. She is also practicing with an electronic communication system. Her IEP for physical education is as follows:

Performance Area: Motor Skills

Present Level of Performance

Nadia can bat a beeping ball from her wheelchair off a batting tee with physical assistance at the hands three out of five times with proper grip and follow through.

Annual Goal

Nadia will improve her motor skill of batting.

Short-Term Objective/Benchmarks

Nadia will bat a beeping ball using a batting tee from a standing position with physical assistance at the hands four out of five times, with proper preparation, grip, and follow through.

Assessment Method

Nadia will be assessed using the Test of Gross Motor Development, second edition (TGMD–2) with the paraeducator and physical assistance when needed.

Schedule

Nadia will be assessed on her object control skills every quarter by the adapted physical educator and her paraeducator.

Special Education Program or Services

Nadia will be provided a paraeducator for all classes and a one-to-one trained peer tutor for physical education. She will use a tactile communication system in all classes as well as signs and gestures. When possible she will use the communication system Proloquo2go.

SIDEBAR 3.7 *(continued)*

Related Services

Nadia will receive physical therapy two times every week. She will receive occupational therapy once a week. Nadia will work with the deafblind specialist on communication three times each week.

Testing Accommodations

Nadia will receive physical assistance when necessary and will perform assessment skills from her wheelchair when necessary. She will receive communication through tactile symbols and tactile signs. She will express herself through signs, gestures, and tactile symbols.

Participation with Students without Disabilities

Nadia will be in a separate physical education class with four peers with disabilities and four trained peer tutors without disabilities.

Transition Services

Since Nadia is only 8 years old, she will not be receiving transition services at this time.

2006), although all 60 students with visual impairments knew they had an IEP, only 40 percent knew that they had goals related to physical education, and of that group, only 10 percent knew what the goals were.

Supplementary Aids and Services

The term *supplementary aids and services* refers to additional supports provided in the classroom or other educational settings that a student needs to benefit from his or her education. This is an extremely important component of the IEP for physical education because it provides an avenue to secure needed supports so that students with visual impairments can be successfully included in physical education class with students who do not have visual impairments. The nature and type of support may vary depending on the unique needs of the student.

Two types of support commonly requested for physical education are *personnel support* and *equipment support.* Personnel support ensures that there are enough staff members in the gymnasium to provide a safe and successful program. For example, if Juan has a paraeducator who supports him in his classroom, the IEP may state that the paraeducator must accompany him into all of his physical education classes in order for him to be most successful. Personnel support may include adapted physical education consultants, teacher's aides or paraeducators, interpreters or interveners for students who are deafblind (see Chapter 4), or trained peer tutors (see Chapter 7).

Equipment support ensures that specialized or adaptive equipment needed to allow the student to experience a high degree of participation and success is available. For example, if it is necessary for Juan to use a volleyball trainer (a bright yellow volleyball that moves more slowly than a regulation ball) to serve the volleyball over the net, this piece of equipment needs to be specified on the IEP as one of the required supplementary supports. It is important to review the physical education curriculum to determine any types of specialized equipment that may be needed in order for the student to be appropriately included and successful in the physical education program.

Once these areas of support are agreed on by the IEP team, the district is responsible for supplying the requested resources. Another source of equipment for students with visual impairments is the Federal Quota Program funds administered by the American Printing House for the Blind (see Sidebar 3.8).

SIDEBAR 3.8

Obtaining Equipment through the Federal Quota Program

The need to provide adapted equipment, print materials in accessible formats, and assistive technology for the education of students with visual impairments means that, in general, it is more expensive to educate them than it is to educate students without disabilities. The Federal Quota Program, created by Congress in 1879, supports the provision of educational materials for students with visual impairments. Through this program, which is administered by the American Printing House for the Blind (APH; see the Resources section for more information), "quota funds" are provided through state departments of education, residential schools for the blind, and other agencies to purchase materials for each year, with the amount distributed based on a census of eligible students who are visually impaired.

Quota funds cover equipment, books, and other materials related to physical education and recreation. Although different states may vary in their procedures, equipment and materials purchased with quota funds must be ordered from APH by a teacher of students with visual impairments or O&M specialist. The physical education teacher can coordinate with these professionals to determine what equipment and materials a particular student needs. APH offers beeping balls, kits, books, and curricula to improve the physical activity of children with visual impairments. Information on specific physical education products that can be purchased with quota funds is available on the APH website at www.aph.org/pe.

Examples of specialized equipment might include beep balls, adjustable basketball baskets, modified bicycles, bowling ramps, and switches that when touched can move or propel objects. This equipment can be used by students with visual impairments and severe disabilities who may lack the ability to utilize large muscle groups. Most of this equipment can be purchased through specialized physical activity catalogs (see the Resources section). (See Chapter 4 for more information about equipment used to adapt activities.)

Statement of Participation in Regular Settings

The statement of participation in regular settings in the IEP designates where the student's physical education class will take place. Placement of students with visual impairments into physical education classes is frequently a difficult issue for IEP teams and school districts to determine because they may be afraid the students will get hurt and are not familiar with the methods of including them (Columna, Davis, Lieberman, & Lytle, 2010). The goal is to provide the most appropriate and beneficial placement for each child. In making a decision on placement, the IEP team members need to look at specific variables that will contribute to the student being placed in the least restrictive environment in which he or she can participate successfully in physical education. Some of the variables to be considered include the following:

- the student's sensory needs, for example, the effect acoustics, spatial relationships, and size of the class may have on performance

- the student's individual skill set, such as motor and physical fitness
- behavioral factors, such as the student's ability to work with classmates and to work independently

If a student has severe disabilities, medical conditions, or behavioral conditions that would impede success in an integrated physical education class, documentation must be provided on the IEP to justify a totally segregated placement (Lieberman & Houston-Wilson, 2009).

Because support services are a component of the IEP, teachers who may lack the necessary training to accommodate students with disabilities in their classes should be provided with appropriate support to ensure everyone's success. Support may include assistance from additional team members, as mentioned earlier in the chapter. It can also include offering the teacher in-service training or additional college courses in providing physical education to students with visual impairment and additional disabilities.

The law states that the student must receive at least as much time in physical education as his or her same-age classmates. Additional time would be added if time permits and if the student would benefit. If a child has a more severe visual impairment, the child will often need time for pre-teaching at the beginning of each unit (Conroy, 2012; Perkins, Bailey, Columna, & Lieberman, 2012). Pre-teaching can be implemented by the teacher of children with visual impairments, O&M teacher, adapted physical educator, general physical educator, trained peer tutor, or a paraeducator. It consists of orientation to the playing area, the equipment, and equipment variables, as well as positioning on the field and terms used for specific strategies that will be taught during the unit. This way the child is not behind during the unit of instruction and has full understanding of the lesson. It can be delivered before or after school before a unit, for a few minutes before each class, or during a special prearranged time during school. If pre-teaching is necessary for a student, it should be written with specifics on the IEP.

Other components of the IEP process include assessment, a key component necessary to ensure that students' strengths and needs are understood, and planning for the students' life after secondary school, known as *transition services*, both of which are discussed later in this chapter.

ASSESSMENT

Assessment is an essential part of teaching any subject, and it is also mandated for all students with disabilities by IDEA to make sure that students receive services that are appropriate to their needs. Assessment is needed for all students to ensure that they receive an appropriate physical education experience. Lack of information about students' abilities can compromise physical education programs, because without assessment, teachers do not know what goals to set for a particular student or when goals are reached. Lack of assessment information can be especially harmful for students with visual impairments or deafblindness because many physical education teachers are not familiar with their abilities and may make inaccurate assumptions about them.

Assessments need to accurately reflect what students can and cannot do in relation to the curriculum content. Often, teachers who underestimate the abilities of someone with a disability are guilty of using superlatives to describe the student's skills. For example, if a teacher believes that it is "awesome" that a student who cannot see well is able to run all the way around a track (though slowly), or jump a few inches into a long jump pit from the edge of the approach, that teacher may wrongly lead the student and others to believe the student's skills are better than they really are. Effective assessments—those prepared and administered with a clear purpose, that are related to the curriculum content, and that accurately measure what they are intended to—will assist in the development of appropriate goals and objectives for all students and can really help to shape and develop students' abilities (Henderson, French, & Kinnison, 2001). Sidebar 3.9 gives a summary of the purpose for assessment.

SIDEBAR 3.9

Purpose of Assessment in Physical Education

The following points summarize the purpose of assessment in physical education:

1. Holds the teacher accountable for whether the teacher has adequately guided students in reaching specified goals and objectives
2. Holds the students accountable, as they will be aware of goals and achievements
3. Provides a baseline of performance level
4. Drives instruction and content
5. Is a keystone of the IEP; shows progress by the goals achieved
6. Is a motivational tool for both the student and others involved
7. Determines achievement in meeting the standards
8. Determines whether there is improvement from the baseline
9. Is a program evaluation tool that assists the instructor in determining whether methods or programs are adequate

Types of Assessment Tests

Assessment of skills can be as simple as observation of absence or presence of target skills, but the use of appropriate standardized or ready-made tools that have been devised is recommended. Most standardized tests typically have not been normed on students with disabilities—that is, the expected results or scores were determined using a population that did not include these students—so their results may need to be interpreted based on a different standard. Also, a teacher of students with visual impairments or an intervener for students with deafblindness may need to help administer certain assessments. Suggestions for assessment tools that can be used with students who are visually impaired are discussed in the following sections.

Testing Fundamental Movements

Fundamental or so-called basic movements are those associated with early childhood, such as throwing, catching, skipping, and hopping. A common assessment that can be used with children with visual impairments is the Test of Gross Motor Development, second edition (TGMD–2; Ulrich, 2000). This test covers locomotor skills and object control skills in children from 3 through about 10 or 11 years of age, although it can also be effective for measuring skills in older children who have developmental lags in their skill performance. The TGMD–2 takes about 15 to 20 minutes to administer and provides detailed descriptions as well as illustrations of the following gross motor skills:

- *Locomotor skills:* running, galloping, hopping, leaping, horizontal jumping, and sliding
- *Object control skills:* striking a stationary ball, stationary dribble, kicking, catching, overhand throwing, and underhand rolling

The TGMD–2 has been validated for use with children with visual impairments from 6 to 12 years of age (Houwen, Hartman, Jonker, & Visscher, 2010). It is also being incorporated into an instructional kit, "Count Me in: Motor Development in a Box," designed to enhance motor skills of children from 3 to 8 years old with visual impairments by the American Printing House for the Blind.

Testing Physical Fitness

As already indicated, physical fitness is an important part of life, generally achieved through exercise, correct nutrition, and sufficient rest. It comprises two related concepts: general fitness (a state of health and well-being) and specific fitness (a task-oriented definition based on the ability to perform specific aspects of sports or occupations). The Brockport Physical Fitness Test (BPFT; Winnick & Short, 1999) is a health-related physical fitness test for children with a variety of disabilities, including visual impairments. It was developed to provide standards for what is deemed healthy for youths from 10 to 17 years of age who have disabilities. The items on this test reflect the items in the commonly used Fitnessgram Test developed by the Cooper Institute for Aerobic Research (2004; www.cooperinstitute.org/fitnessgram; www.fitnessgram.net), which has standards for children without disabilities. With this in mind, students with disabilities can be tested with their classmates yet be evaluated in comparison to standards that are appropriate for them. The BPFT covers the following areas:

- Upper body muscular strength and endurance, measured by ability to do push-ups.
- Abdominal strength and endurance, measured by the ability to do sit-ups.
- Body composition, measured as percentage of body fat, estimated using a two-site skinfold technique.
- Cardiovascular fitness, measured by either the 20-meter PACER test (the Progressive Aerobic Cardiovascular Endurance Run used as part of the Fitnessgram) or the mile run, using a sighted guide or tether for students with visual impairments or deafblindness.
- Flexibility of the lower back and hamstring muscles, measured by reaching toward the toes in a sitting position with outstretched legs straight, using a device called a sit-and-reach box.

Measuring each fitness item can be difficult with a child with a visual impairment or deafblindness. Sidebar 3.10 describes these measures in more detail and presents some ways to help children with visual impairments or blindness perform to the best of their ability on each area of the assessment (Lieberman, Byrne, Mattern, Watt, & Fernández-Vivó, 2010).

SIDEBAR 3.10

The Brockport Physical Fitness Test

The following are instructions for conducting the measures used on the Brockport Physical Fitness Test:

Upper-Body Muscular Endurance

Ask students if they know how to perform a push-up. Those who respond affirmatively can be asked to demonstrate their technique to confirm their ability. Students who indicated that they were not familiar with a push-up or who performed it inaccurately should be taught the correct form and technique. Ask the students to lie down with their hands next to their shoulders and push themselves up off the floor. A teacher or teacher aide can position the student's body such that a straight line is maintained between the shoulders, pelvis, knees, and feet. Students can be assessed once they independently demonstrate the proper form and technique. They can be shown the straight-leg push-up or the bent-knee push-up. Once the assessment begins, students are allowed 3 seconds to complete each push-up and should be instructed to complete as many at possible. There is no time limit to this test. The test is terminated when the student can no longer perform push-ups with appropriate form.

Abdominal Muscular Endurance

Ask students if they know how to perform a sit-up. Those who respond yes can be asked to demonstrate their technique in order to confirm their ability. Those who indicate no or who performed it inaccurately can be physically assisted into the position and taught the movement by physical guidance and tactile modeling. (These methods are described in Chapter 4.) All students can begin by lying in a supine position while maintaining 90 degrees of knee flexion, with their hands at their side. They then contract their abdominal musculature until their hands have traveled along the mat to a point below their knees. Students then return their shoulders to the mat in a controlled movement. The test is terminated when the student is no longer able to perform sit-ups with appropriate form.

Body Composition

Percent body fat is estimated using a two-site skinfold technique (Winnick & Short, 1999) on the calf and triceps. All measurements can be taken on the right side, and each skinfold thickness is measured 2 to 3 times (depending upon repeatability of the measurements) using a Lange skinfold caliper. As some participants may be anxious about having the measurements performed, students are encouraged to feel the caliper prior to being measured. The instructor also places the jaws of the caliper on the student's finger so the student can get a better understanding of how the tool will feel on their skin. Once the data are collected, the sum of the skinfold measures is then used to estimate body density and subsequently percent body fat (Siri, 1961).

Cardiovascular Fitness

Cardiovascular fitness can be measured by either the 20-meter PACER test (the Progressive Aerobic Cardiovascular Endurance Run used as part of the Fitnessgram) or the mile run. Either can be used with youth with visual impairments. It is important that students with significant vision loss have a sighted guide for the mile run or a tether or sighted guide for the PACER test. (For more specifics about sighted guide techniques, see Chapter 8.)

Flexibility

Flexibility is measured using a specially constructed sit-and-reach box, which is available commercially or can be homemade. The front end of the box is closed so that participants can brace their feet against it. A ruler or meter stick is embedded in the top of the box to measure how far an individual can reach. Have students initially feel the structure of the sit-and-reach box. Then ask if they know how to perform a hurdler's stretch. Students who respond yes can demonstrate the stretch in order to confirm their ability. Students who indicate that they do not know how to perform the stretch or who perform it inaccurately can be taught how to do so

SIDEBAR 3.10 *(continued)*

correctly using physical guidance and tactile modeling (O'Connell, Lieberman, & Petersen, 2006). With the palms facing downward, the student reaches forward along the measuring line as far as possible, keeping the front knee straight and pressed to the floor. The distance the student reaches along the measuring stick is recorded. Students should practice the test two to three times while being provided verbal and physical feedback to enhance the accuracy of the assessment. Students then perform the sit-and-reach stretch twice on each leg. The highest value measured with no knee flexion is used as their sit-and-reach score.

Measuring Physical Activity

Physical activity is any body movement that works the muscles and uses more energy than is used when resting. Walking, running, dancing, swimming, yoga, and gardening are examples of physical activity. Keeping track of an individual's performance in a physical activity provides an objective way to measure progress and can also motivate the individual to strive for improvement. The BPFT includes methods of measuring a variety of activities. Having a student recall and record his or her physical activity each day is a simple method that requires no equipment. There are also a variety of devices that provide audible feedback such as a talking pedometer or talking heart rate monitor.

The talking pedometer is an accurate, valid, and enjoyable way to measure the walking performance of youths with visual impairments (Lieberman, Stuart, Hand, & Robinson, 2006). The talking pedometer can be worn on the hip opposite the mobility aid and gives automatic feedback every 1,000 steps, and can give verbal feedback on the number of steps when the button is pushed (Holbrook et al., 2009). The minimum preferred number of steps taken per day to be healthy is 10,000 and the preferred number is 12,000 to 15,000 steps per day (Beets, Foley, Tindall, & Lieberman, 2007; Tudor-Locke et al., 2004). Although there are several talking pedometers on the market, they have been shown to be equally effective (Beets, Foley, Tindall, & Lieberman, 2007).

For example, Viva, the student in the opening vignette, could be shown how to use a talking pedometer to see how many steps she walks to get to and around school and compare her total with a target goal of 10,000 to 12,000 steps. Knowledge of one's performance is usually motivating, so having audible output of her performance will likely encourage Viva to take more responsibility for her effort to become more physically fit. Talking pedometers can be easily incorporated into physical education classes with students with visual impairments (Foley, Lieberman, & Wood, 2008).

Measuring Sports Skills

There is no validated assessment to measure sports skills for children with visual impairments. One assessment that has been used at a variety of sports camps is the Camp Abilities Activity Assessment Checklist (CAAAC). This checklist provides task-analyzed descriptors of the following sports that are conducive to including children with visual impairments:

- goalball
- beep baseball
- track and field
- swimming
- gymnastics
- judo
- tandem biking
- bocce

The checklists assist the instructor in determining both the student's level of skill and level of independence. In addition to the qualitative analysis of skills provided in the CAAAC, it has places to document the quantity or product of a skill, such as how far a shot put is thrown, number of laps run around the track and time, or number of miles ridden on a bike. The CAAAC can be found in the Appendix at the back of this book.

Use of Rubrics for Assessment of Skills

Often units are covered in physical education classes for which there are no valid and reliable assessments. In addition, some of the existing assessments for some activities may be too formal or time consuming for everyday use.

In such cases, *rubrics* are often created to reflect the levels of skills being covered in classes. A rubric is a detailed guideline with explicit criteria for assessing performance of a particular task and assigning a score or grade. The specific scoring criteria are then used to assess students' performance and progress. Scoring is generally qualitative rather than quantitative. Rubrics are used in a formal way when levels of achievement are assigned in common sports such as karate, gymnastics, or swimming, where different ranks or levels are established, with specific criteria for each. They can be used to guide skill development in instruction, as they detail the specific skills and abilities required at each level. For example, the sample rubric in Figure 3.1 was developed for a basic aerobics unit in high school. Following this rubric, the teacher can teach an aerobic lesson with several moves in a row and then increase the number of moves taught in a row to increase the class's level of skill and fitness. In another instance, a rubric might guide two classmates in improving their skill development or the number of times they can perform a particular movement. The levels were labeled to correspond to colors of martial arts belts, as these may be familiar to the students.

The teacher should develop and share rubrics with students before the unit is taught so that students know what is expected of them (Lieberman & Houston-Wilson, 2009). Use of a rubric evaluation system gives students a comprehensive idea of how to perform, what to perform, and the number of trials to be performed. When students, including those with visual impairments or deafblindness, know in advance what is expected, they can be held accountable for their own learning. As students chart their own progress and note improvements based on their levels of achievement, the rubric serves as an excellent motivational tool as well. And because students must pass levels in a specific sequence and must possess prerequisite skills to advance, the hierarchy is excellent for ensuring safety.

An additional benefit of the rubric system is that it can cover a wide range of abilities and can accommodate heterogeneous classes.

TASK: AEROBICS: BASIC WORKOUT	
Task description:	Student will participate in a 30– to 45–minute aerobics class
Scale components:	a. Ability to execute the skill that is demonstrated b. Keeping up the specified beat c. Duration of continuous exercise
Rubric level	**Rubric descriptors**
1 White	Student will be able to execute 3-4 aerobic moves, as demonstrated by the instructor, with no music
2 Yellow	Student will be able to execute 5-8 aerobic moves, as demonstrated by the instructor, with no music
3 Orange	Student will be able to execute at least 8 aerobic moves, as demonstrated by the instructor, with music, to a 1/4 count, for 10 minutes continuously
4 Green	Student will be able to execute at least 10 aerobic moves, as demonstrated by the instructor, with music, to a 1/4 count, for 15 minutes continuously
5 Blue	Student will be able to execute at least 10 aerobic moves, as demonstrated by the instructor, with music, to a 1/8 count, for 20 minutes continuously
6 Brown	Student will be able to execute any number of moves, as demonstrated by the instructor, with music, to a 1/8 count, for 20-30 minutes continuously
7 Black	Student will be able to execute any number of moves, as demonstrated by the instructor, with music, to a 1/8 count, for 30-45 minutes continuously
	Optional—student could lead all or part of the workout
Source: Adapted with permission from Lieberman & Houston-Wilson, 2009	

FIGURE 3.1 An Example of a Rubric for a Basic Aerobics Unit in High School

Unique rubrics are created for each lesson plan and class and can therefore be easily individualized. A rubric can be developed to assess the *process,* or quality, of a movement skill; the *product,* or quantity of a movement (how far, how fast, how many); and the *parameter,* the conditions under which the movement skill was performed. In the rubric for aerobics in Figure 3.1, each level is measured using skill level, beat or tempo, and duration, identified here as "scale components." This type of rubric can be used for any unit.

When a rubric or other printed material is to be provided for a student with visual impairments or deafblindness, it needs to be provided in a format that the student can access, whether that is large print, braille, or an audio format. Teachers therefore need to plan ahead and provide the teacher of students with visual impairments with the material and with enough time so that he or she can make an accessible version.

PLANNING A PHYSICAL EDUCATION PROGRAM

In planning physical education activities for students with visual impairments or deafblindness, there are two main aspects to consider:

the specific curriculum or activities taught and the methods or instructional models used to teach them.

Curriculum

The curriculum is the content of what is taught. In physical education the curriculum might be sports skills, adventure-based activities, or lifetime recreational activities. Curriculum guidelines were discussed at the beginning of this chapter. It is important to remember that students with visual impairments or deafblindness should learn all of the same units as their classmates. Modifications may need to be made to the instruction, equipment, or rules, but students should have access to the same units no matter what type of class they are placed in for physical education. As already described, by learning all of the same units their classmates learn, students with visual impairments or deafblindness will have more choices and control over their lives and more opportunities for self-determination (Robinson & Lieberman, 2004).

Regardless of the particular curricular content that is chosen, there are several important components of physical education to keep in mind when planning activities for students with visual impairments or deafblindness. It is important for their curriculum to include a variety of activities that contain both open and closed skills and discrete and continuous skills as well as sports that are particularly accessible to students with visual impairments.

Open and Closed Skills

Every physical education curriculum including a student with a visual impairment should contain a combination of open and closed sports and skills. *Open skills* are those that have variables that change constantly such as trajectory of a ball, offense and defense, speed of the game, and angles of play. Examples of open sports include volleyball, soccer, football, baseball, and tennis. *Closed skills* are those in which

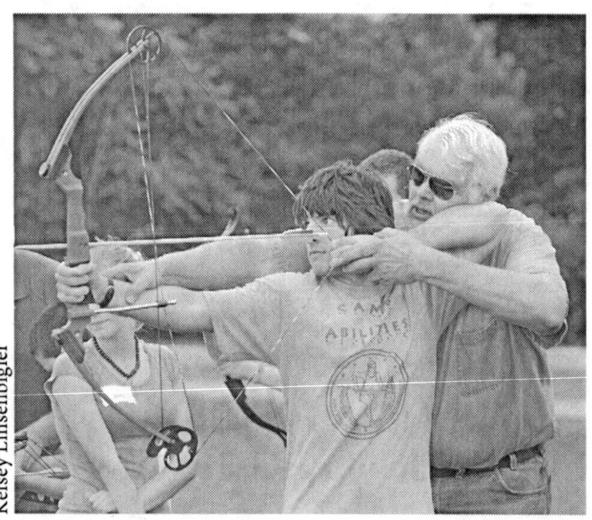

Kelsey Linsenbigler

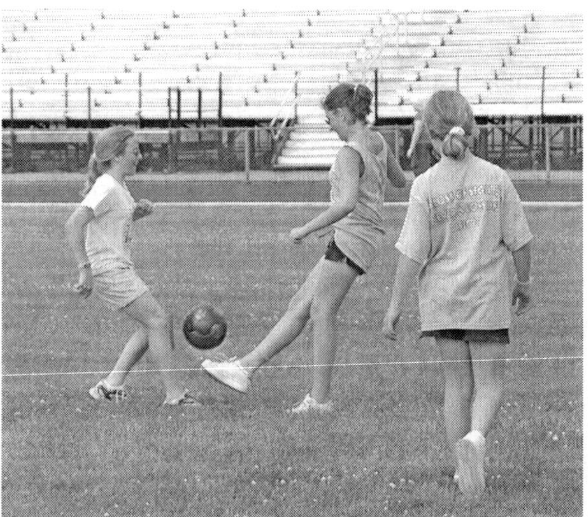

Amanda Tepfer

A good physical education program includes all kinds of activities. Archery (left) is both a closed and a discrete skill. Soccer (right) is an open sport since the speed and trajectory of the ball changes constantly.

the environment is constant and predictable and the student has control of the timing and pace of performance, such as archery, bowling, weight lifting, and running. In many cases the physical education teacher omits open sports because of the varied nature of these activities. Although they may take more time to plan, they are a major part of the curriculum and important to teach to students with visual impairments or deafblindness.

Discrete and Continuous Skills

Every physical education curriculum should also include a combination of activities that are discrete and continuous. A *discrete skill* is one that has a finite beginning and ending in a short period of time. Examples of discrete skills are doing the shot put, bowling, archery, kicking, throwing, and long jump. *Continuous skills* are those that continue for long periods of time and do not have a finite ending. Examples of continuous skills are swimming laps, running, rock climbing, canoeing, and aerobics.

Blind Sports

Physical education curricula should include several units of sports governed by the United States Association of Blind Athletes (described in more detail in Chapters 8 and 9). These include goalball, tandem cycling, powerlifting, track and field (sprint, distance and cross-country running, long jump, high jump, shotput, discus), 5-a-side soccer, wrestling, swimming, judo, and both downhill and cross-country skiing.

Models of Instructional Delivery

A model of instructional delivery is the way the units in a curriculum are taught. Because blindness, severe low vision, or deafness can prevent a student from receiving information conveyed in the usual ways in which instruction is delivered, this topic requires extensive discussion, and the entirety of Chapter 4 is devoted to it. In general, however, there are two major categories of instructional delivery models:

- modification of the instructional methods themselves
- creating a one-to-one "team" with the student and a classmate or a member of the instructional staff

Instructional Modification

Methods of modifying instructional methods to include students with visual impairments or deafblindness are discussed in detail in Chapter 4. To a large extent, such modifications involve the methods used to communicate information or demonstrate techniques. In addition, Chapter 5 provides detailed information on how to adapt activities for individuals with visual impairment or deafblindness, based on the needs of the learner and the situation. It is important to remember that the goal for students with visual impairments is to achieve in sports and recreation, just as it is for their sighted classmates, not just to participate. It is for this reason that teachers need to make modifications and ensure the students do their best and improve each day.

One-to-One Team

In general, students with visual impairments, particularly those who are also hard of hearing, need more specific instruction and feedback than do students with unimpaired vision. Students with visual impairments therefore typically perform better in a one-to-one situation in which they can receive the individualized instruction they need. The one-to-one team model of instruction can be used simultaneously with any modifications used to deliver instruction. Having a person assigned to work directly with the student can relieve concerns that physical education instructors might have about having insufficient time or staffing to address the needs of the student who is visually impaired or deafblind. It is important that this individual be aware of the effective ways of working with a student who is visually impaired, including the need to avoid overprotection to encourage the student's independence and to have expectations for the student that are similar to those held for others.

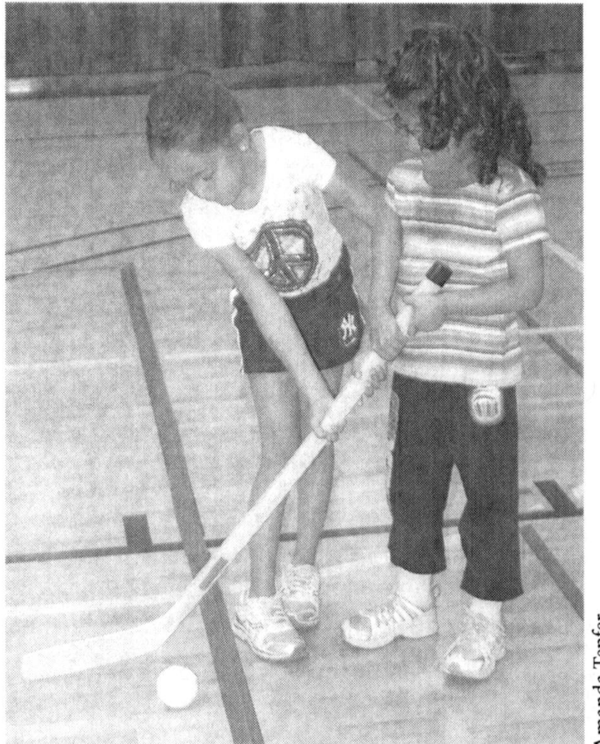

Amanda Tepfer

This student assists her classmate by helping her feel the motion of swinging the hockey stick.

Peer Tutoring

Peer tutoring can be set up so that a sighted peer can help instruct the student with a visual impairment. Research has shown that peer tutoring is effective in improving motor performance of students with visual impairments (Wiskochil, Lieberman, Houston-Wilson, & Petersen, 2007). Peer tutors can be trained to instruct (with tactile means when necessary), give feedback, give directional cues, record performance, demonstrate, encourage, ensure safety, and facilitate socialization (Lieberman & Houston-Wilson, 2009).

Paraeducators

As described in Chapter 2, paraeducators are often a major part of the educational process for students with visual impairments. Paraeducators can be trained to assist in the instruction of students with visual impairments in physical education classes and ensure that they are being truly included in physical education (Lieberman, 2007). However, care needs to be taken that a paraeducator assigned to an individual student does not fulfill the role appropriately assigned to a teacher, nor should a paraeducator serve as a babysitter for a student or encourage a student's dependence on him or her. Typically, the student and paraeducator listen to the instructor's directions, and the paraeducator assists the student with verbal or other prompts (Piletic, Davis, & Aschemeier, 2005). Paraeducators are not often trained for physical education (Davis, Kotecki, Harvey, & Oliver, 2007; Lieberman & Conroy [in press]; McKenzie & Lewis, 2008).

TRANSITION SERVICES AND PHYSICAL EDUCATION

Whether students with visual impairments plan to go on to college after finishing high school or to live in the community, they will need to learn skills and make arrangements that go beyond those needed by students without disabilities. For that reason, it is important to start planning for their adult life early, and that process is built into the law. Under IDEA, *transition services* are a component of the IEP that must commence at the age of 16 and continue until the end of formal schooling. Transition services involve collaboration between education and vocational rehabilitation professionals (those who provide services to adults with disabilities; they are discussed in Chapter 2) to ensure that the student has the skills, knowledge, and experience to survive as independently as possible and succeed after leaving school or at the age of 21. (In some states, educational services can continue through age 25.)

Transition services related to physical education involve ensuring that the student has knowledge of opportunities for physical activity near his or her residence and has adequate skills to take advantage of these opportunities and the daily living skills to access these opportunities as independently as possible.

A student such as Viva, described at the beginning of this chapter, will eventually have transition goals on her IEP. Although she is only 9, she will start working on lifetime activities, recreation, and community programming before she graduates. Her instructors will assist her with the skills she will need for independent travel, using the telephone or computer to research the times and locations of activities, and methods of requesting orientation to a facility or activity when she arrives. She may go to a YMCA on Fridays to try out the fitness equipment and the pool, go walking at a local track, bowl at a local bowling alley, and take an aerobics or kick-boxing class. These types of experiences will give her choices about how she spends her leisure time in the future and how to be physically fit.

CONCLUSION

Physical education is an integral component of all students' education programming, and can be especially important for students with visual impairments, who tend to be less physically fit than others and have fewer opportunities for socializing. With appropriate instruction, students with visual impairments can excel in all areas of physical activity and have a great quality of life. Appropriate instruction includes sound assessment, well-written and shared IEP goals and objectives, and a curriculum with a variety of sports and activities, as well as instructional styles that meet the needs of the student. The following chapters provide more detailed information on how instruction in physical education can be provided to meet the needs of students with visual impairments or deafblindness.

APPENDIX 3A

Sample IEP Form

The following form is presented only as an example of an Individualized Education Program. Individual states and districts have their own forms that school personnel are required to use.

INDIVIDUALIZED EDUCATION PROGRAM (IEP)

Student Name: ____________________ Disability Classification: ____________________

Date of Birth: __________ Local ID #: ____________

Projected Date IEP Is to Be Implemented: __________ Projected Date of Annual Review: __________

Present Levels Of Performance And Individual Needs

Documentation of student's current performance and academic, developmental, and functional needs

Evaluation Results (Including, for School-Age Students, Performance on State and District-Wide Assessments)

Academic Achievement, Functional Performance, and Learning Characteristics

Levels of knowledge and development in subject and skill areas including activities of daily living, level of intellectual functioning, adaptive behavior, expected rate of progress in acquiring skills and information, and learning style:

Student's strengths, preferences, and interests:

Academic, developmental, and functional needs of the student, including consideration of student's needs that are of concern to the parent:

Social Development

Degree (extent) and quality of the student's relationships with peers and adults; feelings about self; and social adjustment to school and community environments:

Student's strengths:

Social development needs of the student, including consideration of student's needs that are of concern to the parent:

Physical Development

Degree (extent) and quality of student's motor and sensory development, health, vitality, and physical skills or limitations that pertain to the learning process:

Student's strengths:

Physical development needs of student, including consideration of student's needs that are of concern to parent:

Management Needs

Nature (type) and degree (extent) to which environmental and human or material resources are needed to address needs identified above:

Effect of Student's Needs on Involvement and Progress in the General Education Curriculum or, for a Preschool Student, Effect of Student's Needs on Participation in Appropriate Activities

---

Student's Needs Relating to Special Factors

Based on identification of student's needs, the committee must consider whether the student needs a particular device or service to address the special factors as indicated below, and if so, the appropriate section of the IEP must identify the particular device or service(s) needed.

Does the student need strategies, including positive behavioral interventions, supports, and other strategies, to address behaviors that impede the student's learning or that of others? ☐ Yes ☐ No

Does the student need a behavioral intervention plan? ☐ Yes ☐ No

---

For a student with limited English proficiency, does he or she need a special education service to address his/her language needs as they relate to the IEP? ☐ Yes ☐ No ☐ Not Applicable

---

For a student who is blind or visually impaired, does he or she need instruction in braille and the use of braille? ☐ Yes ☐ No ☐ Not Applicable

---

Does the student need a particular device or service to address his or her communication needs? ☐ Yes ☐ No

(Continued on next page)

In the case of a student who is deaf or hard of hearing, does the student need a particular device or service in consideration of the student's language and communication needs, opportunities for direct communications with peers and professional personnel in the student's language and communication mode, academic level, and full range of needs, including opportunities for direct instruction in the student's language and communication mode? ☐ Yes ☐ No ☐ Not Applicable

---

Does the student need an assistive technology device (or devices) and/or service? ☐ Yes ☐ No

If yes, does the committee recommend that the device(s) be used in the student's home? ☐ Yes ☐ No

---

Beginning not later than the first IEP to be in effect when the student is age 15 (and at a younger age if determined appropriate):

Measurable Postsecondary Goals

(Long-term goals for living, working, and learning as an adult)

Education/Training: ______________________________

Employment: ______________________________

Independent Living Skills (When Appropriate):______________________________

Transition Needs

In consideration of present levels of performance, transition service needs of the student that focus on the student's courses of study, taking into account the student's strengths, preferences, and interests as they relate to transition from school to post-school activities:

Measurable Annual Goals

The following goals are recommended to enable student to be involved in and progress in general education curriculum, address other educational needs that result from student's disability, and prepare student to meet his or her postsecondary goals.

Annual Goals *What the student will be expected to achieve by end of year in which IEP is in effect*	**Criteria** *Measure to determine if goal has been achieved*	**Method** *How progress will be measured*	**Schedule** *When progress will be measured*

Reporting Progress To Parents

Identify when periodic reports on the student's progress toward meeting the annual goals will be provided to the student's parents:

Alternate Section For Students Whose IEPs Will Include Short-term Instructional Objectives and/or Benchmarks:

Measurable Annual Goals

The following goals are recommended to enable student to be involved in and progress in general education curriculum or, for a preschool child, in appropriate activities, address other educational needs that result from student's disability, and, for a school-age student, prepare student to meet his or her postsecondary goals.

Annual Goal *What the student will be expected to achieve by end of the year in which IEP is in effect*	**Criteria** *Measure to determine if goal has been achieved*	**Method** *How progress will be measured*	**Schedule** *When progress will be measured*

Short-term instructional objectives and/or benchmarks (intermediate steps between the student's present level of performance and the measurable annual goal):

Annual Goal	**Criteria**	**Method**	**Schedule**

Short-term instructional objectives and/or benchmarks (intermediate steps between student's present level of performance and measurable annual goal):

Annual Goal	**Criteria**	**Method**	**Schedule**

Short-term instructional objectives and/or benchmarks (intermediate steps between student's present level of performance and measurable annual goal):

Reporting Progress To Parents

Identify when periodic reports on the student's progress toward meeting the annual goals will be provided to the student's parents:

(Continued on next page)

Recommended Special Education Programs and Services

Special Education Program or Services	Service Delivery Recommendations*	Frequency *How often provided*	Duration *Length of session*	Location *Where service will be provided*	Projected Beginning/ Service Date(s)
Special Education Program:					
Related Services:					
Supplementary Aids and Services/ Program Modifications/ Accommodations:					
Assistive Technology Devices and/or Services:					
Supports for School Personnel on Behalf of Student:					

*Identify, if applicable, class size (maximum student-to-staff ratio), language if other than English, group or individual services, direct and/or indirect consultant teacher services, or other service delivery recommendations.

12-Month Service and/or Program: Student is eligible to receive special education services and/or program during July and August: ☐ Yes ☐ No

If yes:

☐ Student will receive the same special education program/services as recommended above. OR

☐ Student will receive the following special education program/services:

Special Education Program or Services	Service Delivery Recommendations*	Frequency	Duration	Location	Projected Beginning/ Service Date(s)

Name of school/agency provider of services during July and August:

For a preschool student, reason(s) the child requires services during July and August:

Testing Accommodations (to be completed for preschool children only if there is an assessment program for nondisabled preschool children):
Individual testing accommodations, specific to student's disability and needs, to be used consistently by student in recommended educational program and in administration of district-wide assessments of student achievement and, in accordance with Department policy, State assessments of student achievement

Testing Accommodation	Conditions*	Implementation Recommendations**
☐ None		

*Conditions—Test characteristics: Describe the type, length, and purpose of the test upon which the use of testing accommodations is conditioned, if applicable.
**Implementation recommendations: Identify the amount of extended time, type of setting, etc., specific to the testing accommodations, if applicable.

Beginning not later than first IEP to be in effect when student is age 15 (and at a younger age, if determined appropriate):

Coordinated Set of Transition Activities

Needed Activities to Facilitate Student's Movement from School to Post-School Activities	Service/Activity	School District/Agency Responsible
Instruction		
Related services		
Community experiences		
Development of employment and other post-school adult living objectives		
Acquisition of daily living skills (if applicable)		
Functional vocational assessment (if applicable)		

(Continued on next page)

Participation in Statewide and District-Wide Assessments

(To be completed for preschool students only if there is an assessment program for nondisabled preschool students)

☐ The student will participate in the same statewide and district-wide assessments of student achievement that are administered to general education students.

☐ The student will participate in an alternate assessment on a particular statewide or district-wide assessment of student achievement.
Identify the alternate assessment:

Statement of why the student cannot participate in the regular assessment and why the particular alternate assessment selected is appropriate for the student:

Participation with Students without Disabilities

Removal from the general education environment occurs only when nature or severity of disability is such that, even with use of supplementary aids and services, education cannot be satisfactorily achieved.

For Preschool Student:
Explain the extent, if any, to which the student will not participate in appropriate activities with age-appropriate nondisabled peers (e.g., percent of the school day) and/or specify particular activities:

For School-Age Student:
Explain the extent, if any, to which the student will not participate in regular class, extracurricular, and other nonacademic activities (e.g., percent of the school day) and/or specify particular activities:

If the student is not participating in a regular physical education program, identify the extent to which the student will participate in specially designed instruction in physical education, including adapted physical education:

Exemption from language other than English diploma requirement: ☐ No ☐ Yes - Committee has determined that the student's disability adversely affects his or her ability to learn a language and recommends the student be exempt from the language other than English requirement.

Special Transportation

Transportation recommendation to address needs of the student relating to his or her disability

☐ None

☐ Student needs special transportation accommodations or services as follows:

☐ Student needs transportation to and from special classes or programs at another site as follows:

Placement Recommendation

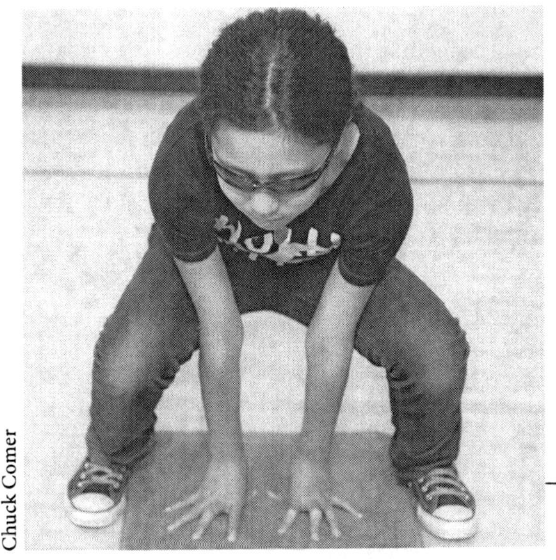
Chuck Comer

PART 2
Modifications and Adaptations for Teaching Physical Activities

Modifying Instruction to Meet Students' Needs

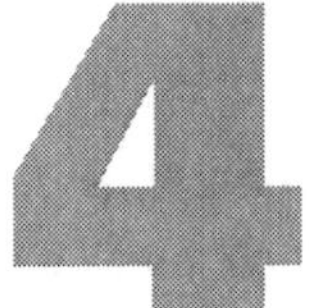

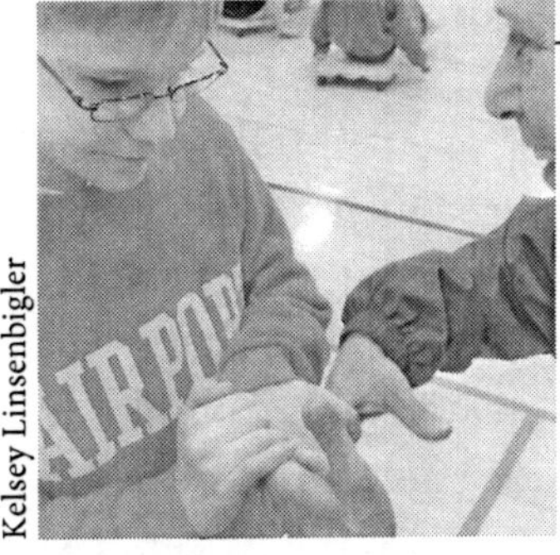
Kelsey Linsenbigler

IN THIS CHAPTER

- **Working with Students with Visual Impairments**
- **Instructional Modifications for Students with Visual Impairments**
- **Instructional Modifications for Students Who Are Deafblind**

Ms. O'Brien, an itinerant teacher of children with visual impairments in a cooperative school district, has a strong interest in sports and recreation and enrolled in a class on adapted physical education and visual impairment during her graduate studies. She works with Mr. Hwang, an adapted physical educator assigned to a large middle school in the district, who has a good deal of experience working with children with visual impairments.

One afternoon, Ms. O'Brien received a message from a therapist in the school district asking for information or materials on how to teach students who are visually impaired how to jump or run on behalf of a physical education teacher who is trying to teach introductory track and field skills to Felipe, a student in his class with no functional vision. "The physical education teacher said Felipe tends to slap his feet on the floor instead of jumping or stomps his feet down instead of running. I'm not sure how to explain to the student how to jump."

Ms. O'Brien knew Felipe well and was able to explain to the therapist the source of the problem in Felipe's lack of basic physical skills, including running, jumping, and throwing, because he had not been privileged to have early childhood interventions related to such skills. She guessed that the foot slapping and stomping were an attempt on his part to duplicate the sounds he heard while the other students were performing jumping and running activities. Ms. O'Brien added that she and Mr. Hwang, the adapted physical educator, would be happy to work with the therapist and the physical education teacher to introduce these skills through a series of step-by-step activities. She promised to e-mail the therapist activity plans that included information on how to teach basic skills, including track and field activities, to students with visual impairments, so the therapist could review them before Felipe and the therapist began working together.

Learning can be defined as behavioral change in individuals that results from their experiences (Merriam & Caffarella, 1999). Children generally experience or learn the physical skills required to carry out everyday life tasks and participate in basic sports, such as running, jumping, throwing, and kicking, by watching their parents, brothers and sisters, or other role models and by listening to them describe how they are doing the tasks. In other words, they learn these skills through visual demonstrations and descriptions that are paired with visual experiences. As described in previous chapters, children and adults who have visual or hearing impairments also learn through demonstration and description, but their visual or combined hearing and visual impairments may act as barriers to the usual pairing of observation and description in the learning process. Their learning may therefore depend more on direct communication and individual instruction between teacher and learner.

This chapter and the one that follows focus on methods for helping students with visual impairments or deafblindness learn the skills needed for physical activities, and, in particular, the modifications and adaptations commonly used when teaching these students. The present chapter covers the interaction between the teacher and the student, while Chapter 5 covers the interface between the student and the activity to be performed. This chapter offers techniques primarily focused on how to modify day-to-day teaching techniques to overcome the barriers inherent between a teacher with vision and a student with too little vision to enable learning through demonstration and observation. Chapter 5 presents principles for systematically analyzing a given physical activity and then devising adaptations that decrease or eliminate the access barriers that generally keep students with visual impairments or deafblindness from participating. Later chapters provide more detail about lessons and teaching methods. Taken together, these materials provide readers with the information needed to teach students who are visually impaired or deafblind effectively and successfully. For the purposes of this book, the term *modification* generally refers to changing one's usual teaching methods, while *adaptation* usually relates to changing some parameter of an activity to make it accessible to students with visual impairments or deafblindness.

This chapter uses school-related learning situations as a basis for presenting how one might begin to modify instruction in physical skills for learners of any age with visual impairments or deafblindness. These methods can be of equal assistance in teaching any activity, including sports or recreational activities for adults (whether running sprints, bowling, skiing, or swimming) and wherever the instruction takes place (track, bowling alley, ski slope, or pool). As noted earlier, the emphasis is on modifications to communication between the physical education teacher and the student with a visual impairment or deafblindness.

WORKING WITH STUDENTS WITH VISUAL IMPAIRMENTS

When teachers have a student with a visual impairment or deafblindness in their class for the first time, they often feel unprepared to work with him or her. As stressed in previous chapters, however, each student with a visual impairment is a unique individual; the visual impairment is just one aspect of who he or she is. The first principle of interacting with a student with a visual impairment or deafblindness is to remember that the student is a child first, more like the other children in the class than different from them. Sidebar 4.1 offers some other suggestions about working with students with visual impairments in a physical education class, most of which also pertain to students with deafblindness. The second half of this chapter will have more information about working with students who are deaf or hard of hearing in addition to being visually impaired.

It is important for a teacher to get to know a student's specific needs and abilities, as even individuals who have the same visual condition with the same visual acuity may experience it differently and have different functional vision (see Chapter 2). Individuals may also have vision that fluctuates at different times of the day or under different environmental conditions. The teacher of students with visual impairments can be a primary resource for information on a student's visual impairment and other health conditions, if any, as well as for specific suggestions about meeting each student's unique needs and helping the students participate in the class.

Part-to-Whole Learning

It is helpful for teachers who work with students who are visually impaired to understand how a visual impairment affects the way children or adults with visual impairments learn (Ferrell, 2011). Without vision, learners do not necessarily grasp concepts, such as how a basketball game is played, simply by being present when a game is going on or by hearing an explanation. For individuals with visual impairments or deafblindness, concrete, hands-on experience with objects and the physical experience of performing a movement is a crucial aspect of learning.

In addition, instruction may need to be more specific and systematic. For example, although typical vision enables individuals to see and comprehend an entire object or scene all at once, before examining the individual

SIDEBAR 4.1

Tips for Teaching Students with Visual Impairments

The following are some suggestions for interacting with students with visual impairments in any class and including them in physical education classes in particular:

- Treat the student as part of the class. The same disciplinary rules should apply to everyone. Make exceptions only when necessary, just as you would for any other student.
- Address the student directly, not through a companion or guide.
- State your name when approaching a visually impaired student. Voices are not always easy to identify, particularly in crowds or stressful situations. Also, introduce others in the room, especially if they are newcomers or people who are not usually in the classroom.
- Do not raise your voice so that a student who is blind will understand you better, unless the student is also hearing impaired.
- Speak naturally when you talk. Do not be afraid to use words that refer to seeing. However, words like *here* and *there* are too general to be descriptive. Be specific; label objects and give direction and location.
- In a group setting, call the student by name when you want a response from him or her. Gestures are not always enough.
- Use sound to help the student. Your voice leads and directs a visually impaired student within the environment. Get the student's attention before giving instructions. A moving speaker confuses a student with a visual impairment. Describe with clear directions and in a normal speaking voice where you are and how the student can reach you.
- Help make the sound environment meaningful for the student with a visual impairment. Eliminate confusing or conflicting sounds. The sorting of sounds is a difficult skill which takes time, experience, and explanation to develop.
- Orient the student to the classroom and equipment in the gym. Let the student know if you have changed the room around. Independent mobility is important and sometimes difficult for students who are visually impaired.
- Explain what is happening around the student. Show from where sounds and smells are coming. As the student explores, describe everything with variety, quality, and richness.
- Avoid overprotection. Remember that all children get bumps and scrapes occasionally. Safety is important, but overprotection can be just as detrimental to a child as underprotection.
- Encourage independence. Let the student do as much as possible for himself or herself.
- Build the student's self-confidence by letting him or her try. Take the student through an activity or game a couple of times before requiring independent movement. For a sighted student, motor imitation is a visual skill, whereas a student with a visual impairment needs to experience the activity physically.
- Answer questions simply and naturally. The other students will ask questions about a student with a visual impairment.
- Consider the available light sources. Light can be distracting for some children with low vision, while for others indirect lighting may be inadequate.
- Teach the student through the remaining senses. A student who is visually impaired cannot learn by observing and imitating the actions of others. You may need to physically put the student through an action or allow the student to experience the actions you are performing.

SIDEBAR 4.1 *(continued)*

- Relay accurate information to the student in order to maintain a sense of trust.
- If you are talking to a student who is blind and you have to leave, tell the student that you are leaving! People look silly talking to themselves thinking you are there.
- Clear the gym and locker room so they are free of clutter and loose objects.
- Make sure doors are completely closed or completely open. A half-open door is a hazard to a person who is blind. Drawers and lockers should also be kept closed when not in use.
- Do not be a servant. Do not do things for a student that the student can do for himself or herself; instead, do things together.
- Tape ropes to the floor to help visually impaired students to identify activity boundaries.
- Occasionally blindfold the sighted students and play a game. This increases empathy for and acceptance of the student who is blind.
- Do not think of your students as blind children. They are children who happen to be blind.

Source: Adapted with permission, from L. J. Lieberman and J. F. Cowart, *Games for People with Sensory Impairments: Strategies for Including Individuals of All Ages* (Louisville, KY: American Printing House for the Blind, 2011).

pieces, learning for individuals with visual impairments often works the opposite way: because they can touch or see only a limited part of an object or a room at one time, they have to build a concept of the whole out of these parts (Ferrell, 2011). Doing so is a process that is likely to be incomplete and, sometimes, inaccurate, and students who are visually impaired may therefore need repeated experiences and detailed explanations. It is consequently important for teachers to consider how to convey the totality of a piece of equipment, a sports field, or a game to a student who cannot see it all at once. (This concept is also discussed in Chapter 7.)

The Role of Communication in Activity Instruction

Communication is key to instruction in any subject area, but because physical education involves movement, teachers often rely heavily on demonstration or nonverbal communication. In most physical education classrooms, teachers may present demonstrations of a basic skill, such as jumping, by standing in front of their students and performing the jump while describing its important aspects. They are communicating with students both nonverbally, by demonstrating the jump, and verbally, by describing it and giving cues. In some cases, particularly if the skill is simple, it might be taught exclusively verbally, such as by saying the instruction "Run around the cones" or "Jump rope with two feet 10 times."

The communication between teacher and student is not unidirectional, however. Rather, it is bi-directional, from teacher to student and back to teacher again; communication from student to teacher indicates the extent to which the skill has been learned. For example, when the instructor presents the basic jump and accompanying description in front of the class, the communication loop is not complete until the students perform the jump, which conveys information to the teacher, so he or she can evaluate the extent to which they have learned it.

The barriers to communication between a teacher with vision and a student with a visual impairment result primarily from a significant loss in the nonverbal or demonstrative communication aspect of instruction. However, it is important to note that the barrier exists in only one direction, from teacher to student, not vice versa. This means that the teacher needs to modify the usual technique of demonstrating a skill to overcome the barrier, but in general with the students discussed in this book, no modification is needed in the communication from student to teacher because the teacher can observe the student's performance and the student can ask questions if needed.

In contrast, the barrier between teacher and student with severe hearing and visual impairments interferes with both the verbal and nonverbal aspects of communication. Here again, the difficulty with the nonverbal aspect of communication is only from teacher to student, because the teacher is able to observe the nonverbal or demonstrative language of the student. The barrier to verbal or descriptive communication can be either in one or both directions. If students are hard of hearing but have verbal skills, the barrier is only from teacher to student, because the student can speak to the teacher but cannot hear spoken instructions. For these reasons, it is important for teachers to consider the communication style of their students, consult with the student's teacher of students with visual impairments, intervener, or other related professional, if appropriate, and determine a way to work with the student most effectively and understanding his or her behavior.

The next section of this chapter describes techniques for adapting the nonverbal aspects of instruction for students with visual impairments. The latter part of the chapter describes the methods for adapting verbal instruction for learners with dual sensory impairments.

INSTRUCTIONAL MODIFICATIONS FOR STUDENTS WITH VISUAL IMPAIRMENTS

In many instances, instructing someone with a visual impairment in physical education is much like teaching anyone else, because issues relating to nonverbal communication on the part of the teacher are evident only under certain instructional circumstances. If the amount of instruction required is minimal, such as when introducing basketball, a table tennis paddle, or a baseball bat, the instruction can be just a matter of handing the object over to the student for a tactile inspection before proceeding to explain how the equipment is used. Similarly, if instruction involves a simple movement, such as taking two steps forward or placing hands on hips, this type of instruction can be accomplished through simple statements, regardless of the student's degree of vision (assuming the student with a visual impairment is able to follow directions and has unimpaired learning ability).

The circumstances in which barriers to instructional communication are most evident are likely to be less common, but are extremely significant. They include the following:

- describing complex apparatus or equipment related to a lesson
- describing the dimensions of a court, field, or other playing area and positions related to the sport

- describing a room or activity area
- assisting students in moving smoothly from place to place
- teaching complex physical movement skills

Situations such as these will generally call for modifications of the teacher's teaching or presentation style when working with students who are visually impaired. Each situation is covered in detail in the following sections.

Describing Complex Apparatus or Equipment

Issues in Describing Complex Equipment

When introducing a new apparatus or type of equipment that is too complex to be identified quickly by touch or remaining vision or by a simple description, the teacher needs to restructure the lesson to introduce the equipment in an alternative way. In most cases, such as when introducing a basketball goal, a trampoline, or a long jump pit, conveying to the student knowledge of its shape, dimensions, and the materials it is composed of is a prerequisite to teaching the activity associated with it. The basketball goal (including backboard, goal ring and net), the trampoline (with its mat, springs, and framing), and the long jump landing pit made up of runway, board, and sand pit are too complex to describe with only words. Imagine standing beside the long jump pit with a student who is blind from birth and coming up with the language needed to establish the concept of how to use the pit without any means of demonstration or actual participation. As is true in most lessons, understanding this concept needs to be established as a prerequisite to developing a particular targeted skill, before the activity itself can begin. In essence, the principle for providing such a description is to create a concrete image for the student, through detailed haptic investigation of the long jump pit or other equipment, equivalent in the brain to a visual image, as explained in Chapter 2 (Merabet, Pitskel, Amedi, & Pascual-Leone, 2008).

A teacher's usual method of describing a new device or piece of equipment to a student with vision might be to physically point at the parts and verbally explain the name of each part and its function. As a result, those new to teaching students with visual impairments often start with that method and attempt to modify it in one way or another. For example, a teacher might guide a student who is blind to each part, and provide explanations related to that part while the student is touching it. This approach is flawed in two major ways. First, the student may not get an image of the "whole" before starting, especially when the piece of equipment is large. Instead, each part is learned separately and then must somehow be painstakingly mentally put together like puzzle pieces back into an understanding of the whole, without the student knowing exactly what the whole should be. Second, the teacher who relies on verbally explaining objects or environments is providing a kind of lecture in which each part is named, and while its function explained, the student is expected to memorize the information without any concrete experience. In the case of a relatively small object or activity area, such as a long jump pit, hands-on experience with the apparatus can be provided by allowing the student to investigate the pit area either haptically or with limited vision.

Raised- or bold-line drawings or tactile scale models of an object can also serve as effective graphical representations for some students. One method of creating a raised-line drawing is to use a specially designed drawing board that raises the lines that are drawn on paper or other media attached to the board, as explained in Sidebar 4.2. These boards can be constructed or are commercially available (see the Resources section). Scale models with raised symbols or lines created by attaching felt, pipe cleaners, Wikki Stix, or the like to stiff paper or cardboard bases are also effective. (Wikki Stix are thin, waxy, bendable sticks that can be bent into shape and will stick in place.) It is important to note that some students who are visually impaired, especially those with early-onset blindness, may have difficulty generalizing from either a drawing or scale model to real life, so a student's understanding of the drawing or model needs to be verified. Since teachers of students with visual impairments are usually knowledgeable about how to make tactile drawings, models, and maps that best convey information for students with visual impairments, they can be helpful in both creating drawings and models and making suggestions to promote the student's understanding. Sidebar 4.2 describes some principles for the creation of tactile graphics that are more likely to be understood by students with visual impairments.

Instructional Modifications for Describing Complex Equipment

Learner description is a technique that circumvents the communication barrier between the teacher and the student with a visual impairment, and it eliminates both weaknesses of an approach that depends on the teacher's description. In this book, *learner description* refers to the use of the learner's own words to describe the equipment or apparatus of the lesson once the learner is given the opportunity to investigate it. The use of learner description can aid the teacher in determining what the student already knows about the lesson.

For example, during a lesson about the long jump pit, the teacher can introduce the long jump pit by taking students to it and then asking them to investigate it either haptically or with their limited vision and describe its overall shape, its parts, and what materials it is made of. The student might describe the landing area as "a big sandbox with railroad tie sides," which tells the teacher that the student already understands some of the parts and may only need clarification or terminology substitutions. In this example, learner description places the task of describing the long jump pit on the student instead of the teacher. The communication barrier related to a teacher's need to verbally explain all the components is avoided, because the description is from student to teacher, where no barrier exists. The student can use nonverbal communication, such as pointing at parts, and use familiar language to describe parts, such as the "jump board" or "the sand." Also, memorization is enhanced by requiring students to find each part and think through its possible use. Using learner description avoids the student's having to put the pieces of the long jump pit he or she has explored together into an image of the whole. If the teacher presented each part of the long jump pit, the student may not conceptualize how the pit comes together and how each part is used. The use of the scale model of

SIDEBAR 4.2

Creating Tactile Drawings and Maps

A variety of products exist for making tactile graphics (see the Resources section at the end of this book). The teacher of students with visual impairments is likely to have access to such materials and experience in using them, as well as knowledge of how individuals with visual impairments may interpret a raised-line drawing, so collaboration between this teacher and the physical educator is advisable.

One method is to adapt a line drawing by transferring it to heat-sensitive paper and passing it through a thermal copying process that raises any black lines or images (Presley & D'Andrea, 2009). This method is quick but requires special machinery. Another method is to make the drawing using a raised-line drawing board.

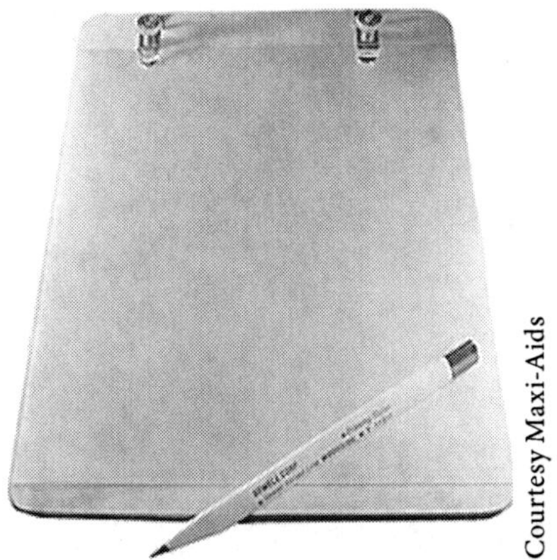

Courtesy Maxi-Aids

A commercially available raised-line drawing board with stylus.

Raised-Line Drawing Boards

One version of a raised-line drawing board is a sheet of rubber, approximately ¼ inch thick, glued to a firm backing of pressed board, plastic, or wood on which a disposable sheet of paper-thin plastic is placed. Writing on the plastic with a pen or stylus produces raised, rather than engraved, lines that can be perceived haptically (Bentzen & Marston, 2010; Ponchillia & Ponchillia, 1996; Presley & D'Andrea, 2009). Commercially available drawing boards (see the Resources section) come mounted on a clipboard that can hold the plastic sheet to be written on in place on the pad under two screw-driven clips. Aluminum foil or plain paper can also be used on it effectively (Ponchillia & Ponchillia, 1996).

A homemade screen drawing board can be made by fastening a sheet of aluminum or steel screen onto the flat surface of a thin Masonite board or a commercial clipboard. The edges of the screen are folded under and sandwiched between the front board and a backing board to protect users from being scratched. It can be used with either a plastic or paper sheet to produce raised images (Ponchillia & Ponchillia, 1996). A raised-line drawing board is a handy addition to the teaching kit of any instructor who works with students with visual impairments.

Tips for Creating Effective Tactile Images

- Figures should be drawn in only two planes. Attempts to add depth, as in visual representations of three-dimensional objects, can confuse tactile readers.
- The writing instrument used on a raised-line drawing board should have a broader writing head than a standard pen.
- The drawing instrument used on a raised-line drawing board should be held at a more slanted angle than when writing on paper to help raise the tactile lines.
- Tactile images must be reproduced in large enough size to allow fingertips and hands to detect detail.
- Raised-print letters should be in an enlarged font for clarity.
- Some individuals may need an in-depth orientation to the tactile graphic, particularly raised-print letters.

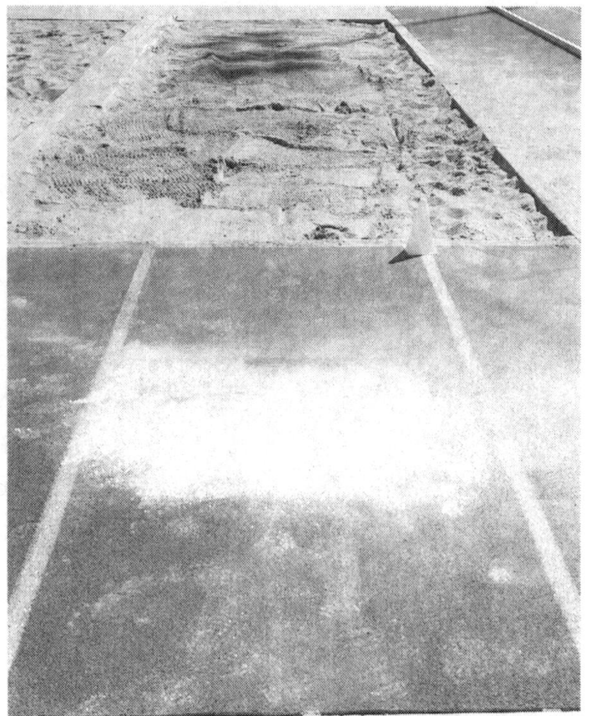

Chuck Comer

A long jump pit, showing the runway, takeoff board, talcum powder used to show the jumper's footprint, sand pit, and wooden edging around the pit.

the long jump pit also helps with these concrete concepts.

At the end of a successful introduction using learner descriptions, there in general have been three major accomplishments:

- Students have a visual image of the long jump pit.
- Students have memorized its major parts and their functions.
- A vocabulary of terms has been established between the teacher and the student.

The teacher can now proceed with the activity portion of the lesson knowing that prerequisite communication has been established.

It is important to note that the organization of a lesson using learner description is not left to chance or to students' ability to find all the parts of an item or a piece of equipment. Rather, the teacher's lesson plan includes notes about all the parts of the equipment or setting, and the teacher needs to ensure that each part is found by the student (or pointed out if missed) and discussed (see Sidebar 4.3). One technique to accomplish this that fits well with learner description is for the teacher to use a "question" rather than "statement" approach. In the long jump example, if the student was investigating the takeoff board and simply said, "This is the takeoff board," the teacher could prompt further exploration by asking, "Can you tell me the shape of the board? Is it wider than long, and how far is it from the sand pit?" An example of how a lesson plan can be organized to use learner description and a question approach to cover all the requisite information is provided in Sidebar 4.3, which contains the instructional portion of sample lesson plans for introducing the long jump pit and the game of basketball to students with blindness or low vision.

Description of the court or field used in a game or activity and the positions related to a sport also needs to be addressed. If a student is blind or has low vision, it is likely that the student has heard of volleyball, archery, or soccer but without understanding the complete activity. It is very important to take the time to ensure comprehension. This will be most effective if it is done outside of the physical education class in which the student with a

SIDEBAR 4.3

Sample Lesson Plans Using Learner Description

The portions of the lesson plans presented here would have been preceded by plan objectives, description, and purpose of the long jump or of the plan game of basketball, and materials. Thus, the student would have an understanding of how the activity is accomplished and what role the pit or the backboard and goal play before the equipment is introduced.

Introducing the Long Jump Pit

1. Discuss the purpose and general layout of a long jump pit.
   a. Composed of a runway, takeoff board, and sand landing pit
   b. General dimensions of the area
2. Take students to the end of the pit opposite the runway and identify their position.
3. Ask students to use touch or remaining vision to investigate the perimeter of the pit and to describe everything found there.
   a. If missed, point out: sand pit, concrete or wooden edging, takeoff board, runway, and distance from takeoff board to sand pit.
   b. If missed, point out characteristics of takeoff board (width, length, and material) and visibility (if learners have enough vision to see it).
   c. If missed, point out important characteristics of runway (width, length, any underfoot safety threats, and visibility if applicable).
4. Ask students to give an overall description from memory.
5. Evaluate by asking students to locate parts and point out characteristics.
6. Evaluate by having students walk down runway, across board, and through and out the end of the pit.

Introducing a Basketball Backboard and Goal

1. Have students climb a ladder and feel basketball backboard, rim, and net.
2. Take students to a lowered backboard and goal (or to a sporting goods store if a backboard cannot be lowered).
3. Ask students to use touch or remaining vision to describe the overall shape and structure of the apparatus and its individual parts.
4. If missed, point out the overall shape.
5. If missed, be sure all parts are found (goal and framework for attachment to standard).
   a. If missed, point out the important characteristics of the goal (goal ring, attachment to board, reinforcement rods for the attachment and ring, net, and visibility if applicable).
   b. If missed, point out the important characteristics of the backboard (where goal is placed on it and visibility and contrast to ring and net if applicable).
6. Ask students if there is a way to make a basket by hitting the backboard with the ball first; demonstrate a bank shot (in which the ball bounces off the backboard and into the net) if necessary.
7. Evaluate by asking students to give an overall description from memory.
8. Evaluate by asking students to locate parts and point out characteristics.
9. Evaluate by asking students to describe a bank shot.

visual impairment is included. The class will move quickly, under the assumption that all students are aware of the dimensions of a court and basic positions. Time is needed to help a student conceptualize the playing area, positions, and goal of a game or sport in order for the student to participate and succeed.

Describing a Room or Activity Area

Issues in Describing a Room or Activity Area

The challenge of describing an activity area is essentially the same as that of describing complex equipment, except the scale and complexity have been increased significantly. Instead of establishing a visual image of a table tennis tabletop, a vaulting horse, a basketball goal, or a long jump pit, for example, the task becomes conveying the image of a recreation room filled with ping pong tables, the school gymnastics room with multiple stations, a basketball gymnasium with bleachers and various basketball courts, or an indoor track facility with its many competition areas. When dealing with the need to enhance a student's concept of space and orientation, the student's orientation and mobility (O&M) instructor is a helpful resource for consultation and instructional techniques.

The barriers to instructional communication are also similar in this task, because the way to introduce students who have vision to these areas consists of either taking them there and having them look around or possibly showing them a schematic or map of a facility. The sighted student can stand in one place, get a view of the entire area, and then begin to investigate each part from that viewpoint, an opportunity that is not available to students with visual impairments.

Again, a teacher's natural inclination might be to modify the approach used with sighted students, perhaps by trying to describe an area or facility verbally to students with visual impairments as the teacher and students stand together at the entry door or gate. As with describing equipment, however, that method does not give students with visual impairments a grasp of the whole before being confronted with the parts; it is also based on rote memorization of multiple objects in space, rather than creating memories through experience.

Instructional Modifications for Description of an Activity Area

There are two major instructional modifications used to describe the size and complexity of an activity area. If the activity is to be taught in a relatively simple space, *room familiarization* is suggested, but if an activity is taught in a complex facility, the use of *tactile or bold-line maps or diagrams* is indicated.

Room Familiarization

The technique of room familiarization is similar to the technique described previously for introducing the long jump pit. *Room familiarization* is a term used by O&M instructors for describing a specific technique taught to individuals with visual impairments. Assuming that students are older than preschoolers and are cognitively able, they can be taken to the room, given a quick general verbal description of its layout, and then asked to explore it. Bozeman and McCulley (2010) suggest that the exploration involve a *perimeter search,* a *grid pattern* exploration of the interior, and the use of *reference points* to establish the layout of the whole and the parts that make it up. The teacher would help the student determine which technique to use.

If the room is simple, such as a wrestling room containing only padded mats from wall to wall, a perimeter search is all that is needed, since the room's shape and the location of its doors are its only distinguishing characteristics. The student would walk the perimeter, noting the location of mats and outside doors or stairways. On the other hand, if the area is a recreation room filled with ping pong tables, the perimeter exploration would not show the room's most important features, in this instance, the tables. In this case, students can use a grid search pattern in which they place their backs to the wall and walk straight across the room and back to the starting point, move down the room a few feet, repeat the crossing, and continue this pattern until the complete interior has been investigated (Guth, Rieser, & Ashmead, 2010). The grid pattern exploration would soon reveal that the ping pong tables were set in rows that form a natural grid to follow. The students then walk around the tables, and then they will know where they are located.

Using a single reference point as a base from which to explore the room is effective if there are one or two significant objects in the room. Ponchillia & Ponchillia (1996) describe a technique based on the learner's knowledge of the six dots in the braille cell, which may assist those familiar with the braille cell concept and who are able to generalize it to larger spaces such as a workout facility. Essentially, the student imagines the six dots superimposed over the layout of the room, and the teacher then describes what is located near each dot.

Sometimes perimeter search and grid pattern exploration do not work. For example, in the aquatics area, a perimeter search would show little except the locker room and exit doors, and a grid pattern would not be feasible because the pool would interfere with walking across the area. However, in the aquatics area, the swimming pool and a hot tub might take up 90 percent of the floor space. In that case, a useful approach might involve moving along the edge of the pool until something of significance is encountered, such as the entrance ladder or the attachment point of a lane marker, then *squaring off* with the pool at that point (putting one's back against the pool or anything that is flat and square) and walking out to the wall to identify any relationship that might exist between the object at the pool's edge and any objects at the wall. If a student uses a long cane for mobility, the cane is a useful tool for exploring areas such as aquatics.

Tactile or Bold-Line Maps

When a facility is too large, is too complex, or poses a danger to students exploring them, they are often introduced first in the form of a map made with tactile markings or extra bold lines and sometimes large print (Bentzen & Marston, 2010), using the methods described earlier for making raised-line drawings or tactile scale models (see Sidebar 4.2). When such maps are used with students who are blind or have low vision, it is important to keep in mind that reading maps by touch differs significantly from reading them with vision. The creation of maps for people with visual impairments is a complex subject in itself, and specialized techniques and guidelines are involved, a key principle is simplicity: a map should include the minimum information necessary for the particular purpose (Edman 1992; Bentzen & Marston, 2010). As was the case with raised-line drawings and tactile scale models, some students may not be able to use tactile maps to learn about movement within a larger environment such as a complex activity area, because they have difficulty spatially interpreting something on paper and relating it to the location of their body within the area being portrayed. Therefore, it is important to assess students' map concepts before attempting to use tactile maps or diagrams to describe an activity area (Bentzen & Marston, 2010). Again, collaborating with the teacher of students with visual impairments is important to ensure the effectiveness of the presentation of materials, as well as to help assess a student's comprehension of maps and their purpose.

If students are able to conceptualize them, tactile maps or tactile scale models of complex activity areas can provide the students with information about the layout of such sites much more quickly than actual exploration, so they are useful tools in a teacher's instructional arsenal (Long & Guidice, 2010). For example, a tactile model of a volleyball court can be used to show a student who is blind the dimensions of the court; the position of the net; the serving area; and the positions and rotation of players during the game.

Assisting Students in Moving from Place to Place

Issues in Assisting Students in Moving from Place to Place

Although it is technically not an instructional technique, one of a teacher's more common tasks is assisting a student who has little or no vision in moving from one place to another. In an everyday situation in which students are sighted, a teacher might simply point and say, "We'll continue the lesson over there at the black tumbling mat." The initial impulse might be to modify that practice by offering an elaborate verbal description of how to get "over there." For example, the teacher might attempt to tell a student who has a visual impairment, "Uh, go to your right four steps, then take a 45 degree turn left, and walk about 20 feet, but don't run into the parallel bars that are on the left about halfway there." Because the route in this example is relatively complex, the student might get there or might not, but the teacher will most likely be uncomfortable with the ambiguities inherent in such a description. Barriers to success when trying to use language to direct a student to a location include the following:

- Spatial language, such as "left," "ahead," "next to," and "under," is not precise, and the terms and can mean different things to different people.
- Many people who are visually impaired may have difficulty walking in a straight line for long distances.
- Distance estimation may not always be accurate among people who are blind.

Instructional Modification for Assisting Students in Moving from Place to Place

Assisting students in moving safely and comfortably from one place to another during a lesson can be done in one of four ways, depending upon the distance to be covered and the complexity of the situation:

- verbal description
- placement of sound cues
- human guide
- using a guide wire or wall (see Chapter 8)

Verbal description can be used in simple situations, such as when the distance to cover is small and there are no obstacles in the path. For example, "The mat is just a step or two directly in front of you"; "Reach behind you with your cane and you'll find the edge of the running track"; or "Go straight across the room to the opposite wall and trail it left a few feet to find the water fountain." In the first two examples, the goal is nearly within reach, and in the last example, the wall provides a "straight edge" and a physical guide to follow leading to the water fountain.

Placing a sound cue at the objective refers to an audible signal placed near the objective being sought that can give a hint as to its location. Either the teacher or another person can give an audible cue from that location or a sound beacon of some sort can be placed there. An auditory cue will assist students with no vision and useful hearing; a cue can also be something that is highly visible to assist students with low vision.

This technique is especially useful if the objective is in the middle of an open area that gives no tactile guidance as to its location or if the objective is placed at an odd angle related to the position of the student. For example, if moving a group of two to three students with visual impairments from a weight bench to a leg press machine nearby, the teacher simply needs to go to the leg press device, slap a palm down on it once or twice, and say "The leg press is over here, folks." Most students will be able to move directly to a sound cue, and it will likely save both words and time (Guth, Rieser, and Ashmead, 2010). This technique does not work well if there are a lot of obstacles or if the level of noise interference is high. In addition, if a student is deafblind, a sighted guide or guide wire or wall is preferable.

The *human guide technique,* a basic O&M technique sometimes referred to as "sighted guide," is used if other methods are not feasible. As its name implies, in human guide the individual who is visually impaired is guided by another person. The guide should first ask the person to be guided if he or she would like to "take an arm" or "take an elbow." The person being guided takes the guide's arm lightly just above the elbow and then walks a half-step behind, following the guide's movements to the desired location. Small children may need to hold the guide's hand or forearm. Most people who have been visually impaired for even a brief time will be able to follow the guide easily. Some individuals prefer to be told of upcoming stairs or they may prefer a brief pause, but it is usually unnecessary to announce turns or stops because the guide's body movement provides that information. Guides should indicate an upcoming narrow passage such as a doorway or path between pieces of equipment by pulling the elbow in toward the body and behind the back, thus signaling to the person being guided to walk directly behind the guide.

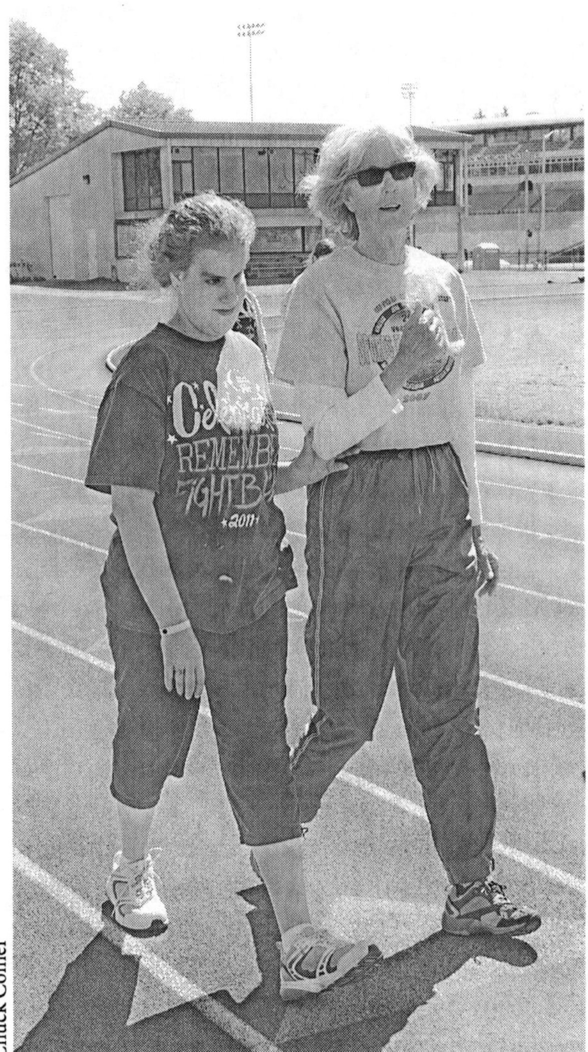

Chuck Comer

Walking on a track using the human guide technique.

Methods of Teaching Complex Movement Skills

Issues in Teaching Complex Movement Skills

The most significant instructional barrier between a physical education teacher and a student resulting from the student's visual impairment occurs when the student needs to learn a complex physical skill. The situation described in the vignette at the beginning of this chapter in which Ms. O'Brien was asked for assistance with a student who "slaps his feet instead of jumping or stomps his feet instead of running" is a typical example and demonstrates the frustration caused by lack of knowledge about this common barrier to physical education instruction. The dilemma exemplified by the teacher's question has its basis not simply in the issue of "How do I demonstrate this skill to a student who can't see me?" but also in the fact that this student has perhaps never acquired the basic skills for jumping and running. The problem has resulted from Felipe's having had little or no meaningful prior education in physical skills, compounded by his current physical education teacher's lack of knowledge of instructional modifications useful in teaching physical skills.

The instructional barriers faced when trying to teach complex body movement skills such as jumping or running probably appear more daunting to a novice teacher than describing equipment or orienting students to an activity area. Thus, a teacher with no knowledge of instructional modifications might attempt a verbal description of the lesson's equipment and of the playing area, but when faced with teaching activity skills to a student who is blind and who imitates the sound of jumping by slapping his feet on the floor might well be daunted by the task.

Instructional Modifications for Teaching Complex Movement Skills

As noted earlier in this chapter, students with significant visual impairments learn by description, observation, and prior experience just as other students do. Therefore, the instructional modifications presented here suggest ways of making the tried and true techniques of observation and demonstration accessible to those with little or no vision using the following:

- verbal instruction
- tactile modeling and physical guidance
- step-by-step instruction

Verbal Instruction

The teacher who requested help from Mrs. O'Brien was surely hoping that there was a simple way to use language in a lesson or two to help Felipe learn to jump and run. In fact, verbal instruction is a powerful tool for some lessons in which the skill is simple or in which students have a good deal of previous experience. The key to using verbal instruction effectively is the use of *precise language* and *common analogies.* If the skill is more complicated or the student has had little previous experience, the skill may need to be broken down into smaller pieces in a process known as *task analysis.*

Using Precise Language. As described earlier in this chapter, it is important to use an extremely specific teaching vocabulary when working with students with visual impairments or deafblindness (Lieberman & Cowart, 2011; Ponchillia and Ponchillia, 1996). There is no place for the general slang words commonly used in our everyday language, such as "thing," "stuff," and "over there," because a student without vision will have no idea what these terms refer to.

It is especially important to be precise and clear when describing movements because of their extreme complexity. Students who have severe visual impairments depend on teachers to use the same precise terms in a consistent manner in order to assimilate definitions of sports equipment and physical movements. The use of general descriptive instructions such as "Just place the crossbar on the high jump standard" or "Place your hands on the vaulting horse" communicate their meaning only to students who can see the accompanying gestures of the teacher or are already familiar with the equipment. In such cases, just a bit more description is required to get the point across to those with visual impairments. For example, "Place the crossbar on the flat bar holder at the very top of the high jump standard" or "Grab each of the two parallel bars at the ends of the vaulting horse like you are shaking hands with them" would clarify the instructions.

Consistency in word usage is also important for effective instructional communication. The use of several different terms for the same behavior is confusing. For example, an *underhand throw* might also be called a softball throw, and the term *jump* can mean many behaviors, such as leaping from one foot to the other foot, leaping from one foot to two feet, or leaping from one foot to the same foot. The term to use should be that which is most accurate, that is, the one used in textbooks or most commonly in the vocabulary of physical educators. In this case, *underhand throw* is a better choice and each of the *jumps* described above actually has a different definition: *step, jump,* and *hop,* respectively. Students who have good vision see the movement being performed when they hear words ascribed to it and therefore can more easily learn to assimilate a range of definitions used for the same behavior. If these terms are to become meaningful to students with extremely limited vision, however, the terms need to be used consistently in the same situation for the same movement.

Shortening the verbal instructions to cues or prompts will help guide the students as well as keep their movements consistent and on task. For example, a dance unit might include movements such as bringing the elbow to the knee for eight counts, stepping side-to-side for eight counts, and moving to the right two steps and then to the left two steps for eight counts. Verbal cues could be "elbow to knee," "side to side," and "move to the right two and to the left two." For a student with deafblindness, touch cues—a signal made on the student's body—would be added to the verbal cues, once their meaning is explained to the student; in this example, a touch cue on the elbow, a touch on the hip, and a touch on the shoulder.

Using Analogies. Assuming that the student has the cognitive ability, analogies can help clarify explanations and descriptions. For example, once a student has mastered the basic underhand softball throw, it is an easy matter to teach a bowling or goal ball throw by drawing an analogy with the underhand throw. Many analogies can be applied to the teaching and learning of physical skills. It is up to the teacher to draw them and use them in the class. Other examples of analogies useful in teaching movement skills include comparing print letter shapes related to arm or leg positions, for example, "Make your legs in the shape of a V"; comparing body movements to familiar ones, such as "a hop is just like a standing long jump, except you jump from one foot and land on the same foot"; or comparing unknown sports to known ones, such as, "Spinning is like riding a bike, but the bike is ridden inside and is stationary." Analogies are especially useful when working with adults, because adults have a great deal of life experience on which to draw comparisons.

If done properly, instructing by using verbal explanations can help all types of people with visual impairments learn physical activity skills. However, verbal explanations work best for individuals with acquired vision loss who most likely have already learned basic physical skills or those with early-onset impairments who have had extensive experience with physical movement. As discussed in Chapter 1, people with acquired vision loss generally have learned the basic skills of running, jumping, throwing, and kicking, so lessons for people with acquired losses generally focus more on teaching them adaptations that make the activity accessible to them. For example, they may only need a beeper placed at the basketball basket to mark its location, as they may already know how to dribble and shoot a basket.

Tactile Modeling and Physical Guidance

Tactile modeling and physical guidance are two modified instructional techniques that can be used to make demonstration of complex physical skills accessible to students who are visually impaired.

Tactile Modeling. *Tactile modeling* is used here to mean a modified adapted demonstration, that is, an exhibition of a motor activity presented by touch so as to make it accessible to students with visual impairments. Modeling can be a demonstration presented haptically to students who are blind or a tactile demonstration that increases the visibility of an activity for those who have low vision (O'Connell, Lieberman, & Petersen, 2006; Ponchillia &

Ponchillia, 1996). Whereas task analysis, or breaking down a skill into its component parts, followed by step-by-step instruction (described later in this section) is a powerful tool of instruction for students with visual impairments who need to learn basic physical skills, tactile modeling is the most common tool used to teach the component parts in step-by-step instruction. It is also the most common instructional method used with individuals with acquired vision loss.

Tactile modeling works well for such activities as tai chi, shot put, goalball defense and offense (see Chapter 9 for more information about goalball), swimming, and many, many others. The following scenarios illustrate how a teacher might present tactile modeling to a student in a variety of instructional situations:

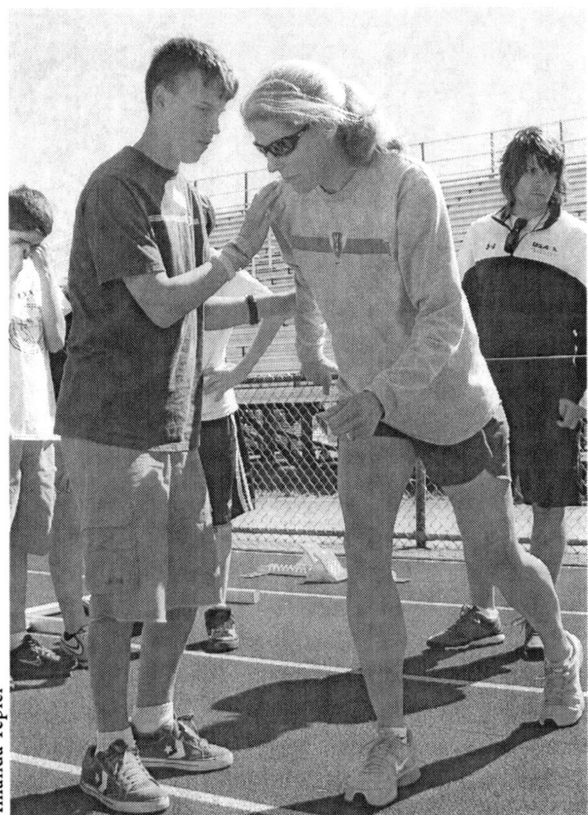

Amanda Tepfer

Marla Runyan, an Olympic gold medal winner who is legally blind, uses tactile modeling to demonstrate proper running form for a student.

- "I am in proper goalball blocking form, so I want you to feel the position of all the joints in my body, including wrists, elbows, shoulders, waist, hips, knees, and ankles."
- "Okay, I'm in the ready position, so use your hands to check out the angle of my knees, waist, and neck, and I want you to also check out where my arms are."
- "I want to demonstrate how much effort I have to put into the final move of the shot put, so touch me here on the small of my back with your fingertips while I let it go, but stand back enough not to get hit by my body when I jump up."
- "I want you to see the proper backswing of a volleyball serve so you can see the proper hit, form, and follow-through."
- "I want to show you how high you need to jump here on the trampoline by having you follow my jumps, so while we're holding hands, just begin to follow my jumps until I tell you we're at the correct height."

Physical Guidance. Tactile modeling is distinguished from the teaching technique called *physical guidance* by the fact that during tactile modeling, the learner touches or observes a model who is demonstrating a skill. Physical guidance, by contrast, involves manipulation of the student; that is, the teacher actively touches and moves the student in some way.

Physical guidance is a powerful part of a teacher's instructional toolbox, because there are some physical activities for which it is the ideal teaching technique. For example, in fast-moving one-to-one sports such as wrestling and judo, there is no better way to demonstrate "moves" than by physically guiding or manipulating the student through them. Sidebar 4.4 provides some key points related to tactile modeling and physical guidance. It is important to remember that each point needs to be coupled with a verbal explanation (or signs for students who have a dual sensory impairment).

Whenever physical guidance is used, however, it is imperative to discuss its use with the student before doing so. People who are blind are understandably often extremely sensitive to being touched or to being urged along by an arm or elbow. Indeed, one of the first principles given when teaching someone to guide people who are blind is "Do not grab or push a person who is blind." This sensitivity to being pushed along is not unique to people with visual impairments, but it is broadly human in nature and may stem from a need for the locus of control to remain within each of us. It is particularly noteworthy in a discussion of instructional modification in physical education, however, because many students with visual impairments may react to physical manipulation with a degree of emotion that can become a barrier to learning. For example, exclamations such as the following, overheard at sports camps for students with visual impairments,

SIDEBAR 4.4

Key Points Related to Tactile Modeling and Physical Guidance

The following are some important points to keep in mind when an instructor or peer is engaging in tactile modeling or providing physical assistance or guidance for a student with a visual impairment:

Tactile Modeling

- Allow the student to feel a peer or the instructor execute a skill or movement that was previously difficult to learn using verbal description.
- Tell the student where and when to feel the instructor or a peer executing a skill.
- To avoid possible misunderstanding or misinterpretation, document how much assistance was given and when and where the student felt you or a peer.
- Repeat tactile modeling as many times as necessary to ensure understanding.
- Combine tactile modeling with the other teaching methods to increase understanding.

Physical Assistance or Guidance

- Make sure the student is not averse to physical touch and will accept physical guidance assistance.
- Forewarn the student before giving physical assistance, to avoid startling the student.
- Assist the student physically through the movement.
- To avoid possible misunderstanding or misinterpretation, record which skills require physical assistance, including how much and where on the student's body assistance was needed so that the teacher can explain if asked when, where, and why the teacher touched a student.
- Fade assistance to minimal physical prompts as soon as possible.

Source: Adapted from M. O'Connell, L. Lieberman, and S. Petersen, "The Use of Tactile Modeling and Physical Guidance as Instructional Strategies in Physical Activity for Children Who Are Blind," *Journal of Visual Impairment & Blindness,* 100 (2006), pp. 471–477.

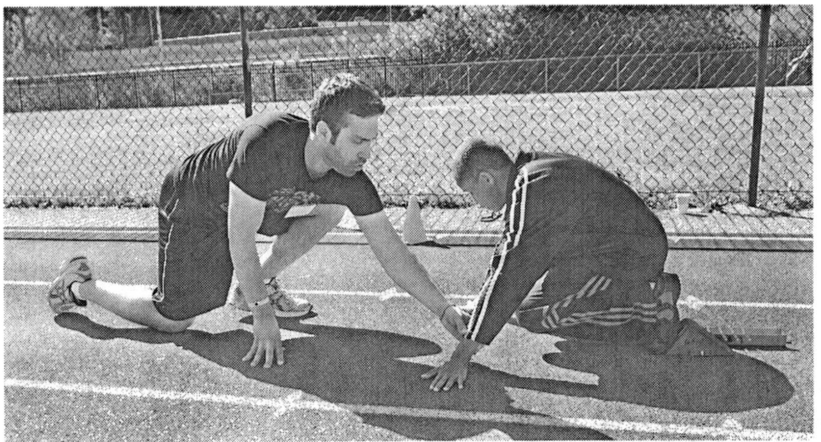

Chuck Comer

An instructor uses physical guidance to show a student the proper placement of the hands when on the starting blocks for a sprint start.

are typical: "When someone grabs my elbow, I just can't think about anything else!" and "Today when that teacher was swinging my arm over my head with the softball, all I could think was, 'Please let go of me!'" In the authors' experience, adults are particularly sensitive to being "handled" and generally prefer tactile modeling.

Physical guidance can be appropriate and effective, but students need to understand that they can ask to be taught by either method if one is preferred. In general, then, when teaching physical skills to students who have no significant intellectual or cognitive difficulties, the general rule is to consider tactile modeling first, and then move to physical guidance if that is the most effective method. The student should have the choice, but the teacher can also consider what usually works best for a given skill or activity, as one method is often most effective in a given situation.

Step-by-Step Instruction

Verbal language alone is not sufficient to teach complex physical movements, such as hopping, skipping, dribbling, or throwing a discus, to students with no previous experience or with limited basic skills. As discussed in previous chapters, some students with visual impairments or deafblindness have physical skills well below those of their classmates and require remedial instruction before they are prepared to play games such as those found in physical education classes or offered at the authors' sports camps. Teaching such students a simple skill, such as the ready position—the stance commonly assumed when preparing for such activities as beginning a distance race, taking up an infielder's stance, or starting a wrestling match—is not necessarily achieved by verbal instruction or by having a student haptically investigate someone demonstrating it. Often, the stance that results from a tactile investigation appears stiff and the knees and head are not held at the proper angle.

Task Analysis. The sports camps the authors have operated have had considerable success using an approach based on *task analysis* to teach activity skills to students who did not

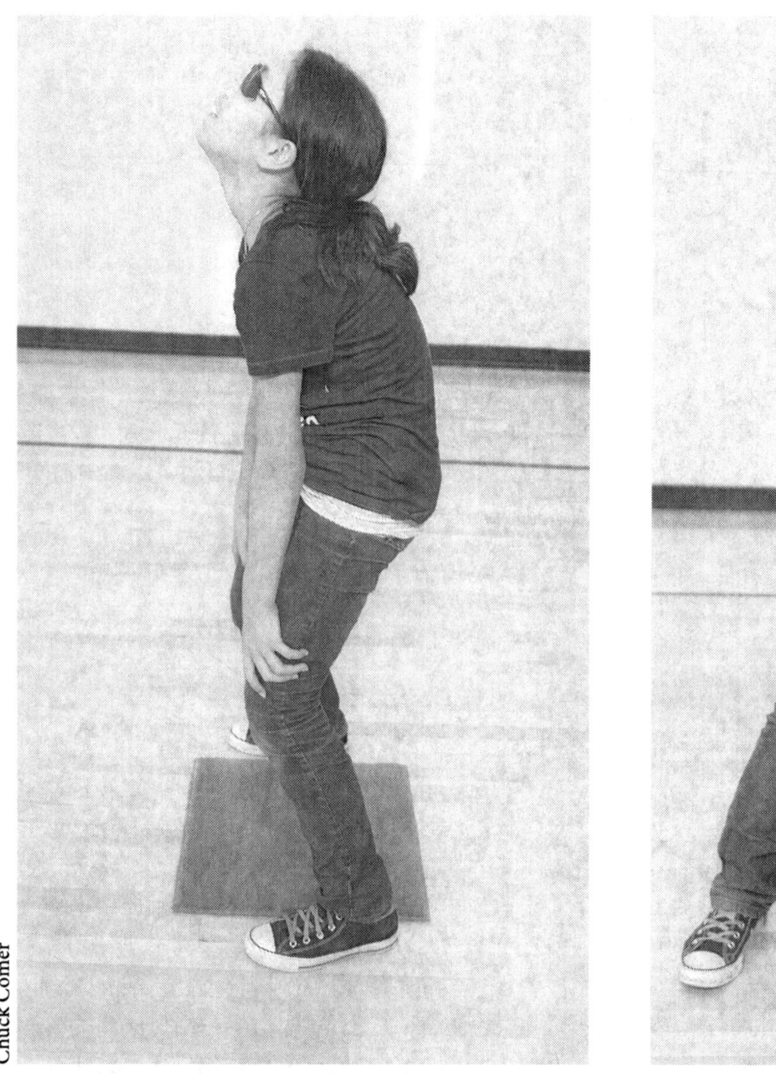

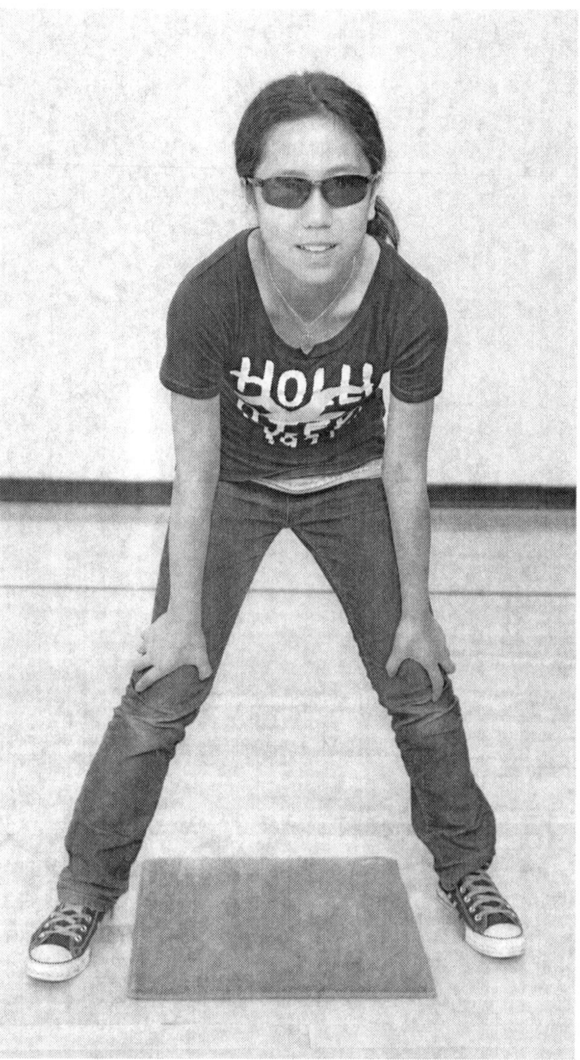

Chuck Comer

When students attempt a ready position after verbal explanation and tactile investigation, they often appear stiff and hold their knees and head at wrong angle (left). A correct ready position (right).

acquire them during early childhood development. Task analysis (based on the work of behaviorists such as Skinner, 1974) is the process of breaking an activity down into its smallest integral parts so that each smaller segment can be taught and the correct behavioral response promptly rewarded. As the steps are mastered, they are linked together until the entire task is learned (Lieberman & Houston-Wilson, 2009).

When used in a physical activity setting, task analysis helps the learner progress through smaller portions of a complex activity, such as learning to throw a ball underhand, rather than needing to master larger parts of the skill involving multiple subtasks. Task analysis also gives the teacher a detailed list of objectives that can be used to measure learning progress that might otherwise go unnoticed.

However, teaching such skills using traditional task analysis requires more time than is typically available in a physical education class or at a short-term workshop such as a sports camp. As a consequence, the authors have used two systematic training techniques used in elementary physical education to teach basic physical skills and to add structure and fun to learning, including a step-by-step method using carpet squares (Debra Berkey, Professor, Physical Education Teacher Education, Western Michigan University, personal communication, May 2000) and another using parachutes (Strong & LeFevre, 2006).

Step-by-step teaching with carpet squares has been used most often in settings in which only students with visual impairments or deafblindness are being taught, while parachutes are an excellent tool for teaching basic skills in an inclusionary setting alongside sighted classmates. Parachutes have also been used successfully with groups at the sports camps, but their exclusive use with students with visual impairments or deafblindness would be difficult in most school settings simply because six or more students are required to handle a parachute.

Because there is little literature describing the use of these techniques with students with visual impairments or deafblindness and because the authors have had outstanding results with them, they will be discussed in detail in this book. Parachute instruction, which lends itself so well to inclusive settings, is discussed in Chapter 7 on elementary education. Teaching on carpet squares is introduced here and discussed further in Chapter 7.

Step-by-Step Instruction on Carpet Squares. Step-by-step instruction on carpet squares uses a carpet remnant, either square or rectangular in shape, to provide orientation and limited structure on which to teach physical skills to students. This method is primarily designed for one-to-one instruction, but can also be used with small groups. (Carpet samples or remnants are often given by carpet stores free for the asking or can be purchased for a few dollars each.) The carpet squares serve to orient students and to help define the range and direction of their movement. The squares need to be affixed to the floor with loops of gymnasium tape (which does not pull up the finish or leave a residue on a gymnasium floor) to prevent them from moving around.

The student is first familiarized with the shape of the carpet remnant and then with the positional terms that will be used during lessons, such *as middle, on/off, edge, front,* and *side,* and with the terms that will be used to refer to his or her body parts and positions, such as *kicking/nonkicking foot, V arms and legs,* and *knees a little bent versus a lot bent.* Once the student is familiar enough with these terms and the positions they refer to that they respond to them automatically, the skills are taught in a sequence that starts with the simplest (such as the basic ready position), moves on to the next simplest (usually jumping jacks), and ultimately proceed through jumping, hopping, underhand throwing, overhand throwing, skipping, triple jumping, and any other skills deemed appropriate or necessary. Teachers can also move from completion of the ready position directly to long jump, underhand throw, or overhand throw. However, a few skills require prerequisites and are best taught in the proper sequence. For example, because a skip is a series of step-hops, hopping should be covered before skipping is introduced.

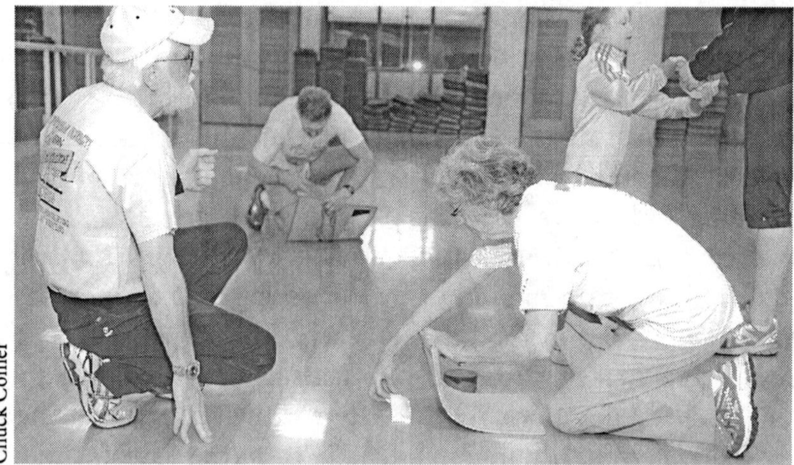
Chuck Comer

Taping down carpet squares before a step-by-step lesson to prevent slipping.

The teacher stands about 10 feet away on the floor, faces the student on the carpet square, and describes the next step to be learned on the way to the next skill in the hierarchy, for example, "Now I want you to stand in the middle of your carpet square and step off the front with your kicking foot. Okay, ready, step!" The teacher then gives feedback on the accuracy of the movement and makes corrections if necessary. The student is given time to practice replicating the movement until the instructor is satisfied that it is being performed at an acceptable level. Once the step being taught is mastered, the teacher introduces the next step, repeating the process of teaching, observing, and replicating until the overall skill is mastered. At the same time, the student is taught to memorize and say three to four words aloud that correspond to the major steps in the skill. This establishes a link between the movements and the words, so that the words, referred to here as *operative language,* can be used as memory tools later when the skill is being put into practice. A good deal of practice time is also allowed in order to implant the relationships between words and behaviors into memory. Sidebar 4.5 offers some guidelines for teaching with step-by-step instruction plans.

Two examples of activity lesson plans are presented in Appendix 4A to this chapter, including the narratives for teaching the ready position and jumping jacks, along with a description of how to set up the activity. Step-by-step plans for teaching the long jump, throws, and other skills are presented in the Chapter 7 on elementary physical education.

There is no recommended amount of time that a teacher should take to complete these plans with a given student. Ideally, the student should first be assessed to determine which skills might be appropriate for a given school unit of time, establish them as objectives on the IEP, and then progress through the lessons at the speed appropriate for that student, making adjustments to the IEP timelines as evaluation warrants.

The step-by-step procedure can also be used with groups. For example, after initial

SIDEBAR 4.5

Guidelines for Using Step-by-Step Instructional Plans

The following are some general guidelines to keep in mind when preparing to use step-by-step activity plans with students who are visually impaired or deaf-blind who are positioned on carpet squares:

- The plans are written to be offered over a long period of time. They could be used for an entire school year for some students, but may take several days or a few weeks for others.
- The plans are best used with one or two students at a time, because it is extremely important that the instructor observe the student's movements closely and give immediate feedback when the student needs assistance.
- The setting should be somewhat private during early lessons, since some students express embarrassment about having to learn such basic skills, particularly if the students are older, perhaps teenagers.
- Writing a step-by-step plan must be done by actually working through the behavior to be taught and jotting down each step in the procedure. In this case, having the carpet square underfoot and going through the physical steps are required in order to be thorough. It is virtually impossible to write a step-by-step plan simply by sitting at a desk and thinking through the process in a virtual way.
- If the student becomes bored with the detailed and repetitive nature of the lessons, the carpet squares can be "dressed up" as magic carpets, flying saucers, or any other favorite object to add the flavor of a game to the lessons. A great deal of reinforcement is also required. Some students respond to keeping track of personal records and trying to better them over time, so keeping a posted chart of milestones of jump or throw lengths can be a good motivator.
- Give many breaks during these lessons. A lot of tension can build up during early lessons when students are still on hands and knees. When the students show signs of fatigue or boredom, stop and let them relax. A good tension breaker is to stand up and "shake out" arms and hands, to give students a snack break, or to work in information about sports that might motivate young students. This might be a good time to discuss well-known sports figures who have visual impairments.
- If there are multiple students in a class, assign one volunteer per one or two students to assist with the movements. Remind volunteers not to interact with the students until the lead instructor gives the signal to avoid many people talking at once.

sports camp assessments, the first day of the 10-to-12-year-old junior camp begins with a two-hour group basic skills session based on the two plans in Appendix 4A. Teachers who hold group sessions can refer to this plan to determine how to arrange the carpet squares in a gymnasium to maximize safety and instruction. The group session is not ideal for all students, because some students cannot keep up with the pace required to complete the lesson in the allotted time period. However, the group lesson is advantageous in a setting such as a sports camp for other reasons. The teaching staff learns along with the students, and overall instruction becomes standardized as a result. Also, the group setting adds a degree of fun that is not inherent in one-to-one teaching.

The activity plan is designed to give teachers a logical step-by-step script to follow while teaching basic skills. Once teachers become familiar with it, the statements can be modified to fit an individual's style or to make the lessons more entertaining. In addition, once familiar with the concept of the step-by-step approach, teachers can add skills, write narrative plans to be used during instruction, and modify the narrative to fit the characteristics of an individual student.

INSTRUCTIONAL MODIFICATIONS FOR STUDENTS WHO ARE DEAFBLIND

All of the methods described thus far for surmounting the barriers to communication from teacher to student and the instructional methods apply equally to students with both visual and hearing impairments. However, students who are deafblind face the additional difficulty of lacking easy verbal communication from teacher to student. Therefore, teachers of students with these dual sensory losses need to be aware of alternative communication methods and systems that their students might use. In addition, Sidebar 4.6 provides general suggestions for interacting with students who are deafblind. The tips offered earlier in the chapter on working with students who are visually impaired also apply to those who are deafblind.

People who have hearing losses experience a range in the severity of their impairments, just as people with visual impairments do; that is, some people have mild losses, while others

SIDEBAR 4.6

Suggestions for Working with Students Who Are Deafblind

The following are some general suggestions on how to interact with students who are deafblind:

- Take the time to find out what methods of communication will be most comfortable and efficient for both you and the student. If you have difficulty establishing communication, ask for suggestions from other professionals who work closely with the student or the student's family members.
- Identify yourself each time you initiate interaction. It is easier to identify yourself if you have a signal or a designated name-sign that the student who is deafblind will recognize.
- Communicate directly with the student who is deafblind; do not direct your comments through another person.
- Before touching or moving students, be sure to communicate with them so they know you are approaching.
- Contact students who are deafblind on the hand, arm, or shoulder to avoid startling them. Or bring your hand up beneath the student's hand, so the back of your hand touches the student's palm. Use a light touch. Leave your hand in contact with the student until he or she responds to you, to make it easier for the student to know where you are.
- Do not grab the student's wrist. Being grabbed or held is confining for a person who uses his or her hands to communicate.
- If you need to touch students who are deafblind somewhere besides the hand, arm, or shoulder (for example, to point to something on their clothes or face), or to touch something they are holding, let them know what you are doing. One way to do this is to put your hand under theirs and then bring your hand toward them with their hand on yours.

SIDEBAR 4.6 *(continued)*

- Be honest when you do not understand. Also, give the student opportunities to let you know when he or she is not sure what you meant, but do not ask repeatedly, "Do you understand?"
- Avoid placing the hand of the student who is deafblind on objects. Pushing the student's hand onto an object is awkward and can be painful if the object is sharp or rough. Instead, tell the student you are putting your hand on the object while the student's hand is on yours. Then the student can find the object by sliding his or her hand off yours as you remove your hand.
- When students with restricted visual fields are watching you, do not move quickly to the side. If students with visual impairments are trying to follow you or look at your signs and you move too quickly to the side, they may lose you. If they cannot find you, you can let them know where you are by touching one of their arms or hands.
- Do not misconstrue the normal speaking voice of a student who is deafblind as a display of strong emotion. Some people conclude from the unusual voice inflections or the emphatic signs and facial expressions with which many people who are deaf and deafblind communicate that they are agitated or perturbed. It is important to realize that the voice may be the student's normal speaking voice, and that eloquence in sign language usually involves dynamic, intense expressions.

Source: D. Sauerburger, *Independence without Sight or Sound* (New York: American Foundation for the Blind, 1993), pp. 4–5; J. Erin, *When You Have a Visually Impaired Student with Multiple Disabilities in Your Classroom: A Guide for Teachers* (New York: AFB Press, 2004); and K. M. Huebner, J. G. Prickett, T. R. Welch, and E. Joffee (Eds.), *Hand in Hand: Essentials of Communication and Orientation and Mobility for Your Students Who Are Deaf-Blind* (New York: AFB Press, 1995).

are totally deaf. Likewise, there are various combinations of vision and hearing among people who are considered to be deafblind, as described in Chapter 2. However, while some people who are deafblind are able to use augmented verbal communications, the instructional modifications described here are primarily aimed at students whose hearing losses are severe enough to require manual communication systems. Some students who are deafblind are able to respond to teachers verbally (that is, with expressive language), so the barriers to communication may relate only to information from the teacher to the student. In that event, the student can explain what he or she already knows about the activity, but may need the aid of an interpreter or intervener to receive explanations—that is, to overcome a barrier to receptive language.

Communicating with Students with Deafblindness

Before starting to work with a student who is deafblind, it is important to find out the student's preferred method or methods of communicating. The physical education teacher can consult with other members of the student's educational team, such as the teacher of visually impaired students, a sign language interpreter, or an intervener. (The roles of these professionals are discussed later in this chapter.)

People who are deaf commonly use American Sign Language (ASL) as their primary

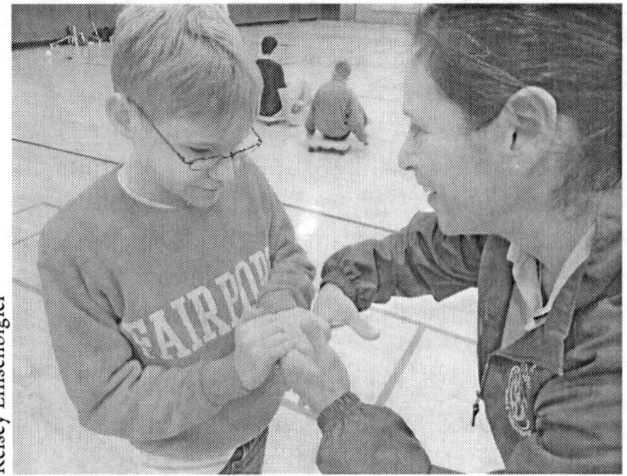

Kelsey Linsenbigler

This student with deafblindness is reading the instructor's signs tactilely. She is signing "Again."

form of communication. American Sign Language is the dominant language of people in the deaf community. It is a separate and distinct language consisting of manual signs and spoken and spelled-out language, as well as gestures, facial expressions, and body movements. ASL has its own grammar, syntax, and lexicon and does not correspond to spoken English (Huebner, Prickett, Welch, & Joffee, 1995; Lolli, Sauerburger, & Bourquin, 2010; Sauerburger, 1993). Someone who has been deaf from birth and who has used ASL for communication is likely to continue using it despite having reduced vision. If an individual does not have sufficient vision to read signs, the learner may rely on reading ASL manually by placing his or her hands over the signer's hands.

Because English is essentially a second language for people who use ASL, a teacher is likely to need the services of an interpreter to communicate fully with students who use it, as discussed in the next section.

If the student can utilize ASL visually, the teacher should use the techniques to increase visibility described in Chapter 2 to augment communication. For example, a teacher can ask the student whether it is easier to communicate in front of a window where lighting tends to be better or whether the use of contrasting clothing might help the student to see classmates better. One student advised her instructor that it was easier to see an interpreter's hands when the interpreter wore a red shirt. Students should be taught using whatever communication method is easiest for them to learn from (Best, Lieberman, & Arndt, 2002).

People who are deafblind often communicate in more than one fashion, and there are other methods that may allow a teacher to communicate directly with a student (Huebner, Prickett, Welch, & Joffee, 1995). Fingerspelling with the American Manual Alphabet (see Figure 4.1), supplemented with some common signs for phrases such as *yes, no, good work,* and *try again*, is the predominant form of manual communication used by someone who is deafblind to communicate with others who do not know ASL, assuming that the individual with deafblindness has the ability to spell fluently. Learning to fingerspell the 26 letters of the alphabet allows student and teacher to communicate back and forth without reliance on an interpreter if necessary.

The American Manual Alphabet has the advantage that most people who have been deaf for any amount of time are familiar with it. Also, from the teacher's standpoint, it is relatively easy to learn. When used to communicate, the letters of the American Manual Alphabet are normally presented to the "reader" near the presenter's mouth, so the word being spelled by the fingers and the word being spoken can be seen simultaneously. However, this

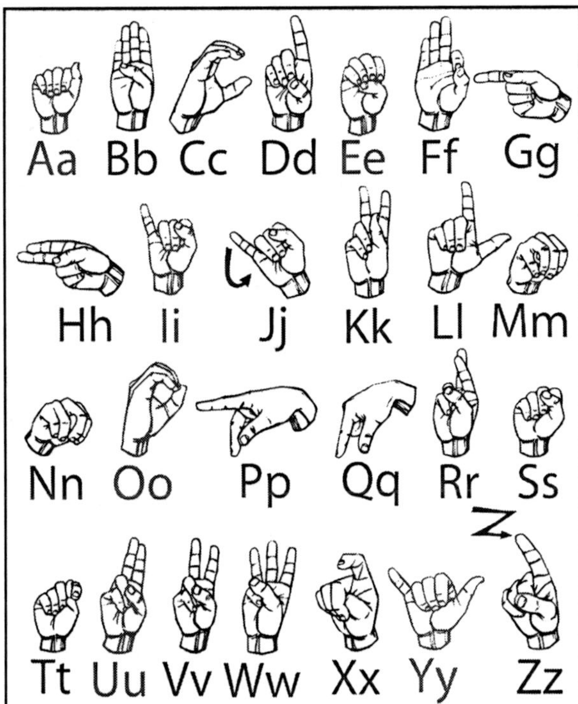

FIGURE 4.1 American Manual Alphabet (fingerspelling) signs
Source: Wikipedia under Creative Commons Attribution

technique is advantageous only if the reader has enough residual vision to see the shape of the mouth and of the fingers doing the spelling. If the person who is deafblind does not have sufficient vision to see the mouth and hand simultaneously, the manual alphabet letters need to be presented in his or her hand, so they can be read haptically. The person who is signing places his or her hands under the hand of the person who is receiving the signs. The important features of each letter must contact the reader's hand in order to make it distinguishable from similar letters.

Palm writing, also known as *print on palm,* is another method that can be used by teachers to get the material of their lessons across to their students who are deafblind. Using palm writing, the teacher draws a block letter into the palm of the student's hand in a specific way. Some tips about using print on palm include the following:

- Print only in palm area.
- Do not try to connect letters.
- Complete a letter, pause, then complete the next on the same palm area.
- Pause longer at the end of a word.

Teachers and their students who are deafblind might also communicate using one or two computers with *refreshable braille output.* Such a device has an electronic tactile display that uses pins to represent the dots in a braille cell, spelling out the text being displayed on the computer or other device. The pins can move up and down, allowing the display to change as the text is read. Using a personal data assistant (such as the BrailleNote) or a laptop or desktop computer with a refreshable braille output device, the teacher can input text on a standard QWERTY keyboard or 6-key braille keyboard, and the student who is deafblind can read the instructions from the braille output device. This method allows instructions to be more explicit, because they can generally be read more quickly than can fingerspelling or palm writing. However, using computers in a physical activity setting could be somewhat awkward. Tactile communication boards containing tactile symbols representing activities or skills may be used with students who are deafblind who do not sign or use print on palm. A communication board can be a board, a collection of pages, or even an electronic device. The student or teacher points to the symbol on the board to convey a message, and students can use the symbols expressively or receptively.

Using Interpreters and Interveners

Under the provisions of IDEA, certified *professional interpreters* are required to be provided for students who are hard of hearing or deaf who rely on sign language to communicate effectively, and the student's IEP team should have included these professionals as part of the student's IEP. The role of an interpreter is to transmit the communications between people who are deaf or hard of hearing and hearing individuals (http://rid.org/interpreting/practice/index.cfm). Interpreting for a person who is deafblind differs from interpreting for a person who is hard of hearing without a visual impairment, however; flexibility is required to enable an interpreter to facilitate communication, including giving visual information and in some instances providing sighted guide (Morgan, 2001).

The use of an interpreter can help overcome the communication gap by interpreting the teacher's explanations and requests to the student and by providing feedback or questions to the teacher from the student if the student does not have sufficient expressive language. Interpreters in physical education classes can increase their effectiveness by learning sports-specific signs before attempting the work, and likewise, it may be beneficial for the physical activity instructor to learn some basic signs related to the activity.

Students with deafblindness are often served by *interveners* (also sometimes spelled *intervenor*) in integrated school settings. Interveners also aid in the communication and learning process. An intervener's role is to intercede between the student and the environment, thereby allowing access to information that is usually obtained through hearing and sight (Alsop, Blaha, & Kloos, 2000). The intervener explains the environment to the student, facilitating learning and the development of skills (Morgan, 2001). (Professionals known as *support service providers* provide a similar service for adults with deafblindness.) While an interpreter is limited to conveying the communications of others, the intervener's role includes more responsibility for aiding a student's grasp of environmental information. For example, during a basketball unit, an interpreter would relay the teacher's spoken commands and relay any questions or concerns of the student to the teacher. An intervener would not only relay the information from the teacher or from the student, but might also tell the student who has the ball, guide the student to the front of the line, and tell the student when it is his or her turn to dribble or shoot.

Communication with students who are deafblind involves a number of considerations. A student may have enough vision to see the interpreter, and thus may be able to use the interpreter the same way a student who is deaf would. However, if the student who is deafblind possesses a limited field of vision, it would be necessary for the interpreter to sign within that limited field. The student's visual field might be so limited that the interpreter may need to stand 8 to 10 feet away for the entire sign to be perceived. Conversely, the student may need all signs to be 1 to 2 feet away. If the student is completely without vision, signs must be communicated by touch in the student's hand. Sometimes the use of a remote alert device that is activated by the teacher, such as a vibrating attachment that is worn on the waistband, can alert the student to turn and look toward the person trying to get his or her attention to communicate via sign or voice (see the Resources section). Sidebar 4.7

SIDEBAR 4.7

Steps to Clear Communication during Physical Activity for Students Who Are Deafblind

Communication is key to including students who are deafblind in a physical education class. The following suggestions will help ensure that communication is clear and the students with deafblindness receive the information they need to participate in the physical activity:

General Suggestions

- When introducing a new activity, try to introduce the activity as a whole before breaking it down into parts, so that it makes sense to the student.
- Take the time to make sure the student and the intervener completely understand the activity and environment before starting, if possible (Morgan, n.d.).
- Use real objects as tactile representations of an activity whenever possible, such as a volleyball for the sport of volleyball or a towel for swimming (Chen, Downing, & Rodriguez-Gil, 2001). Do not use miniature versions of an object, such as a toy roller skate; they seldom feel like the real thing.

Take Time to Get Familiar with the Environment

- Plan how to familiarize both student and intervener with the environment, equipment, and activity (Miles & Riggio, 1999).
- Use tactile maps of the field or court.
- Provide handheld manipulative models of equipment.
- Provide time for exploration for the student; time for exploration is not wasted time (McInnes, 1999).
- Students who are deafblind will typically take longer than other students to understand their environment and the activity. Make sure to factor in this extra time.
- Make sure equipment is in a stationary, safe position.
- Discuss previous experiences with the students who are deafblind and staff who are familiar with them.
- Always ask the students who are deafblind what would support their participation (Morgan, n.d.; Smith, 2002).
- Identify shared goals for the activity with the students.
- Use the expertise available, such as that of the intervener, paraeducator, parents, interpreter, or teachers.

Communication Modes

- Determine the best mode of communication for the student: speaking, visual signs, tactile signing, gestures, or some combination (Bourquin & Sauerburer, 2005).
- The more methods taught to the student, the more choices there are and the easier communication tends to be (Bourquin & Sauerburer, 2005).

Ensure Opportunities for Receptive and Expressive Communication

- Physical activity involves motion and use of the hands and body that can prevent tactile communication. Build in intentional breaks to ensure time for instruction, motivation, and feedback.
- Design and use communication according to the needs of the student. For example, if a student has tunnel vision, the instructor or a classmate may need to sign from 6–8 feet away or more. This distance must be built into the lesson in order to ensure clear directions and feedback.
- Practice the activity with the student's preferred modes of expressive and receptive communication to ensure the student's comfort and your own effectiveness.
- Make sure the student knows the purpose of the activity.

(Continued on next page)

SIDEBAR 4.7 *(continued)*

- Link movement to language, explaining what is happening to ensure the student knows what he or she is doing and why.
- Emphasize the name of, sign for, and description of the skill being taught, such as playing guard in basketball, goalie in soccer, or pitcher in baseball.
- Give students who are deafblind the same information that their classmates receive. Do not leave out information because you think the students who are deafblind do not need to know it (Smith, 2002).

Addressing Terminology That Has No Official Sign

- Preconference: Meet with the team ahead of time to discuss the activity, sport, or skill that has no common sign, for example, showdown, rapelling, or unicycle.
- Review vocabulary related to the activity.
- Create the sign using the student's mode of communication (Chen, Downing, & Rodriguez-Gil, 2001).
- Use videos if possible to share words and methods.
- Come to an agreement with the team on the sign to use.
- Practice the sign during the activity.
- Share the new sign with other key participants.

Make Continuous Activities Discrete

- In general, students who are deafblind better understand activities with a clear beginning and end (Chen, Downing, & Rodriguez-Gil, 2001).
- Discrete activities (such as bowling, shot put, and kicking a ball) allow time for feedback.
- Continuous activities such as running, swimming, and canoeing do not allow specified time for feedback (Arndt, Lieberman, & Pucci, 2004), so make clear breaks in continuous activities to allow time for communication.

Attend to Positioning of All Parties

- Consider where the intervener can be located during the activity to be most easily available for communication with the student.
- Consider what is both comfortable and possible for the intervener.
- Consider how to make both expressive and receptive communication possible for the student.
- Identify the activity as discrete or continuous.
- Preplan what to do about movement or activities that preclude easy communication.
- Review with the student when communication will take place.
- Agree when communication will occur next before beginning an activity.
- Allow flexibility of arrangements in case of an emergency.

Summary

- Be comfortable asking for help from other team members.
- Focus on communication and familiarity with the student's preferences.
- Know the limits of your physical and emotional skills.
- Some activities are easier to set up than others; take the time needed to introduce new physical activity.

Source: Adapted from L. J. Lieberman, "Communication with Individuals Who Are Deafblind during Physical Activity: Eight Steps" (2010), paper presented at the Association for Education and Rehabilitation of the Blind and Visually Impaired International Conference, Little Rock, Arkansas, retrieved 3/12/12 from http://www.aerbvi.org/2010conference/documents/LiebermanAERCommunication.ppt.

provides some additional suggestions for ensuring clear communication during physical activity.

The Educational Team for the Student Who Is Deafblind

In many learning situations, a student with deafblindness will likely have a team of people who can ensure that he or she is receiving enough information about the environment. For example, in physical activity instruction, the team might consist of the physical education teacher, the adapted physical educator, the teacher of children with visual impairments, and an interpreter, a paraeducator, and perhaps an intervener. The student who is deafblind also has responsibility as a team member as do his or her classmates. Sidebar 4.8 lists suggested responsibilities of the team members.

It is important that the physical education teacher coordinate the team in order for the student to receive the best services. Before each unit, the teacher can consult with the adapted physical educator, the teacher of students who are visually impaired, and the deafblind specialist (if there is one). These specialists can offer ideas for communication and modification of activities. Meeting with the interpreter, intervener, or paraeducator before

SIDEBAR 4.8

Responsibilities of Team Members Working with Students with Deafblindness

The following list summarizes the responsibilities of the various members of the educational team when they are working with students with deafblindness in a physical education setting:

Physical Education or Adapted Physical Education Specialist

- Provide the interpreter, paraeducator, and/or intervener with plans for each unit in advance, when possible, including a list of specialized vocabulary so that the interpreter and student who is deafblind can review them and prepare for the new unit before it begins.
- Meet with the interpreter, paraeducator, and/or intervener before the beginning of each unit, when possible, to clarify sport terminology, instructional cues, and idioms that are likely to be used.
- Teach some sport-specific signs to the entire class at the beginning of each new unit.
- Address the student who is deafblind directly.
- Review the location of equipment at the beginning of each class.
- Link movement to language so that students know what they are doing and why. For example, if a student is batting a ball for baseball, explain that he or she is batting a ball so the team in the outfield has to run to get the ball so the student has time to run to the bases. Then another batter has a turn to hit the ball so the student has time to continue running around the bases. Make sure that the concepts of baseball are taught fully before any lesson is started with a whole class.
- Always wear a specific, unique item that can be recognized haptically, such as a watch, a ring, or a whistle, so that the student who is deafblind can easily identify you.
- Check that the student who is deafblind has understood your communications by asking him or her to repeat the instructions, demonstrate the skill or activity, or explain it to another student and repeat instructions as often as necessary.

(Continued on next page)

SIDEBAR 4.8 *(continued)*

- Allow the interpreter, paraeducator, or intervener to stay with the student during games and activities in order to continuously explain what is happening in the surroundings.
- Ensure that "incidental learning" (information that occurs naturally in the environment but may not be communicated verbally, such as thumbs up, a nod from the teacher, or a reprimand for bad behavior) is explained to the student.

Interpreter

- Adapt language to the student's preferred communication style and functional vision.
- Hold information until appropriate stopping points (that is, do not interrupt a game during play).
- Dress appropriately by wearing sneakers and comfortable clothing.
- Occupy positions that facilitate effective visual and communication needs. For example, if an intervener is assisting with a gymnastics lesson, and the student is doing forward rolls on a wedge mat, the interpreter must be in a position to know what the teacher expects and still communicate with the student.
- Be familiar with the rules of the sports being taught, and learn sport signs, before interpreting in physical education.

Intervener's Responsibilities

- Provide the student with environmental information such as what other activity is occurring during lessons.
- Aid the student in communicating with others.
- Developing alternative learning strategies so the student can generalize newly learned skills. For example, a class is learning swimming skills, and the student who is deafblind uses tactile communication.
- Serve as a learning tutor to help reinforce what the teacher is teaching.
- Act as a bridge between the teacher, the external environment, and the student so the student can receive sufficient information about the activity.

Teacher of Students with Visual Impairments and Deafblind Specialist

- Ensure appropriate lighting for the student who is deafblind.
- Teach the physical education teacher, interpreter, paraeducator, or intervener the best positioning for the student in each skill or activity. This will likely differ for each unit. This may need to be done before each unit outside of class so valuable class time is not taken up doing this.
- Make sure that the student has the equipment, products, and modifications necessary for success.
- Conduct in-service training or workshops for the educational team if necessary.

Student Who Is Deafblind

- Participate in class by getting materials and doing the activities just as the other students do.
- Convey communication preferences to the interpreter and what needs to be changed.
- Interact with other students, rather than only with the interpreter.
- Tell the interpreter where to stand so the student can see demonstrations and access communication.
- Seek clarification of skills or points not understood.

Hearing Classmates

- Face the student who is deafblind when talking to him or her.
- Make efforts to learn the manual alphabet or some ASL signs.

Teachers may extend the hearing students' role by allowing them to

- repeat directions and demonstrations
- function as a peer tutor

class to discuss teaching and communication is also recommended. If peer tutors are being used, it is also recommended that the physical educator meet with them before each unit to go over responsibilities and teaching and feedback strategies. During class the teacher needs to monitor the communication, teaching, feedback, and learning process. Any modifications that need to occur can be relayed to the key personnel during class or before the next class. Periodical team meetings to discuss performance are recommended as well.

CONCLUSION

Communication is a fundamental component of all instruction. It needs to be a primary consideration of physical educators when they are working with students with visual impairments or deafblindness in order to remove barriers to learning. Communication with students who are both deaf and blind is an even more central issue because students' ability to understand the teacher and to make themselves understood both must be addressed.

The specific modifications to instructional communication suggested in this chapter—including how to describe equipment and the environment, help students move from place to place, and teach physical skills, as well as methods of communicating with students who cannot hear spoken language—lay the groundwork for teaching students in physical education classes and including people of all ages in physical activities. The next chapter focuses on methods of adapting the physical activities themselves for individuals with visual impairments or deafblindness.

APPENDIX 4A

Sample Instruction Plans for Basic Skills: Ready Position and Jumping Jacks

Activity Site: Gymnasium or other room which has enough open space for throwing and long jumping

Materials: carpet squares, gymnasium floor tape

SETTING UP THE AREA

1. Select a wall in the room that beanbags or balls can be thrown against.
2. If teaching multiple students, place carpet squares facing the wall in a grid at least 10 feet apart and with carpet squares staggered if two rows are required, to keep students from colliding or hitting one another with thrown beanbags or balls. If there is only one student, place the carpet square about 10 feet from the wall.
3. Affix the carpet square to the floor using loops of gymnasium floor tape placed underneath. Test to make sure that the carpet square does not slip on the floor before starting.
4. Assign one student per carpet square.

ORIENTATION TO CARPET SQUARE AND TERMINOLOGY

Teacher's note: The purpose of this section is to establish a common language or terminology between teacher and learner. Position students on hands and knees immediately behind their carpet squares with palms down on the carpet squares. **(Photo A)** Stand at the front of the squares facing students with a carpet square of your own for demonstration.

1. Are you on your hands and knees with your palms on your carpet squares?
2. What is the shape of your carpet square?
3. Please show me the top of your carpet square by slapping it with both hands. [Teacher demonstrates the sound on his or her own carpet square.]

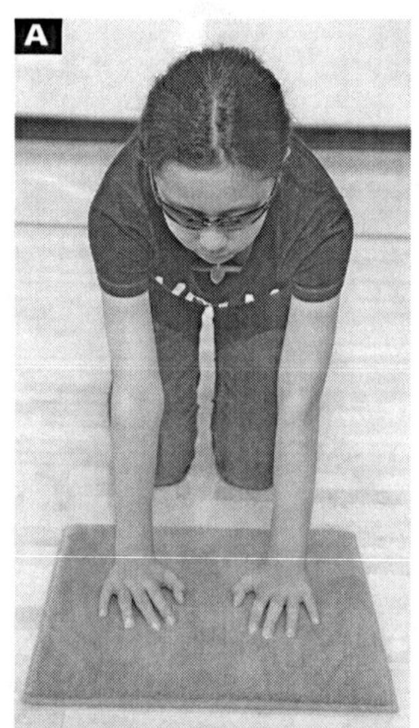

Photos by Chuck Comer

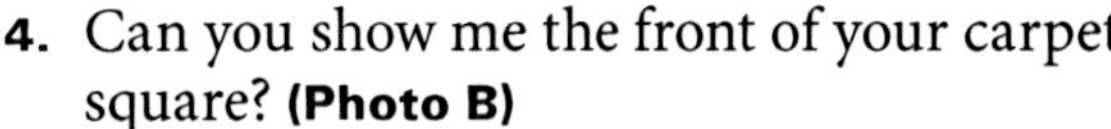

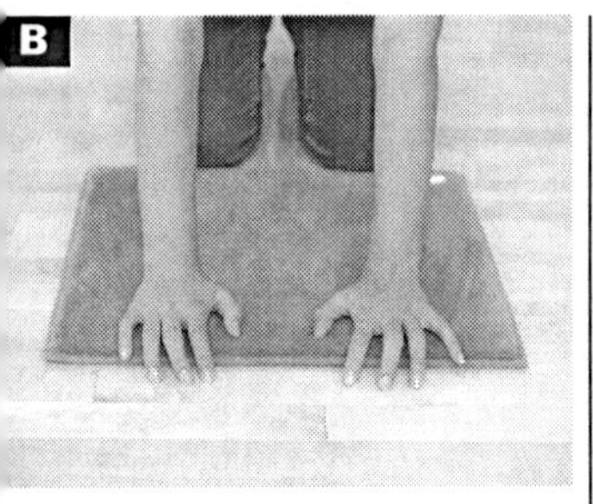

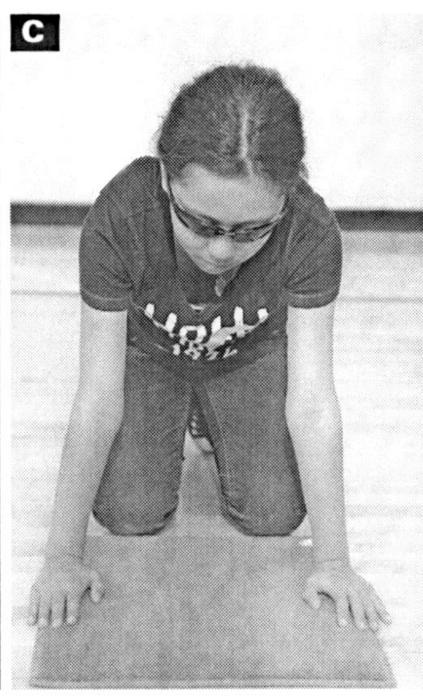

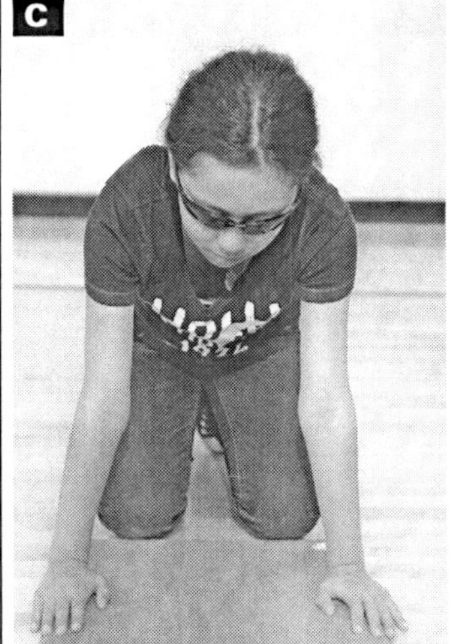

4. Can you show me the front of your carpet square? **(Photo B)**
5. Now let's see you touch both sides at once. **(Photo C)** [If a student does not understand, ask, How many hands does it take to touch both sides?]
6. Can you show me the back?
7. How about showing me the edges of your carpet square?
8. Where is the front edge?
9. Where is the back edge?
10. Where is the side edge?
11. Show me the middle of your carpet square.
12. Super! Where is the bottom?

Teacher's note: When these steps are learned, repeat the commands and questions in rapid succession until the concepts are well enough established that they will not have to be repeated in the next lesson.

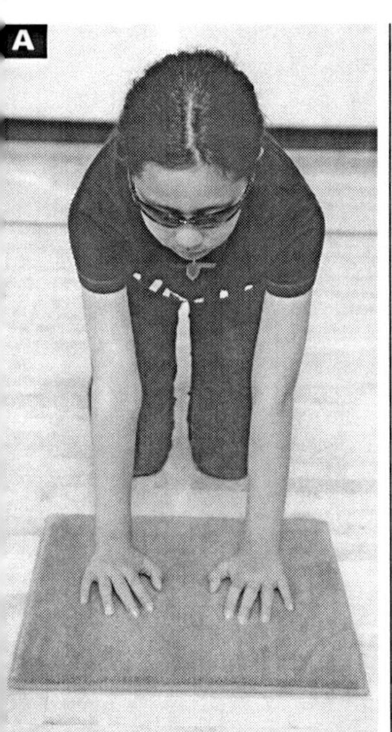

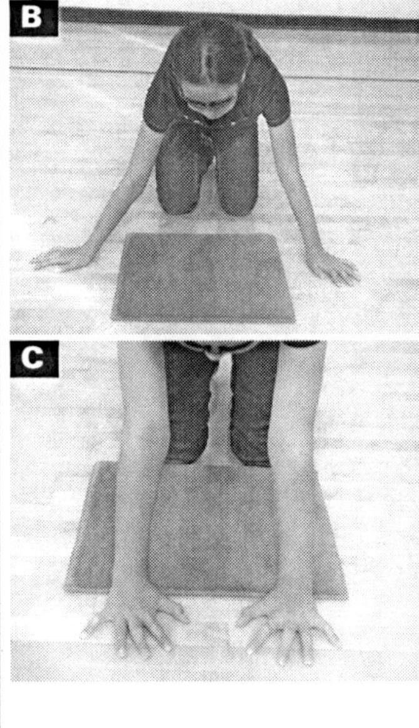

ORIENTATION TO POSITIONS AROUND THE CARPET SQUARE

Teacher's note: An exercise based on commands from the previous lesson can be used as a warm-up for this new lesson.

1. Are you ready? Show me how to put the palms of both of your hands on top of the carpet square. **(Photo A)**
2. Can you use both hands to slap the floor somewhere off the carpet square? **(Photo B)**
3. Use both hands to slap the floor off the front of the carpet square. **(Photo C)**
4. Show me where off the back of the square is by slapping there. **(Photo D)**
5. Put both hands on the middle of your carpet square.
6. Now we'll try something tricky. Can you touch the floor off of both sides of your carpet square at once? **(Photo E)** Great!

7. Let's do middle again. Go!
8. Off both sides again.
9. Here we go: Middle, off, middle, off, middle, off, middle.
10. Hold up the hand you throw with, like you want the teacher to call on you. **(Photo F)**
11. Put your hand down and hold up the hand you *don't* throw with, the one we'll call your nonthrowing hand. **(Photo G)**
12. Now put both hands back on the middle of your carpet square.
13. Now slap the floor in front of your carpet square with your throwing hand. **(Photo H)**
14. Back on the middle.
15. Now, slap the floor off the front with your nonthrowing hand. **(Photo I)**
16. Back on the middle.
17. Off the front with your throwing hand.

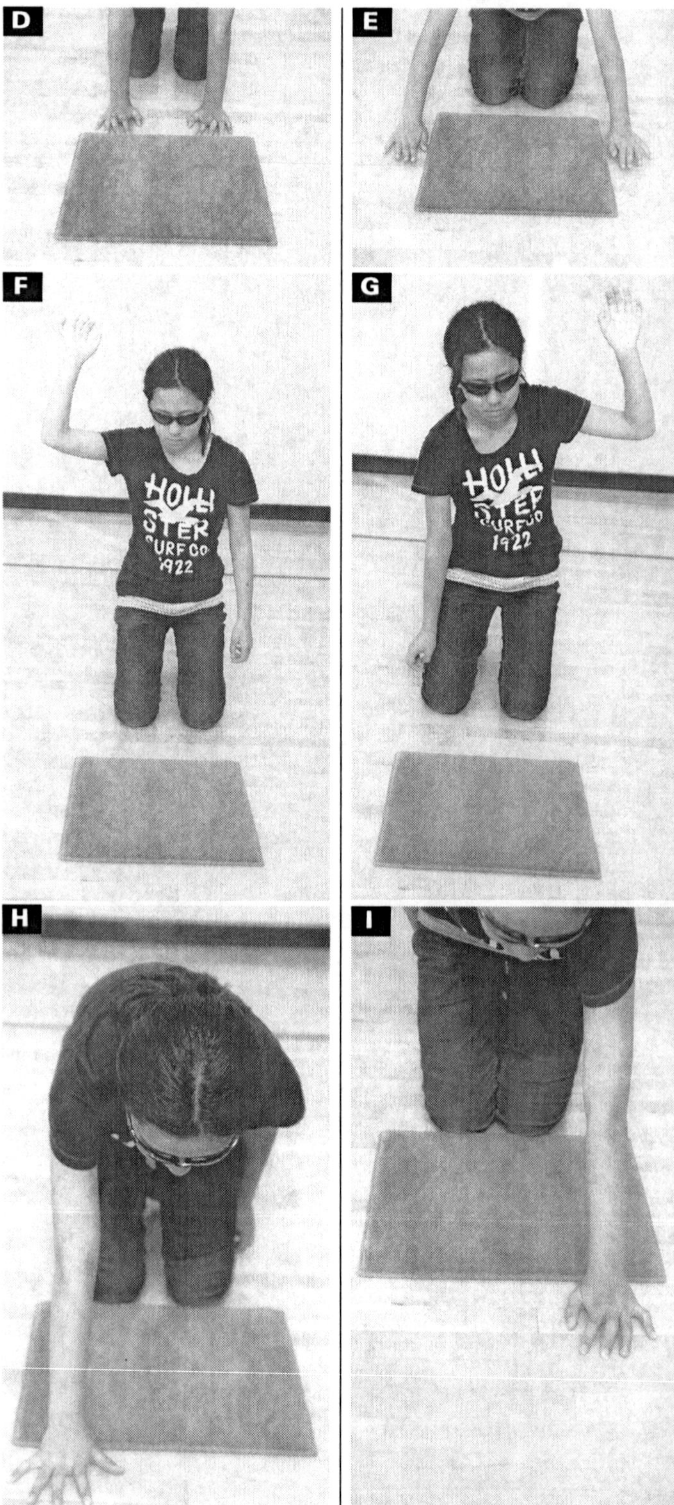

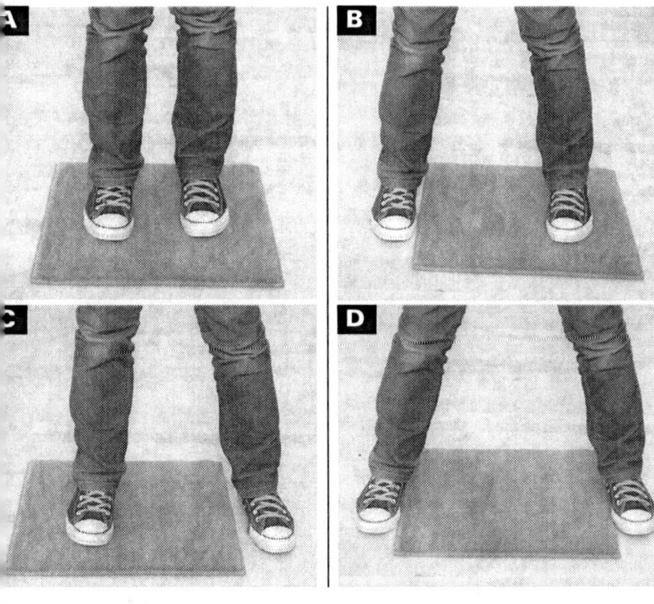

STEP-BY-STEP INSTRUCTION PLAN FOR TEACHING THE READY POSITION

1. Stand with both feet on your carpet square. **(Photo A)**
2. Are you in the middle of your carpet square? If not, get in the middle.
3. Put your kicking foot on the edge next to it. **(Photo B)**
4. Now move it back to the middle.
5. Put your nonkicking foot on the edge next to it. **(Photo C)**
6. Move your foot back in the middle.
7. Think about this: How can you put both feet on the side edges at once? That's right, now do it, both feet on edges! **(Photo D)**
8. Now put them back to the middle both at once.
9. Edges, middle, edges, middle, edges, middle.
10. Put both feet on the edges again and stay there.
11. What upside-down letter does the shape of your legs make? Right, a V!
12. Be sure to keep your legs in the shape of a V.
13. Now while standing in the V position, slap the front of both your legs with your palms at once.

14. Show me how you can clap your hands between your knees. **(Photo E)**
15. Slap the top edges of your knees. **(Photo F)**
16. How about slapping the fronts of your knees now? Good.
17. Drop your bottom toward the floor, bend your knees, and reach between your knees until you touch the front edge of your carpet square with your fingertips. **(Photo G)**
18. Are your knees bent or straight? A lot bent or a little bent? Right, a lot bent.
19. Make your knees straight again. **(Photo H)**
20. Are you still making a V? You should be.
21. Reach down and touch the front edge like you did a minute ago, but hold your position for a second when you touch the edge.
22. Begin to straighten up, but when you do, slide your palms up the fronts of your legs and rest your palms on your knees and hold there a second.
23. Are your knees bent or straight?
24. Are your knees bent a little or a lot compared to when you were bent clear down? Right, a little.
25. Stand up straight again and relax a second by shaking out your hands and arms.
26. Now, still in the leg V, drop your bottom, bend your knees, and touch the front edge of your carpet square.
27. Begin to straighten by sliding your palms up the fronts of your legs again, but stop and rest your body weight on your hands as you place them on the tops of your knees. Grab the tops of your knees with thumbs in and fingers out [see hands in Photo K].
28. Lock your elbows straight and relax, placing your body weight on your knees.
29. Stand up, relax, shake out your arms and legs, and take a quick break.

E

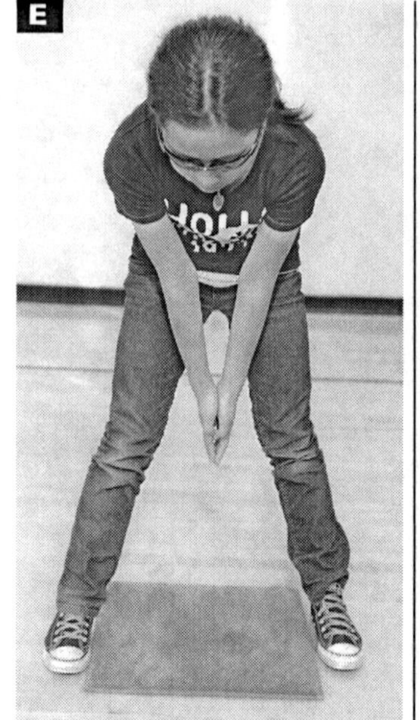

F

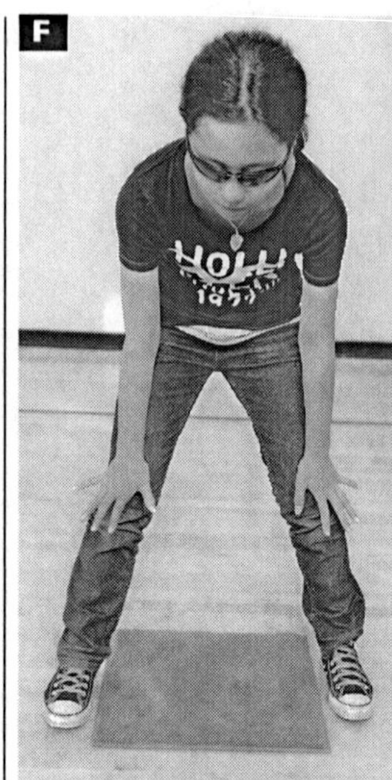

G

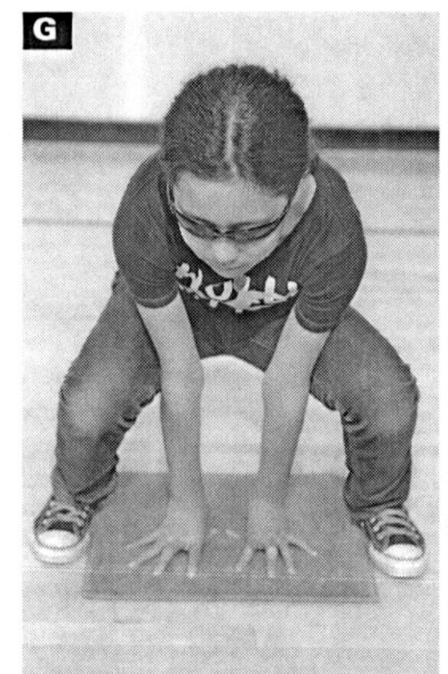

H

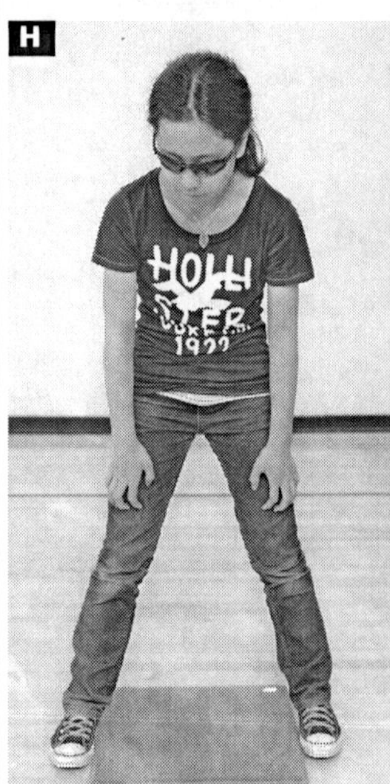

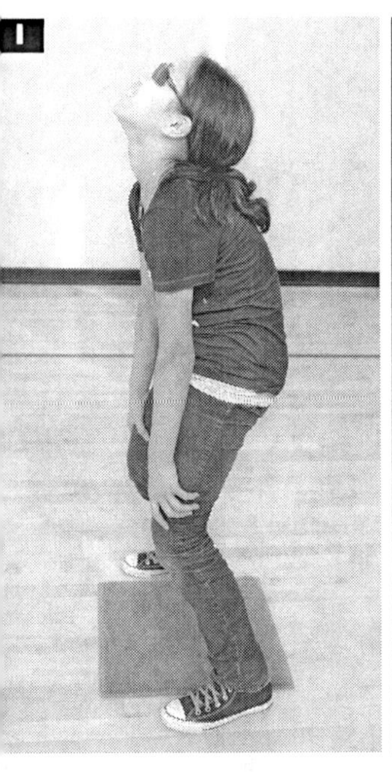

I

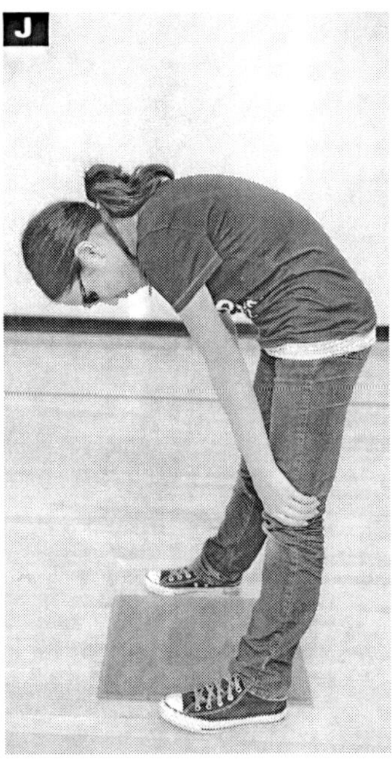

J

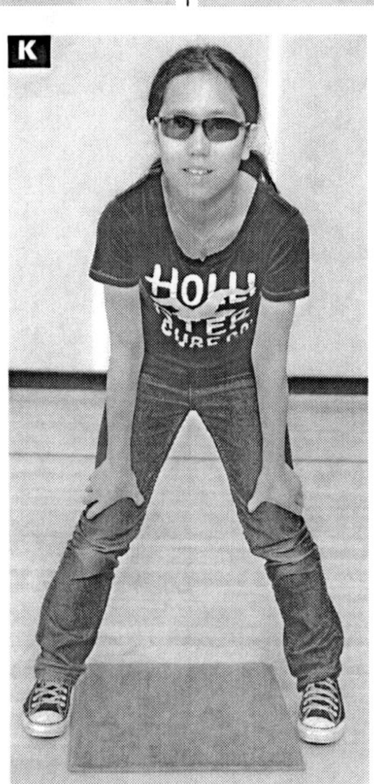

K

30. All right! Here we go again. Make a V, touch the front edge, slide up to your knees, and hold that position.
31. Without letting go of your knees, raise your face up toward the ceiling as far as you can. **(Photo I)**
32. Be careful to hold tight to your knees. Keep your weight on your straight arms and hands.
33. What happens to your bottom and your knees when you look more and more toward the ceiling? Yes, your bottom wants to drop and your knees want to bend.
34. Look more and more down to the floor while holding onto your knees. Yes, your bottom comes up and your knees try to straighten. **(Photo J)**
35. Let your neck relax, but look straight ahead at me, not up or down. This is what you want: look straight ahead, have a medium knee bend, and keep your bottom down and back. **(Photo K)**
36. Congratulations! You are in the ready position.
37. Let's practice getting into the ready position.
38. Step off the back of your carpet square.
39. Get back onto it.
40. We are going to use four words to remind us of how to get in the ready position quickly and accurately: V, touch, knees, face.
41. "V" means make a V with your legs by standing on the edges of the carpet square
42. "Touch" means touch the front of your carpet square between your feet.
43. "Knees" means slide your palms up and then rest your weight on your hands and knees.
44. "Face" means look at me, not up or down.

45. Let's practice until you can do it really fast. Here we go: V, touch, knees, face! **(Photos L, M, N, O)**

Repeat until the student can consistently use the operative language to complete the entire skill independently.

Operative language: *V, touch, knees, face*

Teacher's note: After the skill has been learned, the operative language should always be used when attempting to correct a student's mistakes in the stance. For example, if the feet are too close together, the correction should be "Check your V leg position. Is it wide enough?" If the knees are too straight or too bent, the correction should be, "Check your face position; you have your face too far up [or down]." Students learn the four skills separately and as an entire skill, not in terms of how far apart the feet need to be or how bent the knees should be, so corrections should always be made in terms of the four operative words that they have learned during the lessons.

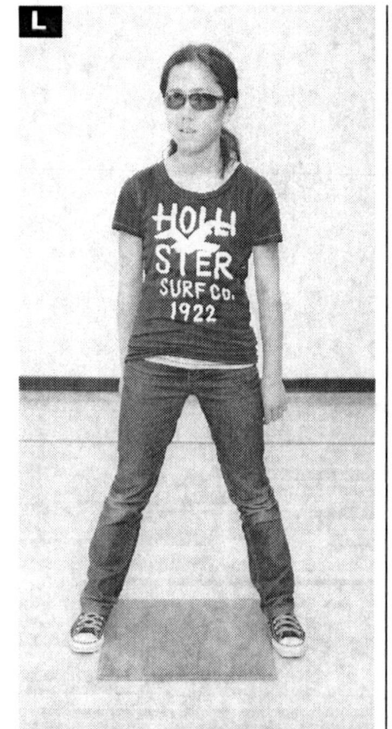

L

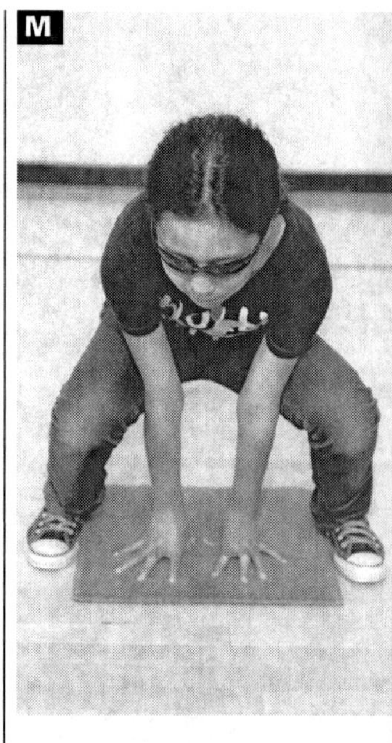
M

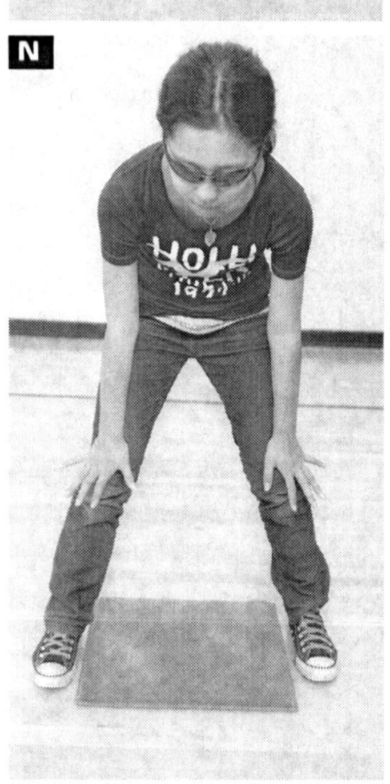
N

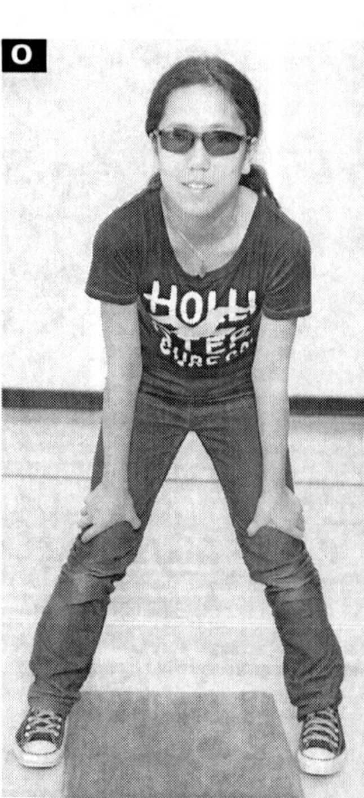

O

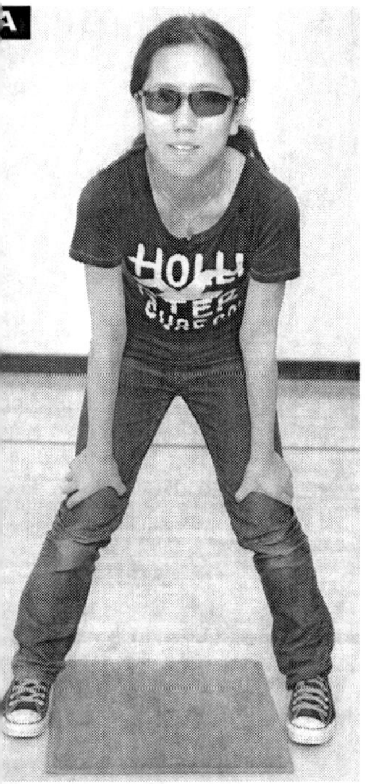

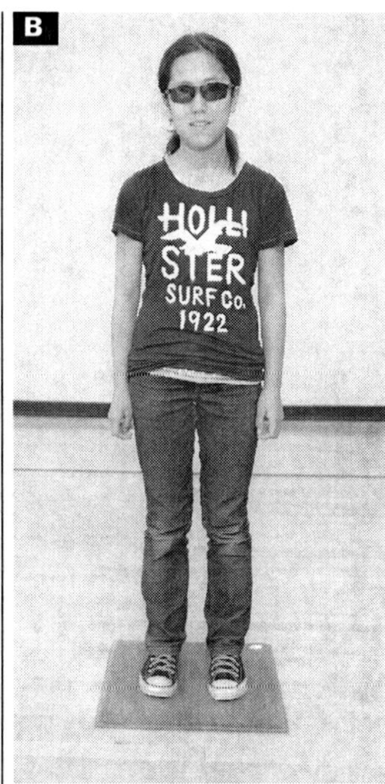

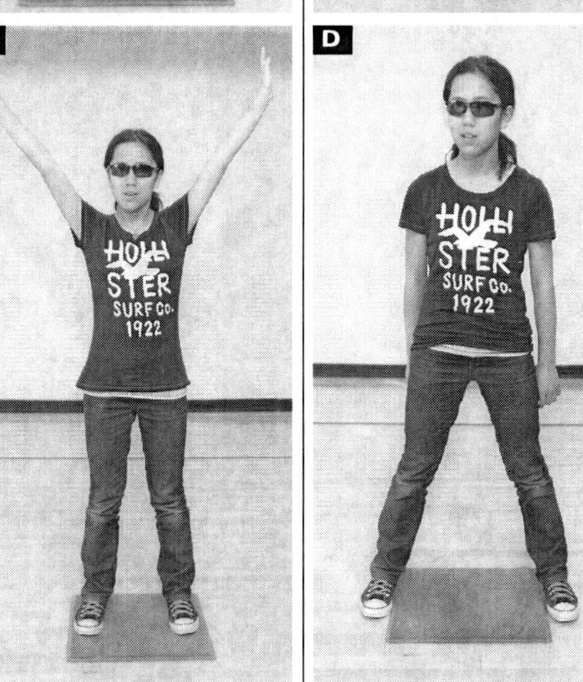

STEP-BY-STEP INSTRUCTION PLAN FOR TEACHING JUMPING JACKS

1. Here we go. Get into the ready position. **(Photo A)**
2. Stand up straight, feet together in the middle. **(Photo B)**
3. Slap the sides of both legs with your palms.
4. Without bending your elbows, swing your arms away and up and make a V over your head. **(Photo C)**
5. Keep your arms straight and slap the sides of your legs again. Is your body straight up and down?
6. Make another V with your arms.
7. All right, here we go: Straight, V, straight, V, straight.
8. Now get back in the ready position.
9. Close the V and bring your legs together and your body straight.
10. Make a leg V, both feet at once. **(Photo D)**
11. Make yourself straight. Erase the V.
12. Make a leg V, straight, V, straight, V, straight.
13. Relax and shake out your hands and arms. Okay, back in the middle of your square in the straight position.

14. Show me how you can make two V's with your arms and legs at the same time. Ready? Go! **(Photo E)**
15. Make yourself straight. **(Photo F)**
16. Now make two V's again.
17. Make two V's, straight, V's, straight, V's.
18. Congratulations! You are doing a jumping jack!

Repeat until the student can consistently use the operative language to complete the entire skill independently.

Operative language: *V, straight, V, straight.*

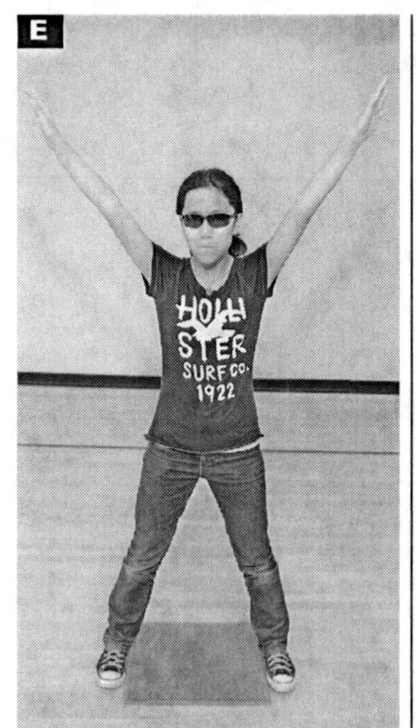

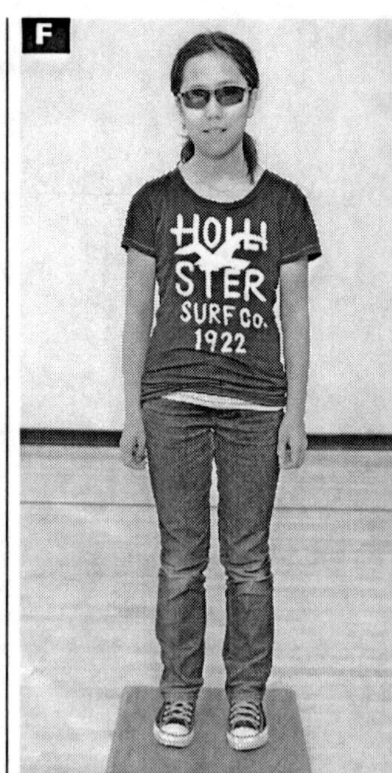

Principles of Adapting Games, Sports, and Related Activities

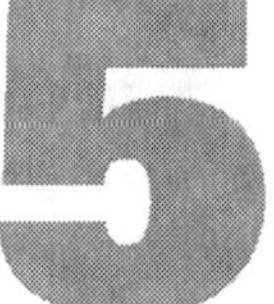

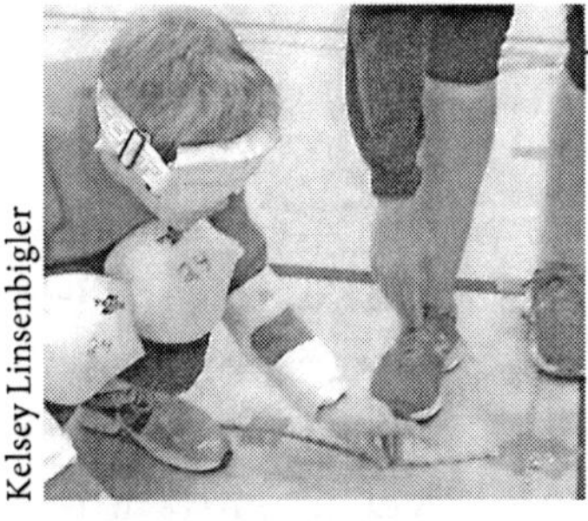
Kelsey Linsenbigler

IN THIS CHAPTER

- **The Purpose of Adapting Activities**
- **Structuring the Curriculum**
- **Sports Designed for People with Visual Impairments**
- **Guidelines for Adapting Activities**
- **The AccesSports Model**
- **Disability Awareness Instruction**

Juanita is a fifth grader who has optic atrophy with light perception only. She loves to move and play with her friends but cannot participate in physical education without assistance and adaptations. Her new physical education teacher, Ms. Myers, understands Juanita's enthusiasm for movement but has a hard time seeing how Juanita could participate in activities along with other students. Although she is a very conscientious teacher, Ms. Myers feels that she has not had enough professional preparation to successfully include Juanita in her class.

When Ms. Myers consulted Juanita's teacher of students with visual impairments, Mr. Vargas, he was insistent that Juanita be included in all physical education instructional units and assured Ms. Myers that it would not be as hard as she thought. He said, "It's important to remember that you have to adapt the activity to Juanita, since Juanita can't change for the activity."

Mr. Vargas went on to offer suggestions such as placing an audible sound source at the basket in basketball, using a sighted guide runner during the track unit, and having a guide wire for relay races. In addition, he helped Ms. Myers learn the game of goalball, a sport for individuals who are blind, so she could teach her whole class to play it blindfolded. The students loved goalball, and since Juanita was very skilled at it, she stood out among her classmates.

As Ms. Myers continued to work with Mr. Vargas and Juanita to make adjustments, her level of comfort increased and her ability to teach all the students in her class improved. Juanita enjoyed participating in all aspects of physical education.

Previous chapters have stressed the importance of involving children with visual impairments or deafblindness in the same or equivalent physical activities as their classmates of the same age. This involvement can improve the competence of a child with a visual impairment or deafblindness in a normal array of physical activities that the child can maintain within his or her repertoire of physical skills. The ability to be involved in the same activities as their peers helps propel children with sensory impairments further along the road to becoming independent, self-determined adults. Likewise, adults whose vision loss has convinced them that they have also lost the ability to participate in their favorite sports or recreational activity may well take their first step toward adjustment as a result of discovering that a simple adaptation makes it possible to continue the activity.

Scenarios such as the one involving Juanita's physical education teacher are common in physical education and sports. As noted in Chapter 3, many physical education teachers do not feel that they have the professional training and preparation to fully include children with visual impairments in general physical education classes (Lieberman, Houston-Wilson, & Kozub, 2002).

Chapter 4 presented a variety of methods for modifying instruction for students with visual impairments or deafblindness. In many instances, however, these students cannot be successfully involved in physical activity without also making some changes to the activities themselves. This chapter provides an overview of the many options for adapting physical activities for children and adults with visual impairments or deafblindness.

THE PURPOSE OF ADAPTING ACTIVITIES

In many units related to sports, fitness, and recreation, individuals with visual impairments or deafblindness will need some variable in a game or activity altered so that they can participate successfully. Older students and adults with visual impairments may also need some variables in a sport or recreational activities to be altered in order for them to participate successfully. These adaptations, or changes to make an activity, task, or object accessible, are necessary to allow individuals with disabilities to get physical exercise, to enjoy the pleasure of games and sports, and to actively participate with their peers.

Some people may ask, why adapt an activity if it is too difficult for an individual with a visual impairment to do without adaptations? In fact, there are many ways to play any game or sport or do any recreation or fitness activity. Participating in the same activities as their peers is a right all children have. In addition, learning and participating with their peers gives children with visual impairments the opportunity to practice making choices and to build their skills in "self-determination," an important part of self-development for all children (see Chapter 3). Thus, when a classmate asks them if they want to play hockey or tennis or go biking, children with sensory impairments will know how to take part in that activity and they can make an active choice. Likewise, adaptations make it possible for adults who have lost vision, hearing, or both to return to the sports or recreational activities in which they participated prior to the onset of their disabilities, which can help those individuals reenter their previous social circles, such as a bowling league or cycling club.

Specific methods of adapting activities often involve making objects more visible or using audible or tactile cues, based on the principles described in Chapter 2. This chapter presents the AccesSports model for eliminating barriers to the participation of children and adults with visual impairments in physical activities (Ponchillia, 1995), which focuses on adapting a sport or activity's traditional rules, equipment, or boundaries. Determining the best variables to adapt requires the instructor to analyze a given activity, taking into consideration the attributes of all the participants, the abilities of the individual with the visual impairment, the objectives of the class or team as a whole, and, for a student, the objectives on the student's Individual Educational Program (IEP), as discussed later in this chapter (Lieberman, Lytle, & Clarcq, 2008).

In some cases it may make sense to adapt an activity specifically for the participant with a visual impairment, such as providing a sighted guide in basketball or a guidewire for use in relay races. In other instances it may make more sense to modify a game for all the players, for example, playing soccer on a scooter, playing volleyball with a beach ball with bells,

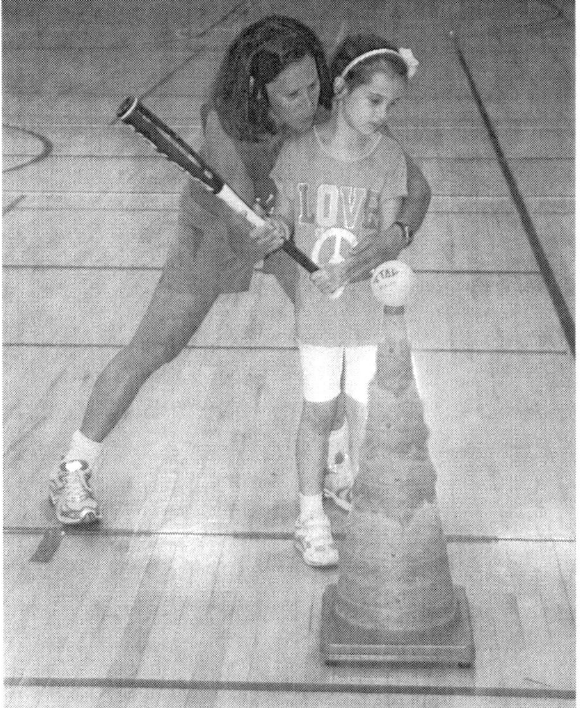

Amanda Tepfer

Adapting activities, such as using a bright red traffic cone for batting practice with a contrasting yellow ball may eliminate a barrier to participation for individuals with visual impairments.

or playing hockey on carpet squares, a game in which each player slides around on two small carpet squares like ice hockey, which slows down the game considerably.

With some careful planning and creativity, teachers, rehabilitation professionals, or coaches can ensure that individuals with visual impairments can be active members of any physical activity program. A valuable side effect is that the others in the class or activity are likely to benefit from getting to know people with visual impairments or deafblindness and learning about their abilities. Especially for students, this exposure will contribute to their overall education and broaden their awareness of diversity as well as the variety of ways to approach a situation. The experience of working with students their own age with disabilities will help students be more accepting of differences among people and create an environment with more respect and tolerance. (See the section on diversity education later in this chapter.)

STRUCTURING THE CURRICULUM

Most students or adults with visual impairments can play virtually any game or sport with appropriate adaptations, although some activities will need more adaptation than others. Although this chapter focuses mainly on adapting activities in the physical education curriculum, it is important to note that the principles can be applied to physical activities for individuals with visual impairments or deafblindness of any age. In addition to adapting the activities themselves, there are ways to structure the physical education curriculum that will also help the student with a visual impairment feel included and at the same time minimize the need for the teacher to continually develop adaptations.

Competition versus Cooperation

Games that are competitive often leave students with visual impairments or deafblindness feeling excluded. Although adaptations and support will help in facilitating inclusion into a game, many students focus only on the objective of winning as opposed to inclusion of all classmates. Thus, in a competitive atmosphere, the student with the visual impairment is not likely to be the only person who may feel left out.

To avoid this situation, the teacher needs to ensure that some of the units offered as part of the physical education year are cooperative instead of purely competitive. Examples of these units may include but are not limited to adventure education (activities such as rope courses, rock climbing, kayaking and canoeing, and mountaineering), team building, weightlifting, hiking, fishing, and cooperative volleyball, in which individuals or teams work together. The teacher may also choose to structure the beginning of a unit as skill development and then add a competitive game at the very end. Students are typically not considered developmentally ready for competitive games, however, until after elementary school. Standard practice is to focus on skill development until high school, with games that have fewer players on a side and are cooperative, such as those that require working together to keep the ball in play in volleyball or tennis.

For example, when Juanita's class learned volleyball, all the students learned the basic skills with a beach ball first. Then they played cooper-

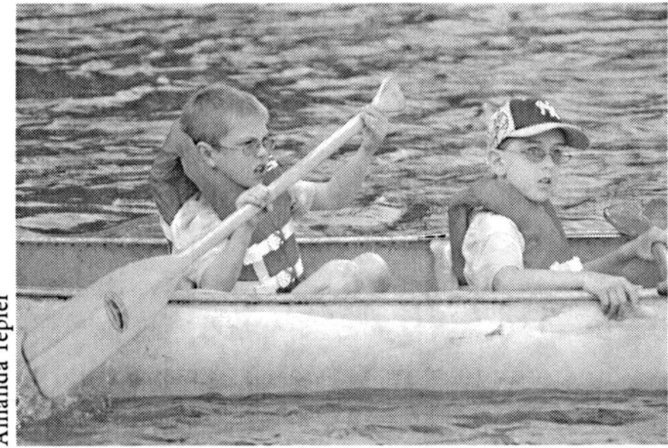
Amanda Tepfer

Including cooperative activities, such as canoeing, in a physical education curriculum or camp setting promotes inclusion for individuals who are not as successful in competitive sports.

ative games to see how many times they could get the ball over the net. Ms. Myers adapted the game to include Juanita by modifying the rules for everyone to allow the ball to bounce before it is returned over the net; allowing a student to catch the ball if the student gives it to Juanita, who then walks up to the net to throw it over; and providing a peer buddy to describe what is happening in the game so Juanita did not feel left out. By creating a cooperative situation with a few simple adaptations, the teacher was able to include Juanita along with the rest of the class in an activity that all could enjoy.

Closed versus Open Skills

Children with visual impairments can frequently participate in closed-skill activities with little or no modification. As explained in Chapter 3, *closed skills* are those that have minimal or no variation in pace, direction, or position. Examples of closed skills are those used in archery, bowling, weightlifting, riding a stationary bike, field events, and running around a track. The environment during a closed-skill activity remains constant. The exercise of *open skills,* in contrast, involves frequent or constant change, such as switching between offense and defense or the changing trajectory and speed of a ball or other object. Examples of sports involving open skills are basketball, volleyball, tennis, and soccer.

It is important to keep in mind that a physical education curriculum should include a combination of open- and closed-skill units for everyone. Interspersing closed-skill units with open-skill units gives the student with a visual impairment or deafblindness a variety of activities in which to experience success. For example, Juanita enjoyed the unit on track and field because she was able to participate with few modifications to the field events and only needed a guide runner for running. (See Chapter 8 for descriptions of track and field events and their adaptations.) In addition, varying units in a curriculum benefits the teacher, who does not have to provide adaptations for every activity the class does.

SPORTS DESIGNED FOR PEOPLE WITH VISUAL IMPAIRMENTS

There are some sports that are specifically developed for individuals with visual impairments, such as goalball, beep baseball, and a game called showdown, which is an indoor competitive table sport. These sports require no adaptation and provide opportunities to increase other people's awareness about visual impairment, since all people can be included in blindness-specific sports. (For more detailed information about such sports, see Chapter 9.) As noted at the beginning of this chapter, for example, when Juanita's physical education class learned to play goalball while blindfolded, Juanita enjoyed a great deal of success, while the other students enjoyed learning a new sport and gained insight about Juanita's day-to-day experiences.

Other sports can be used to "level the playing field" by having all the players simulate blindness and compete on a more or less equal basis with players who have visual impairments. Such sports include track and field events with blindfolds, swimming with blackened goggles, judo with a blindfold, and tandem biking (in this case, only the rider on the back seat wears a blindfold). Students in a physical education class can practice being sighted guides or describing the action to the students who are simulating blindness. Chapter 8 provides more information on the participation of individuals with visual impairments in these activities.

Rules of Competition

When instructors are including a learner with visual impairments in mainstream sports such as track and field, powerlifting, and judo, it is important for the instructors to learn about the adaptations and rules that are used in formal competitions among athletes with physical disabilities, such as the Paralympic Games. (The Paralympic Games are an official equivalent of the Olympics for athletes with mobility disabilities or visual disabilities, amputees, and those with cerebral palsy. They are not the same as the Special Olympics, which primarily involves athletes with intellectual disabilities.) For example, in sprint running a guide runner is required for athletes with severe visual impairments; the guide runner is not allowed to cross the finish line ahead of the runner who is visually impaired. Adaptations and rules for competitive sports are discussed in Chapter 8. Individuals with visual impairments or deafblindness need to learn about and practice using these rules when participating in activities leading up to such competitive sports, just as their classmates or teammates start to learn about the mainstream rules for these sports when practicing basic skills.

GUIDELINES FOR ADAPTING ACTIVITIES

The following section provides a number of concepts to keep in mind when planning for the inclusion of individuals with visual impairments or deafblindness in sports and recreational activities. In analyzing activities and devising adaptations for students or adults with visual impairments or deafblindness, the physical education teacher, coach, or rehabilitation professional can work in consultation with a teacher of students with visual impairments, orientation and mobility (O&M) instructor, adapted physical education teacher, vision rehabilitation therapist, parents if relevant, and the individual or child when possible. Each of these individuals brings a different expertise or familiarity with the individual's needs and abilities that will support the physical educator and contribute to the student's success.

Certain factors need to be considered before adapting any activity, which will ultimately affect the participant's opportunity to perform the activity successfully. These include the following:

- the participant's functional abilities
- the objective of the activity, game, or unit
- the objectives in a student's Individualized Educational Program (IEP)

These factors are discussed in the following sections. Sidebar 5.1 provides some general strategies to guide instructors regardless of the types of adaptations they make. (For suggestions on adapting specific games and activities for students with sensory impairment or multiple disabilities, see Lieberman & Cowart, 2011).

SIDEBAR 5.1

Rules of Thumb for Adapting Physical Activities

The following are some general guidelines and strategies to follow when adapting physical activities for students with visual impairments or deafblindness:

- Include the students in making the adaptations. It is imperative that students with visual impairments are included in the process of adapting physical activities whenever possible. They know best what they can see, how fast they move, and how they prefer to be instructed. In addition, they may have their own ideas about adaptations that might work for them. Allowing them to participate in planning the modification gives them ownership of the activity, and they will be more vested in active participation. In addition, students will learn how to advocate for themselves and suggest other adaptations that might be helpful for full inclusion.

  Example: A teacher is wondering, "How many bells should I insert into the soccer ball to make it audible for my student who is visually impaired?" The best answer is, "Let the student make that decision." The student will not only have the best input about what will work for him or her but also learn more by being involved in the process.
- Make the least adaptation necessary. It is not necessary to change every variable in a game. Change only what has to be changed to ensure the student's full participation.

  Examples: Having the batter hit a baseball off a tee instead of a pitch; tying a guide rope from one weight machine to the next to promote independence in a weight unit; having the student with low vision sit with his or her back to the window and close to the teacher in yoga class.
- Be creative. There are many ways to play a game or activity. Think about the activity as a whole to see what must be modified in order for an individual to participate.

  Examples: In archery, the student needs to know the location of the target; therefore, put a beeper behind the target and add balloons to the face of the target. In Frisbee golf, the student may need guidance on getting around the course, so make a tactile map of the course with relevant distances. In basketball, the student may need an overview of the game; create a tactile diagram of the court and show the student the basket and backboard as well as positions on the court.
- Evaluate whether the adaptations work. The process of designing adaptations is ongoing. Once you have worked with the individual to determine modifications for an activity, be sure to check on his/her success. Do not be afraid to tweak the rules, equipment, or boundaries or even start all over again from scratch. Effective teachers in any subject continually assess the progress of a unit being taught.

  Example: A teacher uses a light beach ball for teaching soccer. The student kicks the ball well, but then asks whether or not he had kicked it. The ball was too light for him to get the proprioceptive

(Continued on next page)

SIDEBAR 5.1 *(continued)*

feedback. The teacher switches to a heavier soccer ball with bells, and the student cheers after he kicks it.

- Use exclusion only as the last option. If the student's IEP says he or she must be included in physical education, then the student must be included. As noted earlier, the student cannot be changed to fit the game; the game must be changed to fit the student. The teacher therefore needs to try everything possible to ensure that the student is included in a physical education class or activity. If a student must be taken out of an activity for some reason—for example, if the student is at risk of a retinal detachment, which could lead to total blindness—the student can be accompanied by several sighted peers so they can all perform the activity together with adaptations. There should be enough students to play the game or do the activity in question and to enable the student with visual impairment or deafblindness to interact with classmates of the same age.

  Example: Bethany has low vision and has a partially detached retina in one eye. She is not permitted to play a regular game of basketball. Her teacher created a three-against-three game on two of the four baskets in the gym. On the other two baskets, the students played Around the World and H.O.R.S.E.—two closed-skill versions of basketball. The student peers rotated among the four options, but Bethany stayed at those two baskets and had a great time playing basketball.
- Educate the class about the student's disability. It is helpful for the rest of the class to understand why a teacher is making adaptations to the activities. The more knowledge they have about the disability and what it is like to live with it, the more likely they will understand the needs of the student with a visual impairment or deafblindness and accept the adaptations made for him or her. (For more on educating classmates about disability, see the section on disability awareness in this chapter.)
- Link movement to language. Whether a student is visually impaired or deafblind, it is important that each skill and activity be explained and the purpose be clear, no matter how a game is modified.
- Retain the original name of the game or sport. No matter how many adaptations are made to a game such as basketball, volleyball, or golf, its name should not be changed when parts are modified. If a different name is used for the game, the student may never know that she or he can play that game or sport, with adaptations, should anyone ask (Lieberman & Houston-Wilson, 2009).

Functional Abilities

It is imperative that the instructor base decisions about adaptations on an accurate knowledge of the participant's functional abilities—that is, what the participant is able to do in a real-world situation. The instructor can obtain this information by observing the participant as well as by asking questions such as the following of the participant, family members, or other teachers:

- What can the individual see?
- What does the individual hear?
- Does the individual have any additional disabilities?
- How does the individual get around?
- Are there any activities that are contraindicated because of the individual's condition?
- What was the individual's previous experience with physical activity?

- What is the individual currently able to do related to the activity being taught? What was the individual's previous experience with the activity?
- How does the individual perform the skills necessary to participate in the activity?
- How does the environment affect how the individual sees or hears? For example, is the individual sensitive to glare or confused in situations with a lot of background noise?

Knowing a person's functional abilities enables the instructor to determine which aspects of an activity will pose a difficulty for the learner and therefore need to be adapted (Lieberman, Lytle, & Clarcq, 2008). For example, in the soccer unit of a physical education class, if a teacher is including a student who has low vision and hemiplegia as a result of cerebral palsy, the teacher needs to know that the student is unable to move the arm and leg on one side of the body. The teacher might therefore decide to have the class play scooter soccer instead to make it easier for the student to participate in the game. Having the student use a chair scooter borrowed from the physical therapist instead of a flat scooter will enable the student to be mobile using only one side of his or her body, and using a larger ball with bells will help the student keep track of the ball's location using his or her hearing and residual vision.

The responses to the questions just listed may point to important adaptations that may be necessary for the safety of a student or for the most successful experience for the participant to occur. It is important to note that a physical education teacher cannot rely on parents, guardians, other teachers, or even a student's physician to determine the degree to which a student can be involved or the type of adaptations indicated; they simply may not know enough about the curriculum and the requirements of the activities in question. The teacher also needs to use his or her knowledge of the activities to make sure safe, appropriate adaptations are provided when necessary, as in the following example:

Mariam's physician, who misunderstood the kind of activity involved in goalball, gave clearance for Mariam to play the sport. However, when the physical education instructor, Ms. Myers, questioned Mariam's classroom teacher, she discovered that Mariam had a shunt (a plastic tube that drained fluid from her head into her abdomen) that would be at risk of being dislodged if Mariam engaged in vigorous goalball defensive movements. As a result, Ms. Myers modified plans and included Mariam in the goalball lesson by teaching her how to throw the ball. Ms. Myers showed Mariam proper defensive form, but did not have her practice the movements vigorously. The goalball throwing activity resulted in increased upper body strength and overall fitness, Mariam had bragging rights to being "an awesome thrower," and she had a better understanding of the sport.

Table 5.1 displays some examples of medical conditions, the concerns they might pose in an activity, and suggested instructional decisions that might be made as a result.

Assessment of the functional abilities of adults with acquired visual impairments or deafblindness differs markedly from that of children in school. Whereas children are still developing physical, social, teamwork, and other skills, adults generally possess well-developed skills. In addition, children have

TABLE 5.1. Medical Conditions That Can Affect Degree of Involvement in Certain Physical Activities: Some Examples

Medical Issue	Concern	Limitations and Adaptations
Shunt	Plastic tube draining fluid from head into abdominal area or heart. Although the tube is not external, no jerking of the head or excessive contact activities with the head or body are permitted	No heading a soccer ball No diving (head first) No contact sports such as wrestling or goalball No forward rolls Emphasize fitness and closed-skill activities
Detached retina	A risk of detaching the rest of the retina of the eye	No vigorous activities No heading a soccer ball No diving (head first) No contact sports
Atlantoaxial instability (often found in children with Down syndrome)	The ligaments between the atlas and vertebrae are loose; thus the student is at risk for spinal cord injury with certain movements such as hyperextension of the neck	No heading a soccer ball No diving (head first) No contact sports No forward rolls No head jerking No high jump, football, or soccer Limitations on warm-up stretching
Photophobia, causing problems with sun glare (commonly found with albinism, cataracts)	Sunlight may cause the student to have problems with vision in a brightly lit room or outdoors	Wear a brim hat Wear sunglasses Wear sunscreen Select indoor or less visual activities on very sunny days
Seizures	The student may have frequent seizures that occur at any time	Always have a buddy when swimming Do not climb to heights that would put student at risk should seizure occur Use low balance beam
Brittle bones	The student is at risk for fracturing and breaking bones during most activities	Avoid high-impact activities Avoid situations in which the student may fall from heights Adapt contact sports

limited experience with physical activities, while adults have developed favorite sport, fitness, or recreational activities. Adults also have the added complication of experiencing reactions and adjustment to their new impairments (see Chapter 2). As a result, the vision rehabilitation teachers, orientation and mobility instructors, occupational therapists, recreation therapists, or others responsible for providing sports, recreation, or fitness services during or following vocational rehabilitation programs must primarily be concerned with assessing individuals' participation in specific physical activities before vision loss, determining their present visual and physical ability to perform the skills required to return to the activities, and, finally, deciding what adaptations will be required for them to continue participation in the activity.

Assessing an individual's sports, fitness, or recreational history is usually done during an interview held at the first or second meeting with the individual, while skills assessment is generally accomplished simultaneously with teaching initial lessons (Ponchillia & Ponchillia, 1996). Required adaptations for a given activity are determined based on the teacher's assessment of the individual's visual and physical abilities and an analysis of the activity using the AccesSports model described later in this chapter.

One additional area of importance in assessing the needs of an adult with an acquired disability is selecting the best activity to be reintroduced first. Activities that require little adaptation and will most likely result in success are generally chosen, because they will more likely promote continued participation, while those that are difficult may be discouraging and inadvertently foster feelings of inadequacy. As already noted, the introduction of activities that require the use of closed, rather than open, skills are commonly selected first for children, because they are considered simpler to adapt and easier to perform. The same is true for adults; closed-skill activities that are familiar to the individual promote success during initial lessons. Such activities might include riding a tandem bike, hiking on an easily followed trail, jogging with a guide, or lifting weights rather than attempting the more complex skills required in such sports as basketball, bowling, or beep baseball.

Activity Goals and IEP Goals

In addition to analyzing the student's functional abilities, before determining what adaptations are necessary, the instructor also needs to consider both the objective of the game or unit and the objectives written in the student's IEP. Is the game or unit objective endurance, upper body strength, or skill development? Do the IEP objectives state that a student needs to work on standing in line, socialization, balance, or perceptual motor skills? The teacher could then determine whether the goal of the activity is appropriate for the student or needs to be modified. At the same time, the teacher can attempt to incorporate the student's IEP goals into the modified version of the activity.

An example of this process can be seen in the efforts of Ms. Myers, the physical education teacher of Juanita, who was introduced at the beginning of this chapter, to adapt the unit on jump rope for Juanita:

▪ *Ms. Myers observed how Juanita moved about, she learned about Juanita's eye condition, and she knew about Juanita's previous activity experiences. The objectives of the jump rope unit were to develop skill with the jump rope and endurance. Ms. Myers's goal for each of the students in class was to be able to jump rope for 10 minutes without stopping. Three of Juanita's goals on her*

IEP were to increase abdominal strength, improve socialization skills, and improve balance.

After considering her goals for the class, Juanita's functional abilities, and Juanita's IEP objectives, Ms. Myers decided to have the whole class begin by doing partner sit-ups with the jump rope, which develops abdominal strength. (In this activity, two students lie on their backs toe to toe with knees bent. They each hold one end of the rope and take turns sitting up and touching the rope to their knees.) Abdominal strength is something everyone needs to work on, and this activity helped Juanita reach the objectives on her IEP. The class also did a fun social jump rope warm-up exercise.

Students then worked on overhead arm movements with the rope and walking over the rope to the beats of music for two class periods. (Students who already knew how to jump rope could jump using the same form, but at a faster beat.) This adaptation was made not only for Juanita but for any student at the beginning level of jumping rope. Juanita was able to meet the goal of walking over the rope for 10 minutes, and progressed to hopping over the rope with one foot. This worked on her endurance as well as balance. She enjoyed the socialization of the warm-up with a friend, and experienced success in her mode of jumping. Thus, the jump rope activity addressed these three IEP goals at the same time that Juanita worked toward the class goals for the unit. ■

(See Chapter 7 for more information on teaching jump rope.)

Analyzing physical activities based on a student's functional abilities and IEP goals and the activity goals for the class allows the physical education teacher to determine the aspects of an activity that need adaptation in order for the student to participate. This information can then guide the use of the AccesSports model, described in the next section.

THE ACCESSPORTS MODEL

Principles of the AccesSports Model

The AccesSports model developed by Ponchillia (1995) is a model for delivering sport and physical activity instruction to individuals with visual impairments. This three-part model can aid instructors who desire to provide high-quality instruction to students and adults with visual impairments or deafblindness but who are not sure how to do so.

Using the methodology of the AccesSports model, an instructor analyzes the abilities of the student and the objectives of an activity that need to be made accessible, as discussed in the previous section, and then examines the following three components of the activity to determine where the barriers to including a student or adult with a visual impairment in this sport or game are found:

- targets and goals (including equipment)—for example, basketball net, soccer goal net, balls
- boundaries—the sides of a playing field or court
- rules of the game

Based on the information gathered, the instructor determines how to adapt the activity accordingly. For example, if a player with low vision wishes to shoot baskets, then the barrier is difficulty seeing the target (basket), and only the target needs modification. If playing the game of basketball is the goal, however, then it is likely that rules and boundaries as well as the target will all need some modification.

Examples of modifications for each of the activity components are listed in the following sections. (See the Resources section for sources of equipment and products referred to.)

Adapting Targets and Goals

Barriers related to targets or goals often have to do with the player's ability to perceive them, although sometimes they may involve the ability to lift or manipulate the equipment. Depending on an individual's degree of vision and hearing loss, the targets or equipment used in an activity can be adapted to increase their visibility—for example, by making them larger or by increasing contrast between the object and the background, as described in the section on environmental adaptations in Chapter 2—or by using auditory or tactile cues.

Besides vision, for most people, hearing is the sense that provides the most information about the environment. Sound sources placed near goals, targets, or boundaries can serve as cues for their locations. In addition, as noted in Chapter 4, sound sources can assist with orientation to a room or playing area by being a constant that allows individuals to monitor where they are in relationship to the sound source, regardless of their movements. Sidebar 5.2 describes a variety of sound sources that can be used as beacons to locate targets or goals for orientation. They may also be used to locate boundaries, as described in the next section.

Some examples of adaptations for targets and goals include the following:

Visual Adaptations

- lowering baskets or nets to make them more visible
- painting the basketball backboard a bright color if it is made of a clear material
- tying a bright ribbon onto a volleyball net
- increasing the size or visibility of the goals by using bright tape, flags, or cones
- making sure the color of a ball or target or other equipment contrasts with the background
- increasing size of bases
- using bright balloons for activities like ping pong, volleyball, or badminton
- using a brightly colored Frisbee instead of a puck or ball in hockey

Auditory Adaptations

- adding a sound source to soccer or other goals
- hanging a sound source from a basket in basketball such as bells, a beeper, or a soda can filled with coins or washers that a teammate can shake during a game
- banging a cane against a basketball hoop to indicate the hoop's location
- tying a string onto an archery target that is long enough to reach to the player with a visual impairment or deafblindness so he or she knows where the target is
- tying a string to hang from a basketball hoop so the player can see or feel where the hoop is
- tying bells onto a volleyball net to emit sound when shaken
- placing sound sources at bases
- using sound-emitting balls

SIDEBAR 5.2

Sound Beacons for Audible Location of Targets or Goals

The following are some of the products that can be used as sound sources or beacons.

Specialized Products

Many products are specifically designed for people with visual impairments, including equipment that can be used in physical activities. These materials are available from organizations such as the American Printing House for the Blind (see the Resources section):

- Specialized beepers or clickers that are sold as assistive devices for people with visual impairments.
- Beeper Sound Tracker (from www.braillegifts.com), a small (2" × 4.5") device that can be purchased with either a constant or an intermittent beep or with music. A remote control is available.
- Motion Pad, a device that senses motion at a 10-foot distance and then emits a prerecorded message. One could record a phrase like "south field boundary" that would be spoken aloud every time an athlete comes within 10 feet of the device.
- Portable Sound Source, Sports Edition, a lightweight (1½-pound) portable sound source that produces variable pulsing sounds (36 to 360 per minute).
- The APH Sound Ball, a colorful electronic ball made of durable foam, measuring 7.5 inches, which features dual speakers, dual volume, and two-tone sounds to accommodate children who wear hearing aids, either "boing boing" or "techno beat." Can be used for activities such as kickball or soccer or practicing sound localization skills.
- The Miniguide, a small, handheld mobility device that emits sound or vibrations when objects are in one's path. Individuals who are deafblind might find the device useful for locating archery targets or golf flags on a green.

Miscellaneous and Homemade Devices

Everyday objects or devices that emit some kind of noise can make easy-to-use sound beacons:

- Devices that emit a constant background noise, such as a portable radio, "boom box," or fan.
- Wireless pet chimes or doorbells, commercial products that allow pets to signal when they want to go out or come inside. They have a receiver that emits a sound—usually either a ding-dong or a barking noise when activated by pressing on a paw-shaped transmitter that can be up to 100 feet away. This signal could be placed on a target and activated by someone who wishes to shoot baskets from a stationary position or to indicate the location of a dartboard or bull's-eye. It could also be activated by the instructor who wishes to give a student an audible cue for long jump or sprints.
- Many brands and varieties of wireless doorbells, including a version with two transmitters and a flashing light indicator, which may be useful for students with low vision or deafblindness with residual hearing and vision. These types of items can be found on the Internet using search terms such as *wireless doorbell* or *remote door chime* or can be found in home improvement stores. Some can be activated with a remote.
- Homemade sources of sound that can make a goal or location audible, such as attaching a bell to basketball net to indicate when the ball makes a basket.

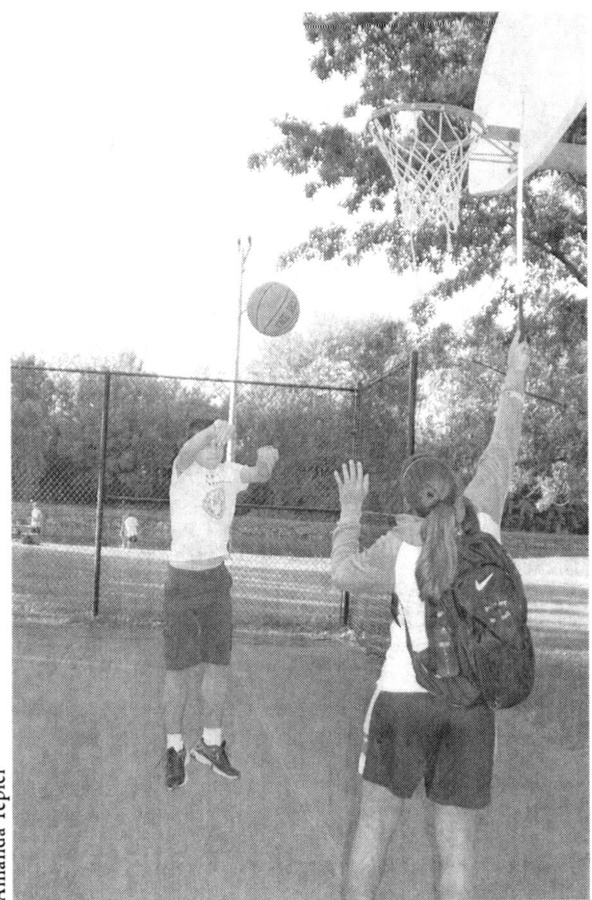
Amanda Tepfer

Tapping on the backboard or basket with a long cane provides an audible target for the student shooting the ball.

Miscellaneous Adaptations

- using softer balls such as Nerf balls or deflated balls to slow down a game
- increasing or decreasing the size of equipment, such as using a larger bat or racquet
- decreasing the weight of a shot put, ball, or goal ball
- using bigger or lighter bats
- using a flat-sided bat
- using Velcro grips or tape to help a player with a visual impairment or deafblindness hold onto a bat, hockey stick, or racquet

Adapting Boundaries

As with targets, boundaries that outline a playing area (such as a tennis court) or mark off particular zones or locations within a game (such as the free-throw line in basketball) may be difficult for individuals with visual impairments to perceive. Boundaries can be adapted by increasing their visibility or adding auditory or tactile cues. Examples of adaptations for boundaries include the following:

- adding highly contrasting gymnasium marking tape to the existing lines on the edges of courts or playing fields
- using large orange cones to mark the corners or sidelines of a playing field
- tying bright tape to the perimeter of a tag area
- placing bright tape over a rope marking a boundary
- putting bright ribbon on nets or baskets
- putting bright lines on the wall
- spray painting a contrasting color on the grass
- placing flags at the corners of fields or courts
- using a guidewire

Auditory beacons can also mark boundaries. Portable radios or beepers can delineate the playing area of outdoor sports like baseball or soccer (see Sidebar 5.2 for sources of sound beacons). Sound cues can be difficult to locate in gymnasiums and swimming pool areas, however, where the sound reflects from walls.

Tactile adaptations include placing a cord under gymnasium marking tape on the edge of a court; it is a good idea to use two or three lines separated by three or four inches, as a single line might easily be stepped over and missed when running. Also, as described in

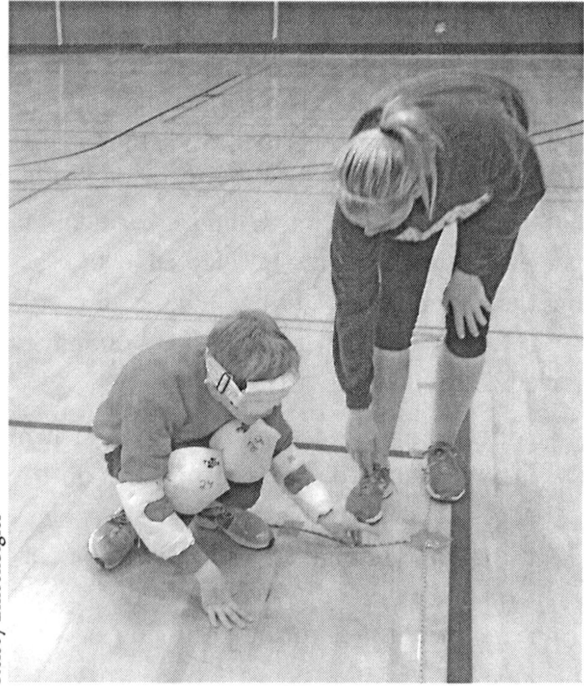

Kelsey Linsenbigler

This student, blindfolded and padded for goalball, is investigating the boundaries made by taping down rope on the gym floor to create a raised, tactile surface.

Chapter 4, creating a raised-line drawing or tactile scale model of the boundaries of a field, court, or playing area on a clipboard or other board of a similar size, with raised felt, Wikki Stix, or Hi Marks (a product that produces raised dots or lines) is a fast, easy way to orient students to a playing area and its boundaries.

Adapting Rules

Adaptations to the rules of a game can affect how the game is played by all the players or can involve special assistance given to the player with a visual impairment or deafblindness, such as verbal description of the play. Adapting the rules or conditions of a game or sport usually simplifies the activity or decreases the complexity of the playing environment by decreasing the number of players, decreasing the difficulty of locating the goal or target, increasing the ease of scoring, or decreasing the possibility of injury. Examples of changes to rules or conditions of a game include the following:

- Allowing the ball to bounce twice before it can be returned in tennis, volleyball, or badminton instead of the usual one bounce, so the players have more time to react.
- Increasing or decreasing the distances involved in games and activities. For example, a player may choose to serve a volleyball at 4 feet from the net instead of at the back service line; a player may stand halfway back to start off in archery.
- Having a player play only offense or defense in a game. For example, in soccer the player may choose to play defense and defend the goal only when the ball is brought down the field by the other team's offense. Defense would be the player's only responsibility. In basketball, defense may only try to prevent the other team from scoring.
- Requiring that each team member has to touch the ball, puck, or Frisbee before the side can score.
- Using a batting tee for baseball so the ball is always in the same place.
- Requiring that everyone on a team go once in kickball instead of switching sides after three players are out.
- Allowing a player to serve the ball closer to the net in tennis or volleyball.
- Lowering the hoop in basketball.
- Allowing an unlimited number of hits on a side before the ball is hit over in volleyball.
- Counting hits or times the ball goes over the net in volleyball instead of scoring points for competing teams.

- Having the instructor pitch in kickball or baseball.
- Throwing the ball over on a serve in volleyball instead of a traditional serve
- Allowing more room between offense and defense to give offensive player more time for a play. For example, in hockey played with a Frisbee (adapted with bells tied across the bottom with fishing string), the student must have a 10-foot boundary with no defender. This rule could apply just to the student with a visual impairment or to all players.
- Using bounce passes or roll passes in basketball instead of thrown passes so the player with a visual impairment can hear the bounce and anticipate the ball.
- Having everyone simulate the same disability, such as blindfolding all or some of the players or one player on each team.
- Requiring that the person with the disability touch the ball before his or her team can score.
- Increasing or decreasing the number of players.

Applying the AccesSports Model

Applying the principles of the AccesSports model focuses on the essential components of activities necessary to meet the needs of individuals with visual impairments or deafblindness. Earlier in the chapter we described how Juanita's physical education instructor, Ms. Myers, adapted the rules for volleyball to offer a cooperative experience for the entire class. The following explanation of how she used the AccesSports model to derive these and other adaptations for volleyball offers an example of how this model can be used to analyze and meet the needs of a player with a visual impairment:

When Ms. Myers introduced volleyball to Juanita's class, she applied the logic of the AccesSports model to consider the targets, boundaries, and rules of the game as well as Juanita's vision level. She was not sure how much Juanita could see inside the gym, so she discussed Juanita's functional vision with Mr. Vargas, the teacher of students with visual impairments. He suggested that Ms. Myers try both visual and audible modifications to the boundaries and targets in the game and that she try them out with Juanita to see which ones worked best in the gym. Sidebar 5.3 presents several adaptations Ms. Myers tried out in the volleyball unit to include Juanita. As noted earlier in the chapter, the rules were modified to make a more cooperative game. These changes also simplified the activity and made it easier for Juanita to return the ball.

Bells and pink tape placed on the net helped all the students get oriented to the playing area. For the skill development part of the lesson, Juanita used a beach ball to make it easier for her to learn the concepts of the volleyball skills. The ball used for the actual game was a trainer volleyball, which is bright yellow and moves more slowly than a regulation volleyball. The ball was allowed to bounce twice for everyone. Players were allowed to catch the ball, but only if they were going to give it to Juanita. Nobody could spike the ball (jump up and hit the ball forcefully down over the net so it hits the ground rapidly). At the beginning there was a rule that Juanita could walk the ball up to the net, but once she understood the dimensions of the court, she chose to throw or hit the ball instead.

SIDEBAR 5.3

Volleyball Adaptations for Juanita

The following adaptations were made for Juanita during her class's unit on volleyball, based on the AccesSports model. These adaptations were used for the entire class. Some students still chose to play with the traditional rules of the game, which was also acceptable.

Targets or Goals

- Bright tape on top of the net.
- Bells on the net.
- Bright beach ball for the skill development part.
- Volleyball trainer ball for the game.
- Ball tied to the net with a string so it does not roll too far. (Once the students got better, the string was taken away.)

Boundaries

- Rope or cord is taped on the floor for boundaries.
- Large, bright cones are placed in the corners of the court.
- Radio is used as a sound source centered just off the court behind the players for orientation.

Rules

- One bounce is allowed before returning the ball over the net.
- The ball may be caught if it is then handed to Juanita.
- Juanita can walk up to the net to throw the ball over.
- The ball can be passed to others on the team from one to five times.
- A peer buddy will describe what is happening in the game for Juanita.
- The ball can bounce off the net and still be in play.
- All players can serve from one of three different distances from the net, indicated by different-colored tape on the floor.

Other examples of how activities such as soccer, golf, and archery can be modified are shown in Table 5.2.

As already noted, some physical activities require few modifications for inclusion of participants with visual impairment or deafblindness. For example, once an individual has been oriented to a weightlifting room, there is little that needs to be done beyond what any novice would be provided related to positioning, amount of weight to start with, or number of repetitions to execute. Other activities that require little or no adaptation include archery, running, canoeing, wrestling, judo, bowling, tandem biking, and fitness stations. When an instructor is faced with the need to modify any activity, however—from parachute games, to scooter racing, or a ball toss game—using the principles of the AccesSports model and working as a team with the player who is visually impaired, the parents or other caregivers, classmates or teammates, and other professionals will make it easier to sort out which parts of the activity need to be modified and in what way.

DISABILITY AWARENESS INSTRUCTION

Sometimes students in local schools who do not have disabilities may be unreceptive to adaptation of activities for students with disabilities who are in their class and may not fully understand the reason for providing them. For this reason, disability awareness is a very important component in any program with students with disabilities. Disability awareness refers to education with the goal of increasing understanding of disability. The means can be quite varied, ranging from guest speakers,

TABLE 5.2 Adaptations for Soccer, Golf, and Archery Based on the AccesSports Model			
Sport	**Targets or Goals**	**Boundaries**	**Rules**
Soccer	Sound source at goal Bright ribbon or tape around goal Tactile cues if student with visual impairment is goalie. For example, a classmate or teacher's aide could tap the student's shoulder and say "Coming left" or "High right." Tapping softly indicates the ball is close, while a harder tap means it is farther away Verbal cues at goal without tactile cues if necessary—for example, "Ball on ground, slight left" or "Ball high left" Larger ball Soft/deflated ball Brighter ball	Bright ribbon around perimeter Large bright cones in corners of playing area Rope with tape on gym floor Radio sound source to provide orientation to field or gym	No defender for the student with a visual impairment. If class chooses to equalize the playing field and blindfold a person on the other team, that person also has no defender Classmate provides auditory feedback to student Play offense only; for example, the student with a visual impairment may stand in front of goal and play the position of offense only and try to score when puck or ball is at scoring end Play defense only; the student with a visual impairment may stand in front of goal and play defense only—only trying to defend goal Verbal cues Fewer players in games
Golf	Sound source placed at hole Bright ribbon or tape around hole Brighter ball Club with grip for orientation Larger ball Auditory ball	Bright ribbon leading from one hole to next Cones at each hole Rope with tape on gym floor	Verbal cues Tactile cues for students who are deafblind One-to-one classmate or scout to give verbal or tactile cues and feedback about what is happening to a student with deafblindness Use cart

(*Continued on next page*)

TABLE 5.2 *(Continued)*

Sport	Targets or Goals	Boundaries	Rules
Archery	Sound source placed at target String tied from target to archer Larger target Bright ribbon or tape Balloons attached to whole target for feedback on shots that hit target	Bright ribbon along boundary Tactile or verbal feedback on shots Contrasting backdrop behind target Bright cones to stand behind Tactile markings so students know when they hit outside white, black, blue, red, or yellow part of target	Verbal cues Bow with grip Allow sighted classmate to point student or arrow to target Verbal feedback by teacher or paraeducator about where arrow hit on target, or if arrow missed, how far target was and if it was too high or too low One-to-one classmate to give verbal feedback about where arrow hit on target, or if arrow missed, how far target was and if too high or too low. In addition, classmate could help student retrieve arrows and describe where on target the arrow hit

books, and articles to videos in the classroom or on the Internet and simulations of a disability.

A three-stage plan for providing disability awareness instruction to facilitate understanding by students who do not have a disability was suggested by Lieberman and Houston-Wilson (2009). This model includes the following three stages:

I. Exposure to the disability
II. Experiencing the disability
III. Ownership

Exposure to the Disability

In the first stage, exposure to the disability, the students learn about a person with a disability. They can learn about the student in their class, another individual, or people with disabilities in general by meeting with them, watching a video, or reading an article about individuals with disabilities. A list of resources focusing on athletes or active people with visual impairments is provided in Sidebar 5.4 to assist teachers in introducing students to the topic.

Experiencing the Disability

The second stage in providing disability awareness involves having the students experience a simulation of the disability such as visual impairment while doing an activity of daily living or a physical activity such as soccer, running, or dancing. Sleepshades or blindfolds

SIDEBAR 5.4

Resources for Introducing Students to Athletes with Visual Impairments

The following are some suggested resources for educating students about the potential of people with visual impairments to engage in sports and physical activities:

Books about Active People with Visual Impairment or Deafblindness

- Marla Runyan with Sally Jenkins (2001). *No Finish Line: My Life as I See It.* New York: G. P. Putnam's Sons.

  Marla Runyan is a world-class runner who competed in the Paralympics and the Olympics in track and field and the marathon.
- Rachel Scdoris and Rick Steber (2005). *No End in Sight: My Life as a Blind Iditarod Racer.* New York: St. Martin's.

  This book is about Rachel Scdoris, a young woman with a visual impairment who competed in several Iditarod dogsled races.
- Erik Weihenmayer (2002). *Touch the Top of the World.* New York: Penguin Group.

  Erik Weihenmayer is the only person who is blind to have climbed the "seven summits," consisting of the tallest peak on each continent. His book has been adopted for many reading programs for youths.
- Cindy Lou Aillaud and Lauren J. Lieberman (in press). *Everybody Plays: How Children with Visual Impairments Play Sports.* Louisville, KY: American Printing House for the Blind.

  Designed to help elementary-age students understand the potential abilities of youths with visual impairments in sports.

Newspaper Articles

Check local newspapers or online for articles about local or national athletes with disabilities.

Internet Videos

Video clips of athletes with disabilities that can be shared with students can be found on the Internet, for example, at the YouTube video sharing website, which has videos about goalball, swimming, track, beep baseball, showdown, and other sports. (Search using terms such as *disabled athletes, disabled sports,* and *blind athletes.*)

Guest Speakers

Individuals who have visual impairments and are physically active may live nearby. Many are willing to visit schools and can demonstrate skills or show their equipment and discuss their experiences.

can be used to simulate total blindness. A variety of low vision simulators can be purchased or constructed (see the Resources section), but instructors should be aware that it is more likely that students simulating low vision instead of total blindness may develop symptoms of motion sickness if they attempt moving around while wearing a simulator. Instructors need to be aware of and sensitive to students' feelings in order to avoid injuries or negative experiences for those who are simulating visual impairment. For example, make sure there is a trained peer tutor to act as sighted guide when students are running or playing soccer. An active, trained paraeducator may also be used.

Ownership

Although not all students reach the level of what has been termed ownership, or actually becoming involved in helping or working with students with visual impairments, it is a goal of disability awareness for all students to reach this level of empathy and responsibility if possible. Students without disability have reached the level of ownership when they are willing to help ensure the welfare of individuals with disabilities. This could be becoming a trained peer tutor, serving a sighted guide in a running race, or explaining the action that is occurring during a basketball game to someone with a visual impairment (Lieberman & Houston-Wilson, 2009). Ensuring that sighted classmates comprehend the student's visual impairment or level of deafblindness will help them understand why modifications are being made and help create an atmosphere of acceptance.

CONCLUSION

People with visual impairments can be actively involved in any activity their same-age peers are doing in a physical education class when their instructors take the time to understand their needs and analyze the activities. Instructors can apply the AccesSports model to determine how adaptations to targets or goals and equipment, boundaries, and rules can best make an activity accessible to all participants. The principles apply equally to children and adults participating in recreation and fitness activities.

Preparing all the participants in an activity to understand the need for adapting the activity is also important. Engaging students by providing disability awareness opportunities and experiences in blindness-specific sports for all students and involving students in determining what adaptations can be made to include all classmates will facilitate successful physical activities for the majority. Keeping these considerations in mind will ensure that efforts to include people with visual impairments or deafblindness into a variety of healthy physical activities are more successful.

The chapters in this part of the book have laid out the principles for teaching and adapting physical activities so that all individuals with visual impairments or deafblindness can participate. Part 3 will investigate the specific needs of children and adults throughout the lifespan, as children develop from birth through preschool, elementary school, and middle school and become full participants in sports in high school. Subsequent chapters deal with participation of individuals with visual impairments or deafblindness in recreation and fitness activities in their daily lives.

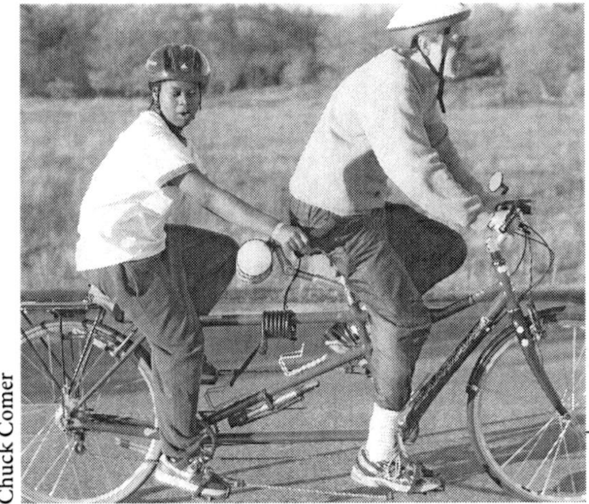
Chuck Comer

PART 3
Teaching Physical Skills throughout the Lifespan

Early Childhood Development

MOVEMENT AND PLAY IN EARLY CHILDHOOD

Tanni L. Anthony

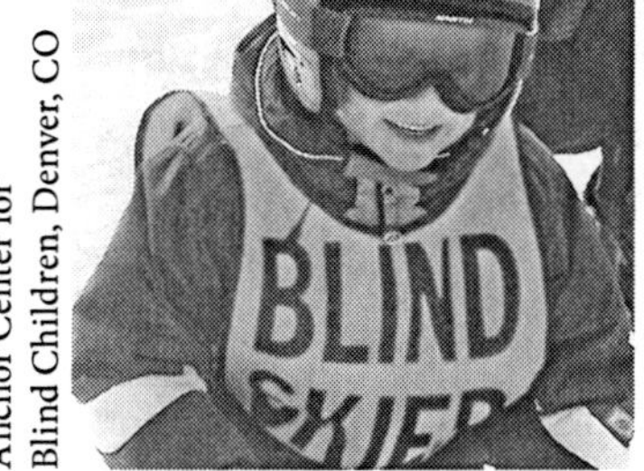

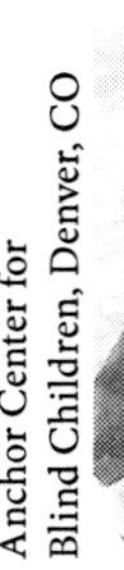

IN THIS CHAPTER

- **Starting Early**
- **Early Motor Development**
- **Development of Play**
- **Preparing for Preschool and Beyond**
- **Recommendations for Using Play to Encourage Physical Activity**

Andrew, a child of about 3 years of age who was blind, surprised his family and his small Alaskan community when he completed a full 5K cross-country ski event (just over 3 miles). His parents put on his skis at the beginning of the race, thinking that Andrew would be able experience the motion of skiing and the fun of his family and others moving forward in the snow tracks together, as they had done on a few previous outdoor excursions. His dad planned to put Andrew in a back carrier for the majority of the race, once his son wearied of the push through the snow. But Andrew persisted and insisted on completing the race. It took longer with a 3-year-old, but Andrew followed his parents' and older siblings' voices and was jubilant at the finish line.

Months later, when it was time for Andrew to enter his village school's preschool program, the teacher of students with visual impairments, who had worked with Andrew and his family since Andrew was 3 months old, met with the first grade children to set the stage for the first child with blindness coming to the school. She asked if anyone knew Andrew and readied herself for the expected questions and possible misunderstandings about his blindness. Instead there were loud proclamations about his accomplishments in the 5K cross-country skiing race: "Andrew is so cool! He was just 3 years old! No other 3-year-old ever did that!"

Andrew's family had high expectations for his full participation in family activities. His parents began to follow through with the recommendations of the teacher who had provided early intervention services to Andrew and his family on how to optimize Andrew's motor development within daily routines of caring for him starting when he was just 3 months of age. There were challenges along the way, but by the time Andrew was 3 years old, his gross motor coordination (the ability to control the large muscles of the body for sitting, crawling, walking, running, and other movement skills) was well developed, and his family expected that he would be able to participate fully in their sports and physical recreation activities. Most important, at a very young age Andrew himself believed that he was fully capable of participating in his family's recreational activities.

STARTING EARLY

Early development of motor and play skills sets the stage for children to participate in movement, recreational activities, and sports throughout their lifetimes. A visual impairment by itself or in association with deafblindness (combined vision and hearing loss of different types and levels) that is present at birth or soon after can have a significant impact on a young child's motor skill development. For this reason, it is vital for families and early intervention personnel to work together to support the development of motor skills and to promote everyday physical activity. (*Early intervention* refers to services provided to promote the growth and development of children under the age of 3 who have disabilities or are at risk of developmental delays, and to support their family, as required under the Individuals with Disabilities Education Act.)

The parents of an infant who has just been diagnosed with a visual impairment or deafblindness are not likely at first to be thinking about what they can do to foster a budding high school athlete or a child who will grow up to be an adult who enjoys lap swimming on weekends, hiking on nearby mountain trails, or doing aerobic and weightlifting exercises in a neighborhood gym. Those images and goals are a very long way away from their small baby, who is still mastering the task of lifting his or her head from a prone (on the stomach) position. However, by encouraging a child to explore the world and the surrounding environment, providing opportunities for physical activity, and promoting opportunities for active play, families and early intervention professionals can contribute greatly to a child's strong and healthy physical and cognitive development.

Physical activity in the early years of life needs to be approached from a developmental perspective that addresses how best to help the young child reach age-appropriate milestones in his or her motor skills. Having a developmental perspective means finding and supporting the beginnings of a skill in the early years. For example, the lifelong swimmer who loves moving in the water began as a child who splashed during the evening bath routine. The mountain hiker was a child who acquired balance and endurance from sitting upright, standing, walking, and eventually moving independently on stairs. The adult who does aerobic and weightlifting routines started out as a baby doing "workouts" on the living room floor, lifting his or her head. With every lift, the baby gained muscle strength in the neck, shoulders, upper back, and chest.

This chapter highlights two developmental areas that are related to physical activity goals for young children with visual impairments or deafblindness: motor development and the acquisition of cognitive and play skills. Motor development is the foundation for strength, coordination, balance, and endurance for physical activities and participation in recreation and sporting events. Play sets the stage for all early childhood learning and supports the development of social-emotional, cognitive, communication and language, and motor concepts and skills. When family members and early childhood personnel understand how a child plays, they can incorporate the child's play preferences into interventions and thus increase the effectiveness of those interventions. Play also serves as a platform for the child to become an individual athlete and a team player and to understand how to play with others and what type of equipment and rules are needed for these activities.

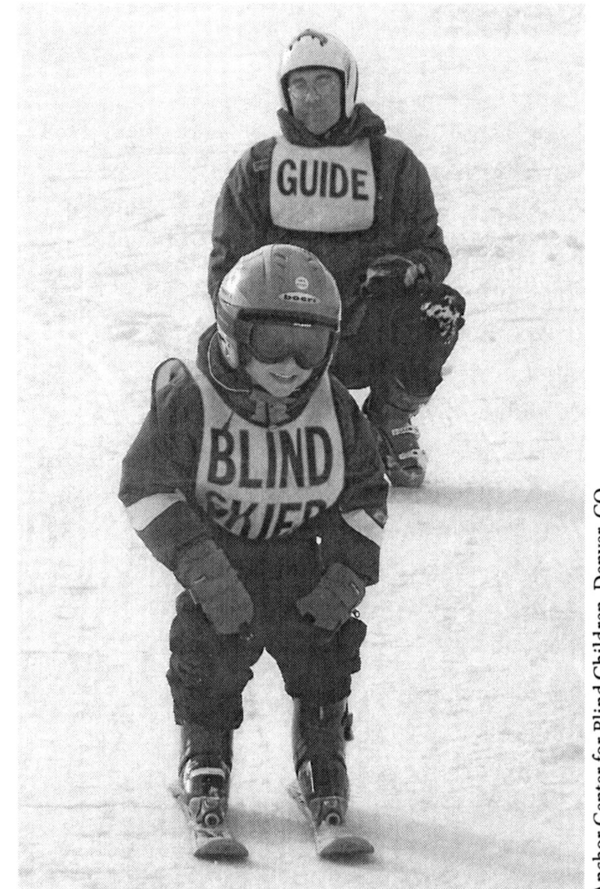

Anchor Center for Blind Children, Denver, CO

Support for early motor development, opportunities for active play, and high expectations that foster confidence can produce a budding athlete, like this young skier.

Although early motor development and play skills overlap and are interdependent in the early years, each topic is reviewed separately in this chapter to examine its unique pattern of skill acquisition and how it helps a child develop into a physically competent and active individual. Suggestions for activities that can help children with visual impairments or deafblindness develop motor and play skills are provided throughout the chapter.

EARLY MOTOR DEVELOPMENT

What should one expect when an infant is born with a visual impairment or both a vision and a hearing loss? The new baby will benefit from early intervention that addresses the child's sensory, physical, and cognitive needs but that is also grounded in the knowledge and expectation of typical motor development. It is important to first understand typical motor skill development and maintain high expectations that the child will engage in age-appropriate, self-initiated, and purposeful physical activities. High expectations come from being aware of the typical skills for children of a certain age range and being prepared for the challenges to motor development that young children with visual impairments or deafblindness may experience.

Typical Motor Development

Motor skills generally develop in a predictable sequence, though at different rates for individual children. Motor development progresses from head to toe (cephalo-caudal) and from the trunk out toward the extremities (proximodistal). For example, infants first master control of the head before they can control their trunk muscles to sit independently. Babies begin to play with their hands at the midline of the body before they can reach out for objects beyond the body. Table 6.1 summarizes the skills acquired during early motor development and indicates the typical age range during which each is milestone attained.

Head control is typically mastered by 3 to 4 months of age, as infants lift their heads while lying on their stomachs, which strengthens the muscles of the neck and upper back and chest. With time and considerable practice, infants become able to prop themselves up on their forearms, look at and interact with their hands, and engage with lightweight objects. Infants need opportunities to practice lifting their heads in order to develop the strength they need to move from a flat position, in total contact with the surface on which they are resting, to a position propped up on their arms. "Tummy time" is important for all infants during their waking hours. "Babies need unstructured free time to play on the floor each day" that is fully supervised by an adult (Stokes, 2002, p. 68).

By 5 to 6 months of age, infants can shift their weight onto one forearm while reaching out for a toy with the other arm. Within a very short period of time, infants gain enough motor control to use both hands for play that involves interacting with more than one object at the same time. At this stage, infants can reach for objects while on their stomachs and are becoming ready to sit upright and move by themselves.

Mastering the skills of supported and then independent sitting gives the child a new vantage point for play. Both hands are now free to reach for and interact with objects. Once upright sitting is mastered, infants are less likely to play on their stomachs or backs (Bundy, 2008). The child's world has moved from a need for body contact and support from a horizontal surface to an upright vertical posture.

As children practice sitting upright, protective responses mature and children have the ability to catch themselves with their arms when they lose balance and fall forward or to either side of their bodies. The trunk muscles are strengthened further in a sitting position

TABLE 6.1 Early Motor Development

The milestones for development of motor skills are not achieved at fixed times; there is an age range for typical motor development, as infants become more proficient in working against the force of gravity, coordinating both sides of their body, and increasing motor precision. This table indicates the sequence in which motor skills are typically attained and the general age ranges within which they appear.

General Age Range	Motor Skills Demonstrated
1 Month	Lifts chin/head when placed on tummy; brings hand to mouth
2 Months	Lifts head and chest when placed on tummy.
3–4 Months	Begins to reach for objects; holds head up steadily when held in adult's lap; rolls side-to-side; plays with two hands at midline
5–6 Months	Sits alone for brief periods of time or propped on hands; turns over when laid on tummy or back; brings feet to hands/mouth
7–8 Months	Pulls self up while holding onto furniture; supports weight and bounces in supporting standing positions; sits independently; propels self by arms, knees, or wiggling movements; bangs blocks
9–11 Months	Stands independently; creeps on hands and knees; walks with two hands or one hand held
12–19 Months	Walks independently; slides down stairs backwards, one step at a time; stoops to pick up toys; climbs on furniture
24–30 Months	Walks with more coordination; jumps off bottom step; pushes self on wheeled toys
30–26 Months	Runs, but may not be able to stop smoothly; alternates feet going up stairs; throws ball overhand, but not always with accuracy; kicks a ball
4 years	Gallops and hops; jumps in place; jumps forward; throws ball overhand with accuracy
5 Years	Stands and balances briefly on tiptoes; skips alternating feet
6 Years	Throws and catches ball with improved accuracy

Source: Adapted from Gross Motor Milestones, Kids Can Do. Retrieved 7/3/12 from http://www.kidscando.org/milestones-grossmotor.html.

as a child reaches for objects located away from his or her body. As a child turns his or her body in order to reach for an object by the child's side, the child learns to master trunk rotation. Trunk rotation involves turning the upper body while keeping the lower body stationary. As the child turns to one side, the child's automatically shifts his or her weight to the reaching side of the body, and the trunk muscles keep the child upright despite the unequal distribution of weight of his or her body.

As sitting is mastered, the child learns to move in and out of the sitting position to other positions. Arms and the trunk are strengthened through these transitional movements, and the child now spends time in a stationary or rocking four-point position in which the child is supported by the palms and the knees. Moving from one position to another requires the child to shift his or her weight, which in turn requires postural stability and the ability to grade, or control, movement from one position to another (Bundy, 2008). Also in this time frame, the child can bear enough weight on his or her legs to stand with less support, "cruise," or move around while holding himself or herself upright on furniture, or walk with someone holding onto the child's hand.

There is a considerable age range of when children first demonstrate independent walking. Babies may begin to walk as early as 9 months and late as 16 months. Following the advent of walking, more independent motor skills are developed, such as climbing into an adult-sized chair and creeping up stairs. By their second year, children can propel a riding toy without pedals.

During the period from 3 to 5 years, movement skills are further refined. The child can maintain coordination as the child's ambulation (that is, moving from place to place) speed increases and can stay balanced when his or her feet have less contact with the ground. Motor skills typically progress to walking and running efficiently, jumping, climbing a jungle gym or the stairs of a slide, and finessing the body to move in and out of spaces of different sizes and elevations (Bundy, 2008). The young child can sit tailor fashion (legs crossed in front) on the floor to play a game. Ball skills have advanced to the ability to kick the ball, retrieve it, lean over to pick it up, and throw it back to his friend. By age 5, most children are learning to skip, hop on one foot, jump from a high step, and throw a ball smoothly and with some directional accuracy (Bundy, 2008).

Effects of Early-Onset Visual Impairment on Motor Development

As just described, all infants face the formidable task of mastering their own bodies and conquering gravity to eventually sit, crawl, stand, walk, and then run. As discussed in Chapter 1, however, when a child is born with or develops a visual impairment or deafblindness or within the first year of life, additional considerations need to be addressed to optimize motor development for movement and physical activity.

Early-onset visual impairment, whether it is a singular sensory loss or accompanied by hearing loss in the case of deafblindness, may affect not only how quickly a young child achieves the milestones in motor development but also the order in which the motor skills are learned and how well the child executes them (Ferrell, 1998, 2011). In young children with visual impairments or deafblindness, milestones that involve ambulation, such as crawling or independent walking, can be delayed in comparison to those developments in sighted peers (Fraiberg, 1977; Sonksen, Levitt, & Kitsinger, 1984; Tröster, Heckler, & Brambring, 1994). Parents of children with visual impairments have noted general delays in all dynamic or movement-based motor milestones (Celeste, 2002). The greatest delays involved cruising around furniture, walking independently, and walking up and down the stairs.

Early intervention from several different professionals can help the family develop and implement strategies to assist with the child's motor development. Under the Individuals with Disabilities Education Act (IDEA), discussed in Chapter 3, infants and toddlers with disabilities are eligible to receive early intervention services from birth to age 3. These services are provided by a multidisciplinary team of professionals, including a teacher of students with visual impairments and an orientation and movement (O&M) specialist, both of whom are trained to work specifically with children with visual impairments. Physical and occupational therapists who have special training in working with young children are also important team members. Speech and language therapists, other early development specialists, and other professionals might be included, depending on the child's developmental needs. The team works with the parents or guardian to produce a plan known as the Individualized Family Service Plan (IFSP), similar to the Individualized Education Program (IEP) discussed in Chapter 3, which details the services needed to support the child's development and includes services that will support the family. Development of motor skills and early concepts about the body and space that inform movement will likely be an important part of the IFSP for the young child with visual impairments or deafblindness.

A variety of factors can influence the motor development of a child with early-onset visual impairment. Three specific possible challenges to motor development examined in this chapter are lack of visual reinforcement for movement, reduced muscle tone, and delays in achieving the concept of object permanence. These issues may overlap one another in their influence on the child's attainment of motor skills, but they are reviewed separately in this chapter, along with intervention strategies designed to mitigate each factor and support the child in his or her path of motor development.

Vision in Motor Skills

Vision plays a role in the motor development skills of children who have sight, including children with low vision. The five primary functions of vision in the acquisition of motor skills (Brambring, 2006) that have been proposed include the following:

- providing an incentive to move
- allowing simultaneous and precise perception of the visible environment and the relationships of the objects within it
- serving a protective function by enabling anticipation of dangerous situations
- enabling control of movement by tracking its performance
- providing feedback to perfect motor performance based on monitoring the quality of executed movements

Two additional secondary functions (Brambring, 2006) are

- obtaining social feedback from seeing others' facial expressions or body language that invite or discourage movement
- observation of others that encourages imitation of movement

Lack of vision to perform these functions in support of motor development may delay the acquisition of specific motor skills or may compromise the performance of the skills.

The first function of vision in motor development—providing an incentive to move—is tied to the development of several early movement skills. An example of early movement that is linked to vision is a reflex called optical righting. This reflex can be demonstrated at 2 months of age when the baby is held an arm's length away from an adult and tilted to one side. The infant is visually reinforced to right his or her head to a position along the body's midline. As the infant works to right his or her head, the infant activates the muscles of the neck, upper extremities, and limbs. When the optical righting reflex is compromised by lack of visual reinforcement, the infant loses opportunities to strengthen head control, which in turn affects the development of neck and trunk muscles (Brown & Bour, 1986).

More frequently, lack of vision may delay the infant's effort to lift his or her head when the infant is lying on his or her stomach. The first obvious sign of motor delay in young children who are blind may be found as early as 3 months of age if the child does not lift his or her head (Prechtl et al., 2001). Vision serves as the lure for a sighted infant to lift his or her head when placed on his or her stomach. It is important, therefore, for caregivers of infants with visual impairments to be aware of how to use other senses to support the baby's desire to lift his or her head and support himself or herself on his or her forearms to strengthen his or her body for the next motor tasks. Sidebar 6.1 provides some suggested strategies. Lifting the head is hard work, so the baby will need to rest in other less-stressful positions.

At this time, and throughout the young child's development, it is helpful to pay attention to what objects and activities reinforce the child's activity. As Stokes (2002, p. 72) noted, "Babies build body-confidence and self-esteem when they follow their curiosity, interest, and desire." Once an object that is of interest to the baby has been noted, it can be used to encourage the baby to move and to assume different positions to play with it. For example, an interesting toy can initially be presented in front of the baby at his or her midline and then moved slightly off center so that the baby needs to shift his or her weight sideways to continue to interact with this toy.

Learning to make movement transitions, such as moving from a sitting to a kneeling position, has also been observed to be delayed or restricted because of reduced visual incentives and opportunities to observe others making such transitions (Brambring, 2006; Brown, Anthony, Shier Lowry, & Hatton, 2004). Sidebar 6.2 describes several strategies that will assist children with visual impairments in mastering transitional movements, including providing incentives to change positions, using physical guidance, using objects for physical support, and offering verbal instruction to guide the child's movements.

Muscle Tone

Another factor in the motor development of young children with visual impairments or deafblindness is muscle tone, which may complicate both the acquisition and execution of motor skills. *Muscle tone* refers to the tension in the body's muscles and provides "motoric 'readiness for movement'" (Rosen, 2010, p. 148) and the support base for independent sitting and mobility skills such as rolling, crawling, and walking (Anthony, Bleier, Fazzi, Kish, & Pogrund, 2002). When muscle tone is affected, a child may have difficulty maintaining a position (static postures) or moving fluidly to another position (dynamic postures).

Hypertonicity, or too much muscle tone, affects the child's ability to control and grade the child's movements (that is, not move too quickly or slowly) from one position to the other. Abnormally high muscle tone, as seen in children with spastic cerebral palsy, results

SIDEBAR 6.1

Strategies for Encouraging Babies to Lift Their Heads

The following suggestions will encourage babies to lift their heads when lying on their stomach, an important precursor to being able to use the hands, reach for objects, and sit independently:

- Place the baby on the chest of an adult who is reclining or lying on his or her back (Cutter, 2007; Stokes, 2002). The baby feels the resonance of the adult's slight body movements and vocal respirations. The baby can be helped to lift his or her head to feel a kiss, nuzzle, or the warm breath of the adult on his or her head or face. The adult can angle his or her body position to help the baby with this action; that is, in a more upright position, gravity will help the baby lift his or her head up off the adult's chest.
- Place the baby on the baby's stomach on a firm, flat surface with a light blanket underneath. Have the adult face the baby and kiss, nuzzle, or talk to the baby to motivate the baby to lift his or her head. The adult can begin by reinforcing the tiniest of movements and then, as the baby gains more motor control, wait for greater head lifts. If the baby has low vision, brightly colored, high-contrast, or illuminated objects can be used to invite the baby to lift his or her head.
- As the baby becomes better at lifting his or her head and freeing his or her hands for play, give the baby different textures and surfaces to stimulate the baby's tactile awareness. Soft squeeze toys may invite play when the baby is on his or her stomach. A scratchboard can be made with two different textures, such a soft bristle toy and a piece of corrugated cardboard glued on to a firm surface, for the baby's tactile pleasure. The idea is to provide something that will motivate the baby's hands to come to midline to play while the baby is trying to stay propped up on his or her forearms.
- Use a resonance board to reinforce the baby's movement. A resonance board is a low platform made of thin plywood raised about an inch off of the floor, which amplifies sound and stimulates movement. Place the baby on his or her tummy or back on the center of the resonance board, surrounded by objects and toys. As the baby moves spontaneously or to search for a nearby object, the baby's body movement will create resonance, or tactile vibration, underneath his or her body (Nielsen, 1992). The resonance board has been used been used very successfully to encourage children with visual impairments or deafblindness to move on their own. Self-initiated movements are critical so that the baby is not just passively responding to people moving his or her body, but is learning how to actively move and is using his or her body to learn more about his or her world (Anthony, 1993; Cutter, 2007).

in restricted movements caused by the stiffness in the child's arms or legs. It may take more time for the child to move his or her arms and legs, and the range of movement may be affected. Children who have visual impairments related to changes in the brain rather than in the eye (see Chapter 2) frequently also have cerebral palsy and resulting hypertonicity.

Infants born with significant visual impairment have been found to have a high incidence of hypotonicity, or low muscle tone (Jan, Robinson, Scott, & Kinnis, 1975; Rosen 2010), which makes initiating movement more difficult. Low muscle tone in young children who are blind or visually impaired and who do not have cerebral palsy or another motor-related diagnosis may be the result of several factors.

SIDEBAR 6.2

Strategies to Assist with Transition Movements

The following suggestions provide ways of supporting babies with visual impairments in learning how to move from one position to another:

- **Provide incentive for the change in position:** A young child will be more motivated to change position when he or she knows what is coming next. Give the child a physical cue such as touching her hand to a favorite ball and announcing, "Let's play with your ball." Or move the object of interest to a location that requires a change in position, such as placing the ball on a higher surface, so she will need to pull up to a standing position to get this object of interest. If the child cannot see the object that has been moved to a new location, allow the child to hold on to it and follow as it is gently moved and placed on the higher surface. With the child still holding onto the ball, it can be tapped on the surface to confirm its new location, as the child works to pull herself upright to continue the play with the ball.
- **Provide motor guidance:** An occupational or physical therapist can assist the family with how to gently guide the child through the incremental movements involved with changing positions. As the child becomes more proficient with these movements, it may still be helpful for the adult to place his or her hand in a strategic place to give stability to the child as he or she changes position. For example, if a child is on her tummy and working to get to a sitting position, it may be helpful to put a firm hand on the baby's hip to stabilize it while she rotates her body to lift upward on her arms.
- **Provide Transitional Support Objects:** A low table, bench, or ottoman can be strategically placed for child to pull up on or hold onto as she moves from sitting to kneeling on one leg to a standing position.
- **Provide Verbal Instruction:** Verbal directions can be offered to the child to guide step-by-step movements from one position to the next. This strategy can be used only when the child has sufficient language skills to process verbal directions, however. If the child is deafblind, it will be important to use a communication mode that is meaningful to the child (see Chapter 4 for a discussion of communication with individuals who are deafblind).

A common theory of low muscle tone with infants with visual impairments involves the lack of "visual tutoring" of the vestibular, proprioceptive, and kinesthetic senses (Brown & Bour, 1986; Prechtl, Cioni, Einspieler, Bos, & Ferrari, 2001). The vestibular system, located in the inner ear, provides unconscious feedback on where the body is in space and helps in maintaining balance. The proprioceptive and kinesthetic senses, located in receptors in the bones, joints, ligaments, and muscles, provide an internal sense of where one's body is in space, where individual body parts are in relation to one another, and the strength of effort an infant uses when moving (see Chapter 2). The vestibular, proprioceptive, and kinesthetic senses benefit from visual reinforcement. Without visual feedback from body movements, the infant may have fewer opportunities to deliberately move his or her arms, hands, legs, and feet. Lack of visual feedback from motor skills reduces the child's reinforcement for practicing proprioceptive awareness and developing muscle tone (Rosen, 2010).

Poor vestibular function may be present in children who are deaf/hard of hearing, including those with deafblindness. In rare instances, such as infants with CHARGE syndrome, which typically results in combined vision and hearing loss (see Chapter 2), the child may also have low or absent vestibular function (Brown, 2007; see Sidebar 6.3).

Low muscle tone can affect the age at which a child reaches milestones in motor development (Brown & Bour, 1986; Jan et al., 1975). Children with low muscle tone often have decreased endurance in motor activity, reduced trunk strength, and out-toeing (turning the feet outward to assist with widening the base of gravity). Low muscle tone appears to have more impact on milestones that do not involve movement, such maintaining an independent sitting position, as opposed to movement milestones such as crawling or walking (Brambring, 2006).

The child's movement may also be affected by low muscle tone. The child may use postural adjustments called "fixing" to support movement or sustain a posture (Rosen, 2010). Postural fixing may offer short-term stability but will limit mobility and the development of true postural stability (Brown & Bour, 1986). Examples of postural fixing in the sitting position include keeping the legs far apart for a wider base of support, sitting with a rounded back to lower the center of gravity, or keeping the hands on the floor to support an upright sitting posture. Postural fixing can also be seen when walking, for example, keeping the legs far apart for a wider base of support, using shuffling or very small steps to maintain more contact with the ground, and locking the knees to help with upright stability. Such body compensations are needed to do what the trunk cannot do because of low muscle tone in the child's core muscles. Although postural fixing enables the child to sit or walk, it compromises and will restrict further movements. For example, when the child is sitting upright, the child risks losing his or her balance when turning or reaching to grab a toy. If the child "undoes the fix" for such actions, the child may lose his or

SIDEBAR 6.3

Effects of Hearing Loss on Motor Development

Poor vestibular function, which affects early head control and overall balance, may be seen in very young children who are deaf, hard of hearing, or deafblind. In addition to children diagnosed with CHARGE syndrome, children at risk for poor vestibular function include those diagnosed with Usher syndrome Type 1, a genetic condition in which children have a profound congenital hearing loss and early-onset visual impairment caused by a degenerative condition called retinitis pigmentosa (see Chapter 2).

These children often have very poor balance that is evident very early in life. It is important for children with deafblindness to be evaluated for their vestibular function by a medical expert recommended by the family's physician if there are any concerns about "weak necks," "floppy heads," or delayed upright sitting and general concerns about balance and equilibrium (Rapin, Korey, Schick, & Kennedy, 1974; Valente & McCaslin, 2011). If poor vestibular function is found, an occupational or physical therapist on the child's early intervention team needs to work closely with the teacher of students with visual impairments and O&M specialist to develop an appropriate motor program that addresses the child's safety and movement needs.

her upright sitting posture. Playing in this fixed position is restricted to objects contained in the child's lap or close to the child's body. The child's ability to play independently with at least one, but preferably two, hands free (Bundy, 2008) is limited if the child is using the hands for support. The postural fixes that are evident when the child is walking restrict the speed of the locomotion.

Low muscle tone also affects the child's arm and leg strength, which is needed for motor milestones involving weight bearing, such as propping up on the forearms in a prone (tummy) position, using arms for transitional movements such as moving from a tummy position to a sitting position and crawling on hands and knees. Strength in the upper extremities becomes important for throwing a ball, carrying items when walking, using a long cane, and using the hands and arms in recreation activities and sports. Lower extremity strength is important for kicking, running, climbing, and jumping.

A variety of strategies that can be used to address low muscle tone, possible compensatory fixing behaviors, and reduced strength in the upper and lower extremities are presented in Sidebar 6.4. In addition to encouraging the suggested activities, parents and other caregivers should be aware of the child's base of support when the child is playing. The height of the table or working surface may need to be lowered or elevated to make the task either less or more physically challenging. For example, toys can be placed on a nearby coffee table where the child must pull up to stand and remain standing to play with the toys.

SIDEBAR 6.4

Strategies for Addressing Low Postural Tone

The following strategies help a child to develop better postural tone and support the development of increased strength in the upper and lower extremities:

- Place the young child on an adult's chest, over the adult's leg, or on a therapy ball as a way to build core strength. As the adult moves gently back and forth or rocks the therapy ball, the child has to use her neck, stomach, and back muscles to respond to the pull of gravity on her body due to the moving ground surface. The same result can be achieved for an older child, by placing the child on a slow-moving horse (known as hippotherapy), which causes the child to use her trunk muscles in response to the weight shifts caused by the horse's movements.
- Play tug-of-war games with the child in a prone, supine, or sitting position. As the child grasps a lightweight toy or facecloth, the adult gently pulls it away and encourages the baby to hang on and pull back. More advanced tug-of-war games can be played in a standing position with a hula-hoop or rope.
- Put the child in play situations that motivate her to move her body. For example, water play in the tub or a kiddie pool will invite splashing with arms and legs. Actual swimming lessons with an adult in a larger pool are also likely to be highly motivating.
- Ask a preschool or older child to help carry items such as a gallon milk carton from the refrigerator to the table or to help to pull out the mats for rough-and-tumble play in preschool.

Object Permanence

A third consideration that should be addressed in the early intervention strategies designed to support the motor development growth in the young child who is blind or visually impaired is the role of object permanence. Object permanence is the understanding that objects continue to exist even when they are out of sight. The average age for sighted children to attain this concept is approximately 9 months of age. Before this point, an infant will reach for objects in view but will stop searching when the object is hidden. Object permanence is attained when the child continues to look for something he or she cannot see or looks for an object where it previously was found.

Achieving the concept of object permanence plays an important role in the self-initiated locomotion of the child with a visual impairment, as discussed in Chapter 1, as it shows that the child understands that objects and people exist beyond the child's body and lures the child toward objects that are out of reach (Bigelow, 1986; Fraiberg, Siegel, & Gibson, 1966). There is a healthy age range for the acquisition of object permanence for children with blindness or visual impairment, and evidence indicates that some children may achieve this concept within the age range for children with typical sight (Fraiberg et al., 1966; Rogers & Puchalski, 1988). However, the median age at which a child who is blind or visually impaired and without any additional disabilities will search for an object that has been removed has been reported to be 13.4 months (Ferrell, 1998). Interestingly, there appears to be no difference in the timetable for beginning to search for an object that makes noise or one that does not for the child who is blind, as both tasks require the concept of object permanence (Fraiberg et al., 1966). The sound of the nearby object does not appear to invite the child to search for it before he or she has attained object permanence.

Typically, before the age of 9 months, or the acquisition of object permanence, neither sighted children nor children with visual impairments understand that an object or person continues to exist when that object or person is out of full view. Both sighted and visually impaired children appear to acquire the concept of object permanence through a comparable cognitive process (Bigelow, 1986). The important difference is that although children with typical sight do not reach for a hidden object prior to the onset of object permanence, they have abundant visual access to the world beyond their body. They begin to lean forward or to the side to stretch, reach, and ultimately move to objects of interest that they can see, even though the objects are not located within touching distance. Sighted children will reach consistently for a visible object at 6 to 7 months, but children with visual impairments do not develop that ability until 10 months or later, when they demonstrate true object permanence (Fraiberg et al., 1966). Therefore, children with visual impairments may have fewer experiences with reaching out to touch and explore objects. Until they understand that people and objects exist beyond what they can reach—that is, until they have the concept of object permanence—they cannot self-initiate crawling or walking. Reaching out in space is the critical link to self-propelled movement for a child who is blind; crawling and walking often follow shortly after the child begins to reach for objects (Fraiberg, 1968). The act of reaching should be considered as "one of the first self-initiated contacts that a child who is blind makes with the external world" (Bigelow, 1986, p. 355).

A general sequence of reaching behavior by young children who are blind or significantly visually impaired highlights the power of touch over sound at this stage of development and provides important intervention strategies

(Bigelow, 1986; Fraiberg, 1968). The first evidence of reaching occurs when a sound-producing object held at midline is removed gently and slowly from the child's hands and the child responds by moving his or her hands in the direction of the object that has been taken away. The child reaches to find the object that was just in the child's hands. With practice, the child is able next to reach at midline to a continuously sounding object that has not touched the child's hands. Touch first, then sound, serves as a cue to the object's existence and location. Sidebar 6.5 presents some activities that encourage the development of reaching behavior (see also Gleason, 2004; Kukla & Thomas, 1978).

Parents and early interventionists can create responsive play environments where the smallest movements will put the child into contact with objects kept in the same places. Availability and consistency of these objects will help the child develop object permanence. An example of a responsive play environment is the Little Room, which is made from three plexiglass wall panels that surround the child (Nielsen, 1992). Various everyday household objects and toys that appeal to the senses are hung from the top of the Little Room and anchored to the two sides. (Care must be taken so the elastic cords securing the objects cannot harm the child.) Whenever the child moves his or her body, the child will come into contact with a nearby object that may invite further manual exploration. The child has many opportunities to come into contact with play objects and begins to deliberately return to the places where the child will find the

SIDEBAR 6.5

Reaching to Sound

The following sequence of activities creates appropriate opportunities for the young baby to learn to reach:

- Choose a variety of squeak toys, rattles, bells, and other noisemakers that produce interesting sounds and are close in size to what the baby can hold. Be careful that the noise is not too scary, shrill, or loud so that it overloads a baby's senses and he or she will "tune it out" altogether.
- Make the sound first at ear level and on the side. Wait for the baby to turn his head toward the sound. If he does not turn his head the first time, make the sound again and gently push his head toward that side; then bring his hand up to touch the toy and make the sound again
- Change the position of the sounds. Once your baby can turn her head to sounds made at the side, move the sound down below ear level. The baby will turn her head first to the side, and then down. Again, coordinate the sound with a reaching movement by taking her hand to touch the object.
- Continue to move the location of sound once the baby has mastered each location. When the baby can localize—that is, identify from where a sound is coming—and demonstrates this by turning his head to sounds below ear level, the next position is above ear level. Use the same procedures you've already used. At this point, you can also start moving the sound out in front of your baby.

Sources: D. Kukla & T. Thomas, *Assessment of Auditory Functioning of Deafblind/Multihandicapped Children* (Dallas, TX: South Central Regional Resource Center for Services to Deaf-Blind Children, 1978). Adapted from K. Ferrell, *Reach Out and Teach: Helping Your Child Who Is Visually Impaired Learn and Grow,* 2d ed. (New York: AFB Press, 2011), p. 181.

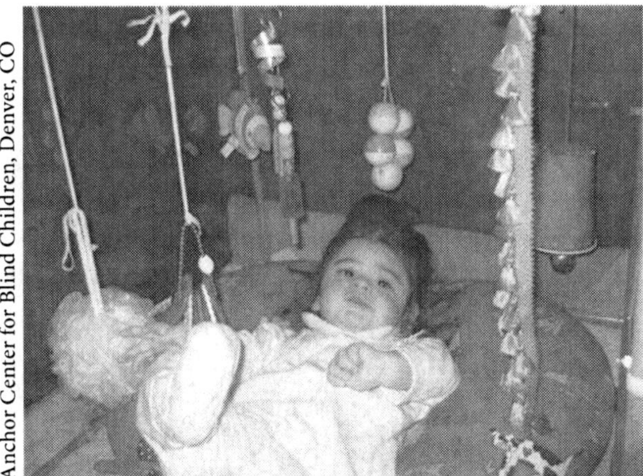
Anchor Center for Blind Children, Denver, CO

A responsive play environment, in which the smallest movement puts the child in contact with an object, helps the child learn about object permanence.

objects that capture his or her interest. As with any play situation with young children, adult supervision is necessary at all times.

All three of the variables just described that can affect the motor development of young children with visual impairments—the effects of absent or reduced visual incentive, low muscle tone, and a possible delay in achieving object permanence—respond positively to well-designed early intervention strategies. Being aware of these challenges enables families and professionals to understand the solutions and address the child's needs. Determining the child's sensory preferences will help ensure that the child receives appropriate incentives for movement. Mitigating low muscle tone and reduced strength in the body core and the extremities can enable the child to develop more postural stability and smoother body movements. Finally, recognizing the link of object permanence to reaching and independent movement can help in creating responsive play environments.

DEVELOPMENT OF PLAY

The intervention strategies that have already been highlighted to support motor development essentially involve the use of play to encourage children with visual impairments to use more sophisticated motor actions or ambulatory movements. If families and professionals understand how play skills develop, they can provide better interventions to encourage motor development.

Play has long been thought of as the "work" of the young child. Early childhood experts agree that play supports ongoing developmental growth and is a window to interpreting a young child's knowledge and skills (Linder, 2008). Through play, children learn to expand, refine, and challenge their physical and movement abilities. In turn, increased physical skills will lead children to more sophisticated types of play, recreation, and sports.

Seven types of play emerge between birth and 6-plus years of age:

- interpersonal play
- exploratory and sensorimotor play
- functional and relational play
- constructive play
- dramatic play
- physical activity and rough-and-tumble play
- games with rules

Each category has a time frame when it is the dominant form of play, builds on the play skills from prior categories, and boosts other developmental domains, including motor development (Linder, 2008). Each play category is reviewed in this chapter with specific guidance on how it relates to a child's budding motor development and preparation to participate in recreational activities and sports.

Interpersonal Play

The social-emotional exchange between an infant and his or her caregiver marks the beginning of a lifetime of interpersonal relationships and the infant's sense of self. The baby engages with the baby's caregivers through touching, looking, vocalizing, and early movements. Caregivers in turn, touch, look, and vocalize back to the child. These reciprocal exchanges, along with predictable care routines, foster an attachment or a base of security for the developing infant. This early security base is critical for the infant's growing ability to interact with others and to initiate his or her own movement within the infant's ever-expanding world. Secure attachment is related to all infants' desire to venture out into the environment to explore and experience it (Warren & Hatton, 2003).

Interpersonal play describes face-to-face interactions, including early social games such as Peek-a-Boo or Pat-a-Cake. As a baby matures, play interactions with other people become more complex and involve skills of imitation and turn taking with both adults and other children. The child expands his or her understanding of cause and effect in physical activity (that is, "I do something and something happens") and deliberately signals to the other person to continue a fun activity, such as by reaching out to his or her daddy's hand to continue a tickling or bouncing game. When the baby is reinforced for touching the daddy's hand to continue the game, the baby is learning the power of his or her actions.

When a baby is blind or visually impaired, early face-to-face games should involve more opportunities for body-on-body contact, such as when the baby is placed chest down on top of the adult, to encourage the baby to lift his or her head. Body-to-body contact increases the intimacy of the play and provides the baby with direct feedback from the adult's movements on the baby's body that is not being provided visually.

When combined with the baby's increasing interest in objects, interpersonal play leads to exploration and sensorimotor play (Linder, 2008). By 3 months, the baby is physically ready to act deliberately with objects. At this point, the baby is more able to raise his or her head and to prop himself or herself up on the forearms, so that the baby's hands are in a better position to interact with objects.

Exploratory and Sensorimotor Play

Exploratory and sensorimotor play is what an infant does to enjoy the sensory input gained from the activity, such as mouthing an object or shaking a rattle (Linder, 2008). Early object use involves early schemes (deliberate motor actions on objects) such as oral exploration of pacifiers or other mouthing toys or lightweight rattles. The infant continues to expand motor actions on toys for a desired sensory result, such as batting at an overhead mobile to watch it move or hear its chimes.

Activities can be designed to encourage the infant to touch new objects. When the infant is lying on his or her back with arms out to the side, the caregiver can add tactile boundaries to the side of the infant for exploration. The blanket underneath the infant can have different textures for exploration. Mylar paper placed underneath or on top of the blanket will provide an interesting crinkle sound when the infant makes a simple arm movement across

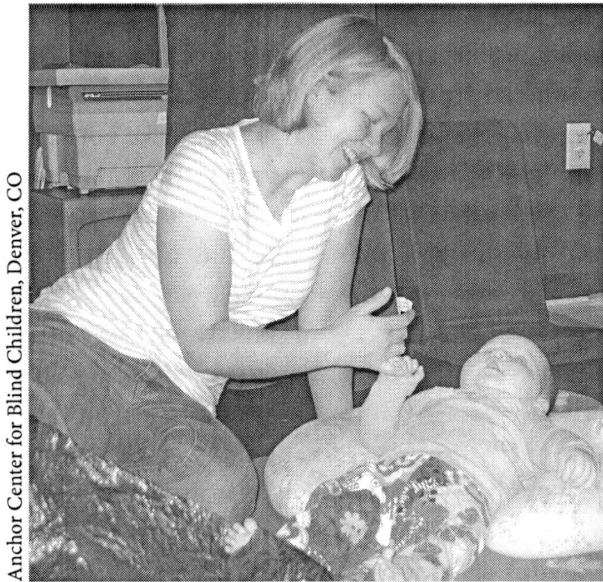

The social-emotional exchange between an infant and his or her caregiver marks the beginning of a lifetime of interpersonal relationships and the infant's sense of self.

the surface or actually grasps the paper. When objects are given to the infant, they should be offered hand-under-hand so the infant has an opportunity to take the object placed under his or her hand.

In addition to encouraging the child to use his or her hands as tools for play, providing other motor strengthening and object interaction opportunities will encourage the child to use other parts of his or her body. Children who are blind, visually impaired, or deafblind may also use also their heads or their feet for exploration (Greeley & Anthony, 1995). With proper supervision, a variety of activities can be designed to encourage a child to use his or her feet. The staff members at one early-intervention center that is designed specifically for very young children with visual impairments have become experts at such activities, which include the following:

- Placing a musical keyboard, Mylar pom poms, or a resonance board next to the child's feet. As the child's random touching to produces a sound or tactile vibration on the child's feet, the child's touching becomes more deliberate.
- Positioning a switch toy, which is a battery-operated toy that can be activated by the child's bearing weight on a pressure switch, at the child's feet.
- Putting tap dancing shoes on the child while the child is in a standing or a supine position. When the child is lying on his or her back, a board can be held perpendicular to the floor next to the child's tap-shoed feet to invite repetitive kicks.

Learning about new objects is reinforced by consistent and frequent play. Opportunities for repetition increase the accuracy of a specific action upon an object and the child's judgment about what action to use on a new object. With practice, the child becomes more proficient in grasping objects positioned on either side of the body and can cross midline and transfer an object from one hand to another. Caregivers and professionals need to be vigilant about ensuring practice opportunities. For some children, especially those with physical restrictions, the use of a Little Room or a play board with objects safely attached will promote active learning.

By 6 to 9 months, new motor actions are added to the child's early repertoire, such as waving, turning objects over, poking, tearing, pushing, and pulling (Linder, 2008). Both the child's thinking and hand skills are becoming more refined and enabling more sophisticated types of object interaction. Actions become more attuned to the features of the object as the child begins to discriminate what object is best to shake, bang, poke, push, or squeeze to get the desired sensory result. This level of discrimination or problem solving is the bridge to functional and relational play.

Functional and Relational Play

Building on sensory exploration and simple manipulation of objects, the child begins to learn how to use objects through observation of these objects in daily routines or, more importantly, through hands-on opportunities to use these objects within daily routines. A cup is recognized visually or by tactile exploration as a drinking receptacle, a brush is brought to another's person's hair, and a ball is used for throwing or kicking.

Highlighting how objects are used by different people and in different environments can help the child understand that an object he or she is familiar with for an intended purpose may be used for that same purpose by another person. For example, the child has a hat to wear for going outside in the sun and so does Dad, and there are different kinds of hats for different places and activities: a knit hat for going out in the snow for sledding and a hat with a brim for outdoor ball play in the summer to keep from getting sunburn on one's face. More functional use concepts can be taught through daily routines; for example, shoes are for feet and mittens are for hands; Dad has really big mittens and Baby Sister has little mittens; and Big Brother has a leather glove different from everyone's mittens that he uses to catch a baseball.

The child begins to show an ongoing understanding of what to do with certain objects based on their physical design and should be encouraged to act independently to figure out how an object works. A choice of objects can be offered from which the child can select the one that is right for a particular task. For example, while playing with a ball, the child can be given a bucket of several objects and asked to locate the ball among the other objects.

Parents and professionals can provide simple suggestions about how to interact with a new toy: "This toy has a pull string like your other toy. Can you find the round ring on the side of the toy? That's right. Now let's give it a pull and see what happens!" This type of guiding language can help the child with further exploration of a toy and is the foundation for directions later on such as explaining the use of equipment in recreational games and physical activities.

Children with a visual impairment or blindness may have an advantage over sighted children in exploring a novel toy, as children who are blind or visually impaired may use more tactile exploration strategies than their sighted peers (Olson, 1983). When adults encourage or allow a child time to fully explore the tactile features of an object, the child with a visual impairment is more likely to discern the features of the toy and how to use it. It is important to avoid immediately giving directions when children encounter new objects and allow them adequate time for exploration (as is also true for older students and adults, as discussed in Chapter 4).

By 8 to 9 months of age, the infant demonstrates understanding that specific actions are needed to use specific toys. The child begins to combine objects in play, such as putting smaller items into a larger container. Early training in echolocation (listening to sounds or echoes to obtain information about physical features of a travel environment) begins during container play, as the child learns to listen to the sound of objects of different sizes and materials when they are dropped into containers with different-sized openings and made from different materials (Daniel Kish, personal communication, April 2011). This activity also provides considerable resonance or tactile-vibratory reinforcement for children who are deafblind.

Predictable storage places for toys and various household objects and defined play environments are helpful for the child who is blind or visually impaired (Lowry, 2004). As Linder (1993, p. 29) notes, "Play is facilitated by an environment where toys and materials are visible and accessible to children." With experience, the child also learns that toys belong in a toy box, dishes in a kitchen cupboard, and clothes in a dresser in the bedroom. Once the child has mastered the concept of object permanence, asking the child to retrieve a familiar object from a familiar place where it is stored teaches early orientation and mobility (O&M) routes within the home (Anthony et al., 2002).

During the child's first and second years of life, the child's ability to relate one object to another object increases. When objects are part of daily routines, the young child can learn how objects interact with one another and where they belong. This is an ideal time for the child to learn about the objects associated with recreation activities and sports, such as a helmet corresponding to the bicycle in the garage for Saturday bike rides with mom. Sara, a 22-month-old child who is blind, announces emphatically, "Swimsuit, swimsuit!" (one of her handful of words) and makes her way quickly to the drying rack in the laundry room when she wants to go to the backyard kiddie pool after her afternoon nap.

Constructive Play

Around the age of 1 year, a child's first constructions often involve stacking cans or blocks. By 18 to 24 months, most toddlers are capable of thinking before acting and inventing a solution to a play situation (Parks, Furono, O'Reilly, Inatsuka, Hosaka, & Zeisloft-Falbey, 1994). For example, the child may begin to build a wall of blocks with a deliberate space in between the blocks for a play car to travel through to the other side. Learning how to use materials to build something becomes a more dominant play skill after 3 years of age. Motor skills are strengthened during this type of play. Floor play such as building with shoe boxes, couch cushions, or other materials lets the child practice moving from one position to another and stretching up as the child makes the structure grow taller and wider (Bundy, 2008). The child should be deliberately exposed to construction toys such as small cushions or large blocks. Early intervention personnel, including teachers of students with visual impairments and O&M specialists, can deliberately model constructive play opportunities with children using everyday household or preschool classroom materials so that their students with blindness or visual impairment may frequently be given or may choose objects that have noise or resonance attributes, sometimes at the expense of constructive or creative art play items (Tröster & Brambring, 1994). Although there is a place for auditory-based playthings, care should be taken to analyze if the toy merely has an interesting sound or truly invites problem solving to activate, stimulates a higher level of play, or encourages active movement. For selecting toys that reinforce movement, parents, other caregivers, and early childhood professionals need to examine how toys with noise or resonance attributes can be used to encourage movement. For example, a sound-making toy that interests the child may be placed in new locations of a room for a child to find, or a beeping ball can be used in a rolling or kicking game as a tool to encourage the child to locate the ball as it moves farther away from or closer to the child.

As the child builds with an end product in mind, he or she prepares for dramatic and symbolic play in the land of "let's pretend." Common objects and the experiences tied to those everyday objects become the fabric for more sophisticated play that involves higher-thinking skills such as imagination and purposeful construction.

Dramatic Play

By 18 months of age, the child shows more imagination in play. Early dramatic play generally emerges just before the second year and continues through 6 years of age. Also called pretend or symbolic play, dramatic play is when objects are used as if they were something else. Symbolic play occurs when an object that is not meant for a particular task is used for a completely different purpose, such as using a block as a pretend cell phone or a twig as a hockey stick, baseball bat, or golf club.

Props encourage children to model activities that the child has observed others do during daily routines, such as eating with chopsticks, sweeping the floor with a small broom, or pushing a toy cart through the kitchen and loading items into it from the refrigerator and cupboards for the next step, a tea party. When families are recreation- or sports-minded, their children will have opportunities to play at bowling, biking, rock climbing, goalball, or ice skating.

Dramatic play offers a wonderful opportunity for children to practice gross motor movements, because pretend play involves characters who dance, chase, run, drive vehicle toys, and make a quick escape to the couch-cushion fortress (Bundy, 2008). Using his or her arms and legs while lying on his or her tummy, the child can propel a scooter board across the gym floor and pretend with the other kids to be driving a car: "Stop, it's a red light. Go, it's a green light." Acting out stories can lead to physical activity, as the child climbs in and out of the baby bear's chair, the mama bear's chair, and the papa bear's chair (Anthony, 1999). The props for acting out the story can involve a host of items that invite climbing, crawling, and jumping activities.

Physical Activity and Rough-and-Tumble Play

Play can build a child's physical endurance, strength, and balance. Movement tasks are inherent in physical activity and rough-and-tumble play. As the child has his or her first experiences with movement within the arms of a trusted person, the child will respond more to other rough-and-tumble play activities. Young children will initiate physical activity for the sake of feeling their body movements and as a way to participate in activity at the hands of another person or with other children. In the first months of life, infants will kick their legs repeatedly in happy pleasure at this self-initiated action. Later, children will rock back-and-forth on their hands and knees to feel the movement of their bodies in this new weight-bearing position. Very young children will enjoy bouncing on an adult's knee, being tickled, or being swung in a blanket. Parts of the child's body can be specifically targeted in games of "I'm going to get your—" (insert the name of a body part), as the adult names the body part to be touched and watches for the child's reaction when the right or the wrong body part is tickled.

Physical play can involve learning how to sequence one action or body movement after another, such as how to get on and off a rocking horse, go up and down a slide, or follow a sounding ball and throw it back to a friend. The game Simon Says is a great way for children to practice listening and following specific and varied directions: "Walk slow; walk fast; turn in a circle; put your hand on the floor, now in the air," and so on.

The preschool child is often especially interested in rough-and-tumble play where children run and chase one another or engage in

SIDEBAR 6.6

Early Rough-and-Tumble Play Activities

The following activities can help young children with visual impairments become used to rough-and-tumble play, starting when they are infants and continuing in more active ways throughout toddlerhood, and prepare them for interacting with other children.

- **Body-on-body play:** A young baby is placed on her tummy on top of an adult's reclining body, as the adult rocks gently so the baby can feel the to-and-fro movements. As the infant's motor control becomes more established, the adult can exaggerate the body movements so that the child is experiencing more of a need to respond to the pull of gravity. Once the baby is able to stay upright, they can play games such as "horsey" with the child positioned on the adult's knee, so that the child feels the up and down of the adult's leg against her body.
- **Mad tickle games:** When the child has the benefit of the floor underneath the length of her body, the adult can play a tickle game where the adult's hands move from one limb to another in a fun tickling fashion. As the child squirms from the tickling hands, she will experience the feel of movement of her body on the ground surface.
- **Hammock Play:** In a swaddled position in a blanket, the child can feel the rhythmic movements of being rocked back and forth by an adult at each end of the blanket.
- **Airplane:** With proper support, the child can feel the whoosh of air as she is lifted up in the air in safe hands.
- **Moving or Dancing to Rhythms or Music:** With the steady tap of a drum, favorite song, or an activity song, the child is given free rein to move to the beat or follow a specified routine of body movements such as raising hands in the air, clapping, stamping feet, spinning, etc.
- **Throwing and Chasing Balls:** The child catches or chases a rolled or thrown ball. As the child becomes more proficient, the distance can be increased. Balls with bells can be used for children who are blind or have a severe visual impairment.
- **Obstacle Course:** Navigating through tunnels, over gym mats, up and down stairs, and the like will build balance, physical strength, and motor planning skills.

roughhousing activities. It is important for children who are blind or visually impaired to be comfortable with fast movement and rough-and-tumble play that occurs in preschool settings.

Developmentally appropriate motor activities for preschoolers include sack-jumping, ice skating (with or without a cone, chair, or bucket or other prop for support), and climbing walls. Sidebar 6.6 lists some activities that can help young children with visual impairments, starting at a very early age, gradually become used to rough-and-tumble play.

Movement tasks that involve bilateral play with both arms and both legs will encourage more coordination, as do movement games that require practice with balance, jumping on a trampoline, or floor games with balls. It will be easier for children to learn how to kick first a static ball and then a moving one.

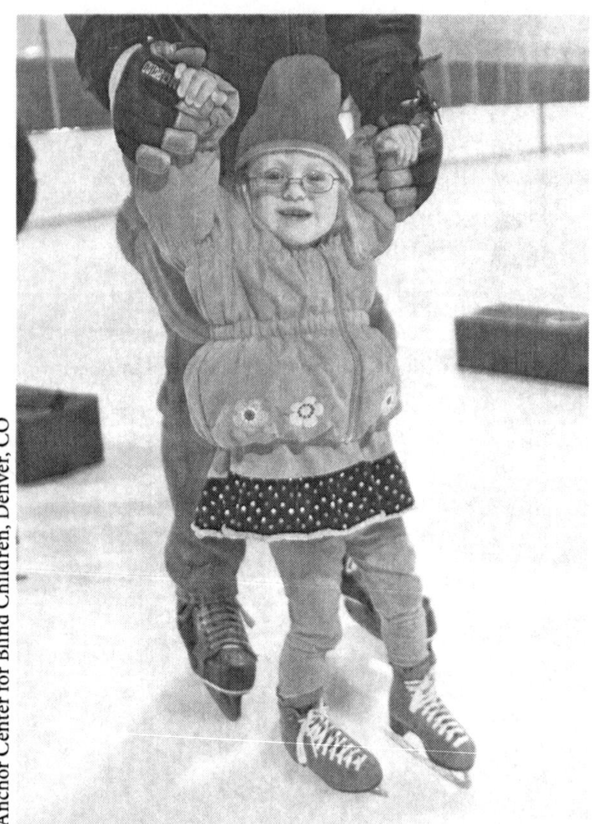

Anchor Center for Blind Children, Denver, CO

Ice skating is an appropriate activity for preschoolers that helps them get used to more rough and tumble play.

As a child develops motor competence and plays increasingly active movement games, the child continues to learn how games are played. Games with rules are the last type of play to develop.

Playing Games with Rules

Children 5 years of age and older recognize that some games have rules that they need to follow in order to play the game with others. Preschool children will have exposure to games with rules in early motor games such as Duck-Duck-Goose or Hide-and-Seek. Such games require some element of shared expectations and a need to comply with the understood procedures of the game (Garvey, 1977). Turn taking is a common feature of games with rules. The games may have preset rules, such as with an established card or board game, or may involve made-up rules by the players. Games with rules also involve concepts of winning and losing.

Motor games with rules need to be explained to children with visual impairments or deafblindness, just as they are explained to their sighted peers (see Chapter 4 for discussion of instructing children with visual impairments and communicating with children who are deafblind). It may be helpful to provide a human guide in the beginning for games that involve circling around a group of children such as Duck-Duck-Goose. Tactile adaptations may be needed in board games.

As the young child with visual impairment or deafblindness expands his or her repertoire of play skills and increases his or her understanding of the world, the concurrent evolution of the child's motor skills also contributes to developmentally appropriate and future recreation and leisure activities. Physical play is the primary avenue for all children to practice gross motor skills (Bundy, 2008).

PREPARING FOR PRESCHOOL AND BEYOND

Children between 3 and 5 years of age are generally very active explorers of their environment and enjoy moving and discovering new ways to discharge physical energy. As children with visual impairments or deafblindness spend more of their time in the world beyond their home, perhaps in a preschool program, it is important that parents, other caregivers, and early childhood professionals understand how to support and expand the child's play and physical skills.

By 3 years of age, a child with a visual impairment or deafblindness may attend a preschool. At that time, the child makes the transition from early-intervention services to educational services, and a team of professionals will work with the parents to draw up the child's first IEP, as discussed in Chapter 3. As part of this process, the teacher of students with visual impairments and O&M specialist should work together with the child's parents or other caregivers and the other members of the educational team to target the child's specific motor skill needs. The IEP should reflect appropriate motor goals and objectives for the child based on an assessment of the child's sensory, cognitive, communication, social-emotional, and motor status needs. The assessment data are used to identify needed accommodations, such as the use of special lighting, specific colors, high contrast, tactile materials, or auditory adaptations in materials or equipment used for early literacy, play, and movement activities; needed wait time between presenting materials and expecting the child to respond; and the use of an adapted mobility device or a long cane for independent travel, if needed.

If the child has both vision and hearing loss, it is critical that the educational team be aware of and fully utilize the child's communication system (see the discussion of communication in Chapter 4). A child may use a picture or tactile symbol board, sign language, or both to communicate. Appropriate pictures, tactile symbols, and signs should be used to help the child prepare for the activities of the preschool day. A speech and language therapist, a teacher of children who are deaf or hard of hearing, and an educational interpreter may all need to be part of the team that oversees the communication program for the child with deafblindness who has communication challenges.

Physical activities can be built into a preschool program, so that all the children have ample opportunities to move, expend energy, and master new motor skills. The preschool program can be designed so that there is at least one physical activity during each hour of its program time. It may be as simple as having the children move from one location to another for the different activities of the preschool day. The children can help gather and set up the materials needed for each activity from cupboards and shelves so that the children are actively reaching, squatting, and lifting. One preschool

SIDEBAR 6.7

Guidance for the Preschool Teacher

The teacher of students with visual impairments and O&M specialist can provide helpful guidance for the preschool teacher that will help address the individual needs of a child with visual impairments or deafblindness, such as the following:

- Concrete information about what the child sees and hears, as well as what types of equipment and materials may help the child to see and hear, as in the following example:

  Meribeth, a child with albinism, can recognize a familiar face from up to 10 feet away and identifies clear, uncluttered pictures of objects that are 1 to 2 inches high. Her vision is less reliable in overly bright lighting, and she is light sensitive outside, which is why she needs to wear her tinted glasses and a hat with a brim when she is outside.

- Information about how the child uses senses other than vision, or other than hearing (if the child is deafblind), for learning. The more the preschool teacher and other team members understand the sensory abilities and needs of the child, the better they can ensure an optimal learning and movement environment.
- Guidance on pre-teaching the concepts and equipment associated with preschool tasks involving motor skills. If the children are going to do a sack hop, for example, it will be helpful for a child with visual impairment or deafblindness to examine the cloth bag before the hop begins. The child can also practice hopping first without stepping inside the bag, to make sure the child has the same level of that skill that his or her classmates do.
- Physical modeling to "motor" the child through a needed motor task (see Chapter 4), including the following steps:
  - Having the child feel the teacher's body as the teacher completes a motor task, for example, how to bend your knees when it is time to jump up high.
  - Working together to practice the motion.
  - Using language that corresponds to the actions that the child can understand to provide cues for the next part of a motor action.

teacher situated the shelves in her room so that reaching a toy involved stretching tall or bending low. She also asked the children to crawl through a tunnel to get to the book mat where a story was read each afternoon. Other motor preschool activities include gross motor play on indoor and outdoor equipment (mats, obstacle courses, swings, slides, and tricycles).

A key guiding principle for children with visual impairments or deafblindness in preschool is the importance of maintaining age-appropriate expectations for the children's physical activities and putting in place customized accommodations and instructional strategies that ensure that the children have the needed information to participate in these activities. (Sidebar 6.7 provides some suggestions about the kinds of assistance and information that teachers of students with visual impairments and O&M specialists can provide to preschool teachers to help them formulate such strategies.)

Sometimes the staff members of a preschool program or other caregivers are overly concerned about the child who is blind or visually impaired getting hurt during physical play activities. One O&M specialist arrived to a preschool program during recess in a nearby playground and noticed that the all children were lining up to take their turn going down the slide except the child who was blind, who was sitting on the ground nearby. When the new person supervising the children was asked what was happening with this boy, she noted that it was too dangerous for him to be climbing the steps up the slide, "because," she confided, "he's blind." The problem was easily solved when the O&M specialist asked the child who was blind if he wanted to join his friends using the slide, which he did; once given permission, off he went, as he was quite familiar with this playground slide.

Adults are responsible for overseeing the safety of young children, and when a child has a visual impairment or combined vision or hearing loss, staff may be overly sensitive about the child's safety. This concern may influence the child to begin to believe that he or she cannot do certain things, try new activities, or take risks. Care should be taken, therefore, to provide sufficient verbal, emotional, and physical guidance to encourage the child through new motor experiences. Staff members need to be trained about the equal expectations for children with visual impairments or deafblindness and typical measures to ensure safety. Tumbles will occur, as they do with all children, but they can be addressed without any unnecessary drama. An adult's "can-do" attitude will reinforce a child's can-do attitude.

Preschool should be a time of joyous romping and refining of motor skills. An educational team, including parents and other family members or caretakers, can capitalize on the natural energy of the child while being deliberate with providing any needed specialized instruction and equipment for movement activities. Developmental checklists that early-intervention personnel use to assess and monitor progress can provide expectations for age-appropriate milestones that will guide such instruction. With a foundation of age-appropriate movement, skills, and activities, the preschooler will have a firm foundation to begin elementary school and

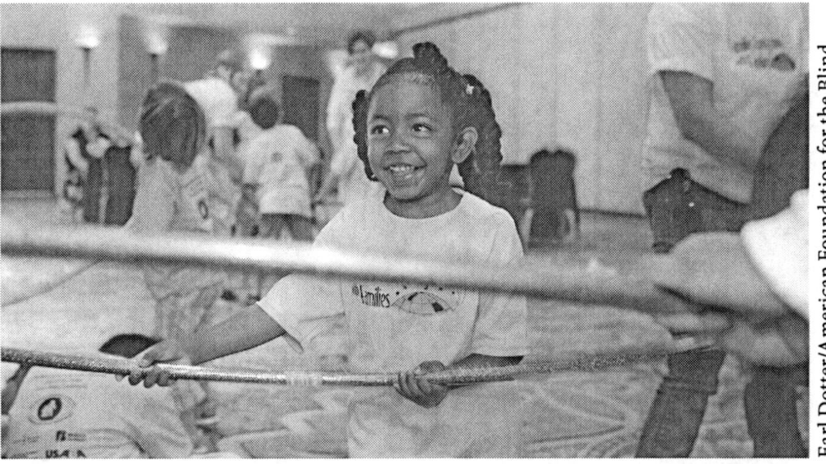

Earl Dotter/American Foundation for the Blind

A foundation of age-appropriate physical activities and skills prepares a child to move into elementary school and formal physical education.

formal physical education activities, as described in Chapter 7.

RECOMMENDATIONS FOR USING PLAY TO ENCOURAGE PHYSICAL ACTIVITY

As noted throughout this chapter, motor development and early play skills are often intertwined in their dependence on and support of one another. Play skills are enhanced by a child's increased physical abilities. Conversely, age-appropriate play activities can and should be used to bolster motor skills. Both knowledge and skill sets support purposeful movement and exploration throughout the early years of life and set the stage for a physically active older child. The following recommendations are for families and early-intervention personnel to collaborate upon when providing physical activity opportunities for young children who are blind or visually impaired:

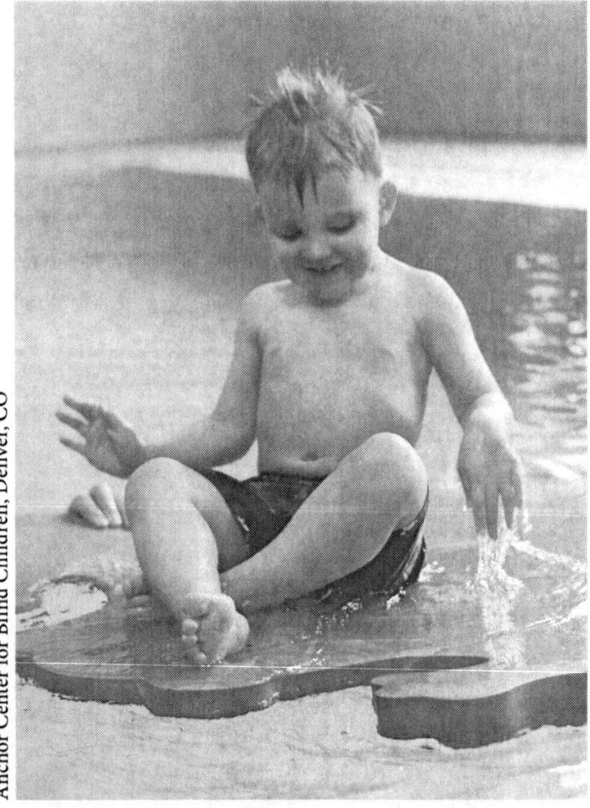

Anchor Center for Blind Children, Denver, CO

Some children love water play and will enjoy movement in a pool or playing with water toys in the bathtub.

Capitalizing on the child's motivation to move. The goal is for the child to initiate the child's own movements as an active learner. The motivation stems from the desire to explore or do a specific task. Knowing a child's preferences will help family members and professionals situate tasks. For example, if a child loves water play, there are many ways to encourage movement with the reward of water: going independently to the bathtub, dumping toys into the tub, standing and shifting weight from one leg to another to stay involved in the activities of a water-play table in a preschool classroom, running through a lawn sprinkler, splashing through puddles on a rainy day, and taking swimming lessons at the neighborhood pool.

Understanding the child's play level. Knowing the play category that the child is in developmentally allows adults to create movement opportunities that are reinforcing to the child. The adult can begin at the play level of the child as a way to invite play, social interaction, and physical activity. For example, the child who is learning relational play can be enticed to move to more than one place to gather two objects that can be used together, such as using a stick to bat a beeper ball.

Expanding play to higher levels of thinking and movement. Once the child is engaged in active play, actions, props, and suggestions can be offered verbally, with physical cues, or in sign language to expand the play routine. The adult can bump up the play level over time by modeling something new with the objects at hand. Using a cup as a container one moment may turn into a stacking task as the cup is turned over and new cups are added to "go higher and higher." The task has changed from relational play to constructive play. The child has to move and adjust his or her body position to add more cups to the growing tower.

Another way to add actions is to build in arm or body movements to rhythms, songs, or action games. Children enjoy repeating actions, which allows for easy practice of movement.

Giving the child chores to support motor skills. Chores and family recreational tasks can be shared, with an adult or an older child modeling how to complete the tasks. For example, the young child can help carry the wet swimsuits from the bathroom to the laundry room or put away the bike helmets in a garage cupboard after a family bike outing.

Using adaptive equipment or physical props. Additional materials or equipment may be needed to adapt a particular activity for a child with a visual impairment or deafblindness and possibly a physical condition. (See Chapter 5 for a detailed discussion of adapting physical activities.) Parents and other family members can help identify the child's needs and contribute to solutions. A physical or an occupational therapist can identify needed equipment for postural support or orthopedic-related ambulation. An O&M specialist can introduce an adapted mobility device or long cane if the child requires one for safe mobility. A teacher of students with visual impairments can help identify how to best utilize color preferences, contrast, positioning of materials for optimal viewing, and lighting needs of the child, as discussed in Chapter 2. Physical props such as furniture, landmarks, toys, or other materials are the shared responsibility of the child's team.

Providing feedback and guidance. Verbal feedback, or, as appropriate for the child who is deafblind, feedback in sign language, provides the child with names for body movements and movement experiences and communicates what is happening with the motor development and play routine. It is important to give children confirmation that their actions were noticed and provide guidance on a next step, but children should be encouraged to do the things that they can do for themselves. For example, a parent may notice a child struggling to get his or her cane around an obstacle and comment, "You are almost to the front door. Just take two steps back and move to the right."

Language can help the child with specific body positioning. As a child matures, he or she will be better able to apply verbal direction to his or her movement. During a swimming lesson, the instructor may say, "Pull your tummy up to the sky," and then gently push on the child's back as the child floats on his or her back in the water, so the child can feel his or her tummy come up out of the water. The next time this command is given, the child will be better able to understand what body movement is needed.

If a child with deafblindness uses another way to communicate, such as tangible symbols, this communication system should be used to provide the child with information about the activity at hand. A tangible symbol, which is selected from the viewpoint of the child for its meaningfulness, may be a piece of the gym mat that indicates that it is time for motor activities in the gym. A pat on the back may be the signal that the child can begin the motor task of crawling through the large tube that begins an obstacle course.

Providing opportunities to expand and challenge motor skills. Problem solving that requires moving the child's body can be encouraged, such as encouraging the child to squeeze behind the couch and the chair in the living room to retrieve a ball that has rolled there. The location of an activity that the child enjoys can be changed. For example, container play, such as dropping pennies into a metal can, can be done on the floor in a sitting position or at a lower table in a kneeling position or at a higher table in a standing position.

Providing opportunities for physical play. Activities within the home, in the back yard, or in a nearby park or school playground can reinforce the child's movement abilities and sense of play. Home activities may include helping to carry something a bit on the heavy side, such as the parent's gym bag, from the car to the front door. A small slope in the backyard may be the perfect angle to roll down the hill in the summer and slide down it in the winter. Monkey bars, swings, slides, and climbing equipment at the park provide opportunities to build strength and coordination. Homemade obstacle courses invite body adjustments to inclines, declines, tunnels, and tight corners. Rhythm games can help a child learn to move to the speed of the beat ("Faster, faster, now slowwwwwly!").

Maintaining high and developmentally appropriate expectations. Age-appropriate independence can be encouraged on movement tasks such as going up and down curbs or climbing onto the sofa or into a grocery cart. Modeling the recreation and sporting activities of the family and older children can increase the child's awareness of specialized equipment and what people do to enjoy their free time.

CONCLUSION

Even though Andrew's family did not expect a child under 3 to finish a 5K cross-country ski race, they gave him the chance to participate in the sport and the event. The result had immediate and long-term effects. That little boy went on to be a successful wrestler in high school, played competitive goalball, and has now grown into an active adult who runs with a guide, goes for long tandem bike rides, and still enjoys cross-country skiing.

Elementary Education Programming

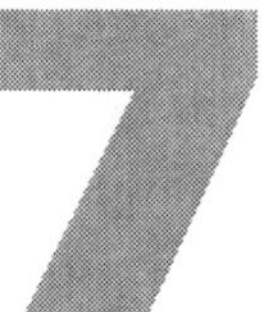

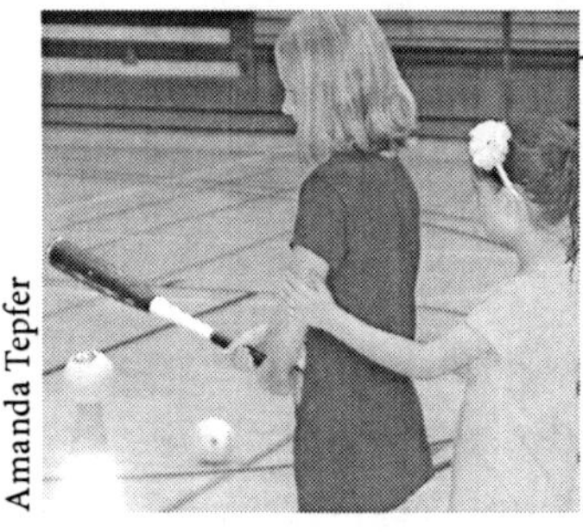

Amanda Tepfer

IN THIS CHAPTER

- **The Elementary Physical Education Curriculum**
- **The Importance of Assessment**
- **Planning Elementary Education Activities: General Considerations**
- **Teaching Basic Skills Using the Step-by-Step Method**
- **Teaching Basic Sports Skills and Concepts with a Parachute**
- **Adapting Common Elementary Games and Activities**
- **Motivating Students**

Brandon is in third grade and has a condition that leaves him with low vision and difficulty distinguishing some colors. He loves to be active and is constantly playing with friends in his neighborhood. He has always looked forward to recess and physical education activities, but they have recently become more and more difficult and frustrating. When his friends play kickball during recess, he loses track of the ball, and when he kicks he misses the ball more frequently than he actually makes contact. His classmates do not make comments about his athletic skills, but he constantly makes remarks about what he perceives to be poor performance on his part. In physical education class, Brandon has trouble distinguishing between the teams in tag and other games, despite the different colored pinnies (pullover vests) that students wear to differentiate the teams, and has occasionally thrown a ball to the wrong team or tagged a person on his own team. His frustration has become serious enough that he has begun sitting out of games at recess and making excuses to avoid physical education.

Brandon's teacher of students with visual impairments, Mr. Hanel, talked to Brandon about why he was finding excuses to avoid activities he had always enjoyed. When Mr. Hanel observed Brandon at recess, he saw that the students were using a faded gray playground ball that did not contrast well against a gray cement playing surface. This made the ball difficult for Brandon to visually track. Mr. Hanel also noted that in physical education class, the pinnies were blue and red. Brandon's functional vision assessment had previously shown that he could not distinguish between darker colors such as purple, blue, red, and green; they all appear to be similarly dark colors to him.

Next, Mr. Hanel met with Brandon's classroom teacher, the physical educator Ms. Myers, Brandon's parents, and Brandon. He shared his findings and asked Brandon what he thought might help him function better in recess and physical education class. Brandon said that he might have less trouble if they used a yellow kickball instead of a gray one. Ms. Myers wondered if having one team wear yellow pinnies would make it easier for Brandon to distinguish teams, and Brandon agreed.

The next week, Brandon was much more successful in his kickball game at recess, and after the pinnie colors were changed to one dark and one light color, he resumed his active participation in games in physical education because he was more easily able to distinguish who was on his team and who wasn't. The two simple adaptations made a big difference for Brandon. In addition, he learned that he could be his own advocate by offering input about what modifications might make it easier to include him.

■

Gabrielle, a fifth grader with deafblindness and hemiplegia cerebral palsy as a result of prematurity, uses some sign language, her remaining hearing, and her voice to communicate. Gabby has been with her fifth grade class since kindergarten. Up to now, her physical education teacher, Mr. Winnick, had always been able to adapt the activities such as parachute games, scooter board, tag games, and obstacle courses for her and her intervener, Ms. Chen. Now that her fifth grade class is working on small-sided games, sports skills, and more organized activities, Mr. Winnick is finding activities such as moving to reach a tennis ball, playing "keep away" in soccer, and cooperative volleyball (trying to hit the ball over the net as many times in a row as possible) harder to adapt.

Mr. Winnick set up a meeting with Gabby's parents; the teacher of students with visual impairments, Mr. Barbera; the state deafblind specialist, Ms. Morgan; and the adapted physical education consultant, Ms. Lopez. He shared his concerns and difficulties with the units in fifth grade and noted that Gabby's IEP required her to be included in physical education. After reviewing the functional vision and hearing assessments, the team agreed that the inclusive setting was appropriate for Gabby and that Mr. Winnick just needed some more ideas for her inclusion into these different units to meet her vision and hearing needs. The team reviewed her successes to date and noted that she does well when the object in use moved slower than a typical soccer ball or volleyball, when it had good contrast with the gym's yellow walls, and when the game was at a slightly slower pace. Ms. Chen, the intervener, also suggested training a classmate to play with Gabby during the games, as Gabby did not feel comfortable in the middle of a fifth grade game. The team agreed to try out some modifications to continue supporting Gabby in her inclusive class.

The next unit was soccer, and the class worked on skill development and a "keep-away" game, in which the team that has the ball tries to keep the other team from getting it by passing it among themselves. Gabby used a soccer ball with 10 ounces of sand inside, which made it move more slowly than a regular ball. Her team wore bright orange pinnies so she could see them. Ms. Chen and Mr. Winnick trained three of Gabby's friends in the signs, guiding techniques, instruction, and feedback that they would need to know to be Gabby's peer tutor. The peer tutors were very patient during the two weeks spent on skill development while Gabby worked on her kicking and ball control skills. They held her hand while she practiced trapping the ball, as she tended to lose her balance at first because of her hemiplegia. During small-sided games she sometimes lost track of where the ball went and became frustrated. Ms. Chen suggested that the peer tutor take Gabby's pointer finger and track the ball during the game so Gabby would know when the ball was coming closer to her. That worked well, as did a rule that all defenders had to stand more than 10 feet away from Gabby.

With the cooperation of her educational team and her classmates, Gabby continued to be included in her general physical education classes. Several more students even asked Mr. Winnick if they could be trained as a peer tutor for Gabby. ■

The elementary physical education class provides a foundation for skill development, physical fitness, and sports concepts; motivation for future involvement in physical activity; and self-concept related to physical activity, as described in Chapter 3 (Pangrazi & Beighle, 2009). The way skills and activities are introduced and taught and the way feedback is given to students form the basis for students' attitudes about their physical skills and abilities. If children enjoy being active and derive pleasure from movement experiences, they are more likely to pursue them for lifelong fitness and recreation. It is particularly important, therefore, that students with visual impairments or deafblindness are able to participate with their classmates in the activities that are offered in physical education classes during elementary school. Success in these activities affects not only students' level of fitness but also their self-image and their relationships with other children. As can be seen in the two scenarios that introduced this chapter, including children with visual impairments or deafblindness may not always be simple, but with some consideration and support, physical education can be accessible to all children.

The scenario featuring Brandon's difficulties in playing kickball reflects both the profound effects of visual impairments on children's experiences and the simplicity of many solutions to problems. It may not always be obvious when a student first enters the classroom what adaptations will be useful. This chapter offers suggestions for adapting activities in the general elementary physical education curriculum so children like Brandon and Gabby can be included successfully.

Key elements in successful introduction of physical education and sports skills at the elementary education level for students with visual impairments or deafblindness are assessment, an instructional plan that incorporates adaptations as needed, adapted equipment as needed, and feedback about performance of skills as they are learned. Taking time at the beginning of each unit to plan, organize, and discuss options can provide the opportunity for the physical education teacher to brainstorm with the teacher of students with visual impairments and possibly the adapted physical educator, parents or other caregivers, and student about the best way to adapt the unit to meet the student's needs.

THE ELEMENTARY PHYSICAL EDUCATION CURRICULUM

The goal of elementary physical education is to give students the foundation of movements and the confidence to be competent movers, and then to start incorporating the basics of sports skills development. In elementary physical education, as noted in Chapter 3, children learn movement concepts, fundamental motor skills (locomotor, non-locomotor, and manipulative skills), specialized motor skills (body management, rhythmic movement skills, gymnastics, game skills, and sports skills), object control, spatial awareness, and simple games and activities (Pangrazi & Beighle, 2009). Some common units may include locomotor control (including running, hopping, skipping, jumping, leaping, and sliding), object control (such as batting, kicking, throwing, catching, and rolling), parachute activities, fitness, scooter board activities, tag games, relay races, cooperative games, and jump rope. The curriculum may focus more on basic movement, spatial awareness, and skills concepts in the early grades and then, about fourth grade, start incorporating more sports skills and concepts into the curriculum. (Playing competitive sports, as noted previously, is not developmentally appropriate in elementary grades.) Although there are recognized national standards for physical education, state standards and district curricula may differ, so that elementary curricula vary in their philosophies and objectives.

THE IMPORTANCE OF ASSESSMENT

The need for assessment is universal; that is, to know how to start teaching his or her students in any subject, an instructor needs to first assess them to see what they are already capable of. Chapter 3 discussed assessment of a student's physical abilities. To consider how to adapt activities and provide appropriate instruction for students with visual impairments or deafblindness, teachers also need to know the students' skills, strengths, and needs. As reflected in the vignettes of Brandon and Gabby at the beginning of this chapter, however, such an assessment needs to be holistic and include direct observation of the student, information about his or her visual and auditory functioning, information about activities the student will be involved in, and input from all parties involved including the student and parents and other caregivers. Every aspect of the student's performance should be considered, including the environment, equipment, family interests, classmates' involvement, and socialization and the student's social and emotional state to give the teacher the whole picture. This type of assessment is ongoing and involves the student's entire educational team in addition to any formal assessments such as those discussed in Chapter 3.

Often, a student with a visual impairment or deafblindness may not have had previous instruction or experience in a basic locomotor or object control skill. Assessment can detect the student's needs in specific skill areas. This baseline assessment, indicating where a student started in a particular skill, provides essential information for program planning and evaluation. A follow-up assessment can be done at a later time to measure the improvement in a student's performance of the newly learned skill. It is important to remember when using standardized assessments that the population from which the norms and standard scores of most such tests were derived were not visually impaired; therefore, these norms and standard scores cannot be used to compare a student with visual impairments to other students or to established standards. If that is the case, a teacher can use the outcome of the assessment only as an individual baseline or starting point for the student to be used in planning and programming, not to compare the student's performance to that of others.

A common assessment that can be used by the physical education teacher or the adapted physical education teacher for students of this age is the Test of Gross Motor Development, second edition (TGMD-2; Ulrich, 2000). As noted in Chapter 3, the test assesses the locomotor skills of running, galloping, hopping, leaping, horizontal jumping, and sliding and the object control skills of striking a stationary ball, stationary dribble, kicking, catching, overhand throwing, and underhand rolling. Each skill is described in detail and has a set of specific performance criteria. Although the TGMD-2 was not normed on children with visual impairments, it has been validated for use with children with visual impairments from ages 6 to 12 (Houwen, Hartman, Jonker, & Visscher, 2010). The scores can also be used to provide a baseline for areas of strength and weakness, along with documentation such as level of vision and any adaptations that needed to be made to conduct the assessment—such as a sighted guide for skipping, an auditory ball for kicking, or batting from a tee.

PLANNING ELEMENTARY EDUCATION ACTIVITIES: GENERAL CONSIDERATIONS

After an assessment has been completed and the teacher has determined the strengths and needs of a student with visual impairment or deafblindness, the results can assist with lesson planning for the student and class. Lesson planning may differ somewhat, depending on whether the student has been placed in a general, modified, or segregated physical education class.

Previous chapters provided information about the needs of students with a visual impairment or deafblindness and suggestions for determining how instruction and activities might be adapted to accommodate them. This chapter and the following one provide suggestions for adapting specific activities in the physical education curriculum. Since instruction at the elementary education level is more basic and builds the foundation for further learning, there are particular considerations the teacher needs to take into account when planning lessons.

Finding Time to Teach

If a student's Individualized Education Program (IEP) specifies inclusion in a regular physical education class, then the teacher needs to plan for including the student in the regular class activities rather than pulling the student out of class to work separately on a particular skill area. Indeed, it is neither legal nor ethical to single out a student in this way. Such separate instruction may make a student feel inferior, and the student's classmates may come to believe that the student cannot participate in the activities.

It is preferable to embed instruction in the areas targeted for a student into existing units of instruction (Kowalski, Lieberman, Pucci, & Mulawka, 2005). For example, if Brandon was having difficulty doing a gallop or skip and his class is working on tee ball, the teacher might have each batter choose to skip or gallop to the bases. This would embed Brandon's goals for improving these locomotor skills into the existing tee ball unit so that Brandon could work on the class's objectives along with his own. Another possibility would be to start the class with a locomotor skill warm-up to ensure that Brandon has an opportunity to work on those locomotor skills. The warm-up will benefit all the students in the class, and no one student is singled out.

If a student needs more time to work on skills than can be provided during the regular class period, the student needs to learn the skills before going to class, or the student will be lost and not know what is happening. Pre-teaching in an additional class in a segregated setting might be added once or twice a week to supplement the student's general physical education class. The student can arrive 10 to 15 minutes early to work on skills that need extra development and to be familiarized with the day's lesson plan along with any new equipment, environment, or terminology. Such pre-teaching classes might also be implemented by the orientation and mobility (O&M) instructor, paraeducator, or teacher of students with visual impairments, based on information from the physical education teacher or adapted physical education instructor. It is up to the physical education teacher and the educational team to determine who has time to teach the concepts and how to work the necessary time into the child's schedule. For example:

■ *Rosita, a student with retinopathy of prematurity, is in seventh grade. She loves physical education, and her class will be working on badminton for the first time. Her teacher, Ms. Chiu, knew that Rosita needed to learn the concept of the net, the dimensions of the court, the service line, the birdie, and the racquet, but Ms. Chiu is the only physical educator for the middle school and had no free periods to work with Rosita. Her school used a large yellow birdie that goes slower than the white one for Rosita's benefit.*

The team decided that the O&M instructor and mobility teacher along with Rosita's paraeducator would take 15 minutes out of two mobility lessons to teach Rosita the concepts of badminton before the first class lesson. Then the paraeducator would work with her on the serve and the other badminton skills during homeroom period, when Rosita usually had 20 minutes when she sat around with her friends. Rosita even brought a badminton racquet home and asked her brother to practice with her once the unit got underway, as she loved the game and was thrilled to be an active part of it.

Time to Learn

Children with visual impairments or deafblindness may take more time to comprehend a skill or activity than sighted children and may need more time to learn the required skills. If the goal is full inclusion of the child, the teacher needs to build in sufficient time for the students with visual impairments or deafblindness to fully understand what is being taught (Lieberman, Houston-Wilson, & Kozub, 2002). Factors such as the assessment of the student's previous learning, the student's previous experience with similar lessons, his or her amount of vision and hearing, and whether one-on-one assistance is available will all have to be weighed when estimating how much activity can be taught in one lesson.

At the same time, however, the additional instructional time required by some students who are visually impaired or deafblind cannot be allowed to interfere with the progress of the general physical education class and others in the class to the extent of preventing them from learning the day's lesson. In that situation, the other students might absorb the negative message that the student's visual impairment was preventing the student from participating fully in the class activities. A better solution is to provide the student with a visual impairment, perhaps through pre-teaching, with additional classes in a small group or to assist the student individually in learning the skill or activity or understanding the dimension and purpose of the environment or equipment, as in the following example:

Extra class time was provided when Brandon, introduced at the beginning of the chapter, was included in learning a dance unit. The class was learning two dances, the Electric Slide and the Macarena, at a fairly fast pace. For Brandon to keep up with his classmates, the teacher taught him the dances in four additional 15-minute classes right before his regular physical education class. All the students were given instruction sheets showing the dance steps so they could practice the dances for homework. Brandon's instructions were enlarged using a copier so he could easily review them at home. In class, Brandon was right on target with his sighted classmates.

Class Organization and Instructional Approach

Some children with visual impairments may have a difficult time understanding how the instructional or activity environment is laid out or may not understand the purpose of certain objects used in the activity. For example, a child new to gymnastics may be aware that a rubber runway mat, a springboard, and a vaulting horse are located somewhere in the gym, but might not understand the physical relationship that they have with each other without getting closer to see them or examining the equipment by tactile exploration. To give the student the opportunity to be oriented to the activity, a "pre-orientation" might be scheduled prior to the first full-class instructional session. This might require some extra time and effort on the part of the physical educator, paraeducator, teacher of students with visual impairments, O&M specialist, or a peer tutor. (See Chapter 4 for a discussion of how to describe apparatus and instructional areas.)

Another aspect of class organization involves the way that the teacher structures the class during lessons and the instructional approach the teacher uses. *Command-style teaching* (also called *direct instruction*), in which the teacher tells the entire class what to do and everyone performs the skills at the same time, is the most common approach to teaching in physical education (Graham, Holt/Hale, & Parker, 2009). However, command-style teaching may not always be successful when a child who is deafblind or visually impaired is included. It is helpful to structure the class at times so that students can explore movement on their own and learn the arrangement of the court or area, the space, and the ability of their body parts to extend, contract, rotate, and move in many other ways. This can be done using such techniques as *guided discovery* or *stations*, or through dance and movement exploration activities. The decision on what type of instructional approach to use depends on the unit being taught, skill level of the class, time allotted, and class objectives. The teacher needs to make the decision ahead of time, although if an approach is not working, the teacher can modify it during class if necessary.

The following are some of the more common instructional approaches used in physical education.

- *Command-style or direct instruction.* The teacher directs the responses of the students by telling them what to do, showing them how to practice, and then directing their practice (Graham, Holt-Hale, & Parker, 2009). For example, when teaching how to kick a ball, the teacher would give every student a ball, show them the four-step approach (run into the kick, step, plant, and kick with weight shift and follow through), and then have them practice that specific approach. The teacher would lead the class through the steps, give specific cues for each one, and have everyone perform the skill at the same time with feedback.
- *Guided discovery,* also called the question approach (introduced in Chapter 4 with regard to describing equipment), is a teaching style in which questions are used rather than statements. For example, the teacher asks students how high they can walk, how many body parts they can balance on, or how far they can throw. To teach the proper way to kick a ball, for instance, a teacher might ask the class, "How far can you kick the ball?" To elicit a proper kicking form, the students pair off, kick the ball as far as they can, and measure the distance. The students discover from their own experiences that the ball goes farthest when they run into the kick, step, plant, and kick with weight shift and follow through.

- *Task teaching* makes use of *stations,* which are different places where students can work on a variety of skills at their own pace and level. Juggling scarves, dribbling a ball, or kicking a soccer ball, for example, can all be practiced at various levels of difficulty during station work. Students get a partner, go from station to station, work at their own pace, and challenge themselves at each station, as in the following example.

Ms. Myers was teaching jump rope to Brandon's class. She has stations set up for the following activities:

- *jumping forward with two feet at five different levels (identified by colors)*
- *jumping with one foot at a time with five different levels*
- *jumping double dutch (two groups get together to do this)*
- *jumping backward at five different levels*
- *jumping over a rope that is slanted at the highest part possible*
- *jumping over a rope on the floor for time and seeing how many times you can do it in a minute*

The class had 28 students, so there were two pairs at each station and one station with three pairs. The students were at each station for 4 to 5 minutes, then the music stopped for 1 minute so they could switch. Each pair did their best and recorded their highest scores at each station. Brandon knew what to expect at each station because his O&M teacher had shown him each station at the beginning of the jump rope unit. In addition, he was paired with his friend Trevor, who knew how to explain to Brandon what was happening.

- *Peer teaching* uses classmates teamed in pairs or small groups to actively teach one another. The teacher plans the tasks and communicates them to the students; the students assume the roles of providing feedback and assessing (Graham, Holt-Hale, & Parker, 2009). For example, to teach kicking, a teacher gives each pair of students a checklist with descriptions of each component of the skill. As one student practices, his or her partner checks off each part of the skill that the practicing student has mastered; then they switch roles. Peer teaching has shown to increase skill levels of children with visual impairments (Wiskochil, Lieberman, Houston-Wilson, & Petersen, 2007).
- *Dance and movement exploration* is the utilization of the motion of children's bodies to music either in a structured way or at their own rhythm.
- *The task analysis* or step-by-step approach of breaking a skill into its component parts, described in Chapter 4, is an excellent technique for teaching skills such as jumping and throwing, as well as for teaching many sports concepts, such as force, time, and extension. It can also be used for teaching group classes, and can be taught with the command-style approach or the guided discovery approach. For example, to teach the backhand throw in Frisbee, the following steps would be taught:
    - gripping the Frisbee
    - turning the body to the side
    - bringing the disc across the body
    - stepping with the same-side foot
- throwing across the body with wrist and arm extension

Cues are used to signal each step: "Grip, turn, back, step, extend." The focus is on the process rather than on how far the Frisbee goes.

One-to-One Instruction

Students with visual impairments or deafblindness who do not seem to benefit from demonstrations of activities in physical education class will often benefit from the use of a one-to-one teaching ratio. As pointed out in Chapter 4, instruction of students with limited vision in physical skills can be facilitated by such techniques as using more specific language, tactile modeling (the student feeling the movement of the teacher, paraeducator, or classmate), or physical guidance (the teacher physically manipulating the student). These approaches often require individual instruction to make sure that the student gets the necessary additional instruction and feedback. The teacher in the one-to-one situation can be the physical educator, the adapted physical education instructor, the teacher of students with visual impairments, a paraeducator, or a trained peer tutor.

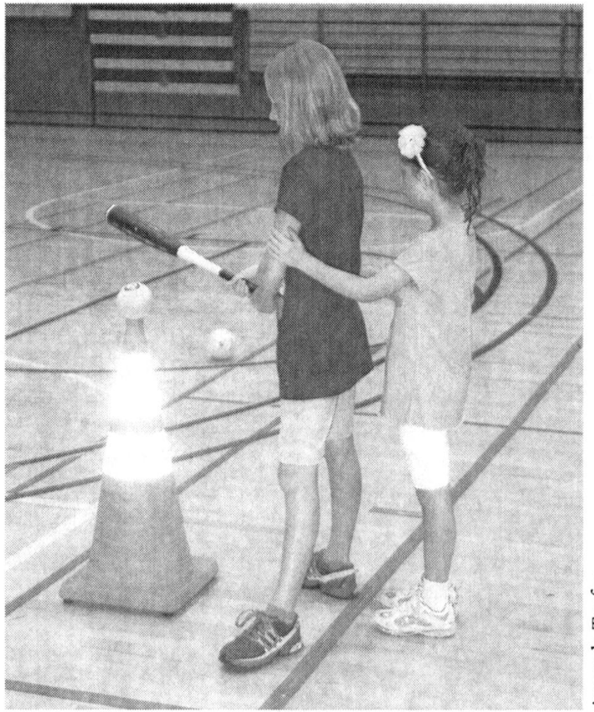

Amanda Tepfer

A peer tutor uses tactile guidance to demonstrate how to hold a bat to hit the ball off the traffic cone.

If a paraeducator or peer tutor is being used as a one-to-one instructor, he or she needs to be trained to provide appropriate instruction and feedback to a student with a visual impairment or deafblindness. Finding the time to gather information about the needs of a student with visual impairment or deafblindness and then train a paraeducator, peer tutor, or adapted physical education teacher may seem a daunting task to an already busy educator. It is important to keep in mind, however, that this kind of training is a process and can be expected to take some time. Again, the physical educator can look to other members of the student's education team for assistance.

Training opportunities for paraeducators may already exist in many schools. The 2004 No Child Left Behind Act requires paraeducators to earn continuing education credits, and many school districts have paraeducator training at the beginning of the school year or on scheduled staff development days. The argument can be made to administrators that offering training related to physical education would benefit the paraeducator, the student with a visual impairment or deafblindness, and the physical education teacher (Lieberman & Conroy, in press). Suggestions for training paraeducators are provided in Sidebar 7.1 (see Lieberman, 2007, for a complete training pro-

SIDEBAR 7.1

Training Paraeducators to Work with Students with Visual Impairments or Deafblindness in Physical Education

Paraeducators require training to provide appropriate instruction and feedback in a physical education class to a student with a visual impairment or deafblindness. The list that follows provides an outline of a training program that can be provided for paraeducators. See *Paraeducators in Physical Education* (Lieberman, 2007) for basic information the paraeducator needs to know about physical education. Information about visual impairment can be taught by the vision teacher, the O&M teacher, or the adapted physical education specialist if he or she is knowledgeable about the topic.

1. Define the basic concepts of physical education.
2. Define the roles of those who are involved with the student and his or her physical education instruction.
3. Review the instructional strategies of the primary physical education teacher.
4. Discuss strategies for including the child with visual impairment in the unit.
5. Discuss strategies for assessing the child's success in the physical education unit.
6. Review behavior management plans for the student.
7. Discuss communication between the paraeducator and physical educator and strategies to resolve conflicts should they arise.
8. Share any resources the paraeducator might find helpful in understanding his or her role.

Sources: Adapted with permission from L. Lieberman (Ed.), *Paraeducators in Physical Education: A Training Guide to Roles and Responsibilities* (Champaign, IL: Human Kinetics, 2007); and L. Lieberman and C. Houston-Wilson, *Strategies for Inclusion: A Handbook for Physical Educators,* 2d ed. (Champaign, IL: Human Kinetics, 2009).

gram for paraeducators in physical education). Even after training, paraeducators will need monitoring and support from the physical educator and other members of the student's educational team to ensure that they have learned the correct techniques for providing explanations, demonstration, physical assistance, and feedback in order to assist the student with the visual impairment throughout each unit of the year.

The training of peer tutors can be approached in a similar way at the beginning of the school year. Students can be asked to volunteer to be tutors for the students with visual impairments. Parents' permission will generally be required for students to take part in a peer tutor program. Many times if the volunteers are in the same class or have known the student with a visual impairment for a long time, the volunteers are already familiar with some of the student's needs. Peer tutors for other students with disabilities, if any, can be trained together. Sidebar 7.2 presents an outline for a peer tutor training program (see Lieberman & Houston-Wilson, 2009, for a complete peer tutor training program). Peer tutors can be trained in two or three 30-minute sessions during recess, during lunch, before school, after school, on staff development days when regular classes are not in session, or during small portions of a physical education class. Just as with paraeducators, the peer tutors will need monitoring and support, especially at the beginning.

SIDEBAR 7.2

Training Peer Tutors for Students with Visual Impairments or Deafblindness

Using peer tutors to provide one-to-one instruction and support for students with visual impairment and deafblindness is a strategy for inclusion that can provide benefits for both students. However, peer tutors need to be trained and supervised for such an approach to be successful. A thorough training program would consist of disability awareness; information about the disability; and techniques for instruction, feedback, assessment, and behavior management. (A complete peer tutor training program is provided in Lieberman and Houston-Wilson, 2009, including sample parental permission forms.) After training, peer tutors require monitoring and support from the physical education teacher.

The following is an outline of a training program for peer tutors:

1. Develop an application procedure for volunteers.
2. Distribute a form to obtain parental permission to participate in the program.
3. Develop disability awareness activities related to the student's visual impairment or deafblindness.
4. Teach communication techniques.
5. Teach instructional techniques related to the child's visual impairment or deafblindness.
6. Use scenarios to aid in teaching.
7. Administer the Test for Understanding, a 10-question written test, to assess the peer tutors' understanding of the training.
8. Introduce methods of monitoring the student's progress.
9. Teach basics of behavior management, motivation, and redirection in case the student gets off task or appears unmotivated.

Source: Adapted with permission from L. Lieberman and C. Houston-Wilson, *Strategies for Inclusion: A Handbook for Physical Educators,* 2d ed. (Champaign, IL: Human Kinetics, 2009).

Active Participation

Children in general will benefit from any sport, skill, or activity offered in which they are active participants, and this is also true for children with visual impairments or deafblindness. In order for active participation to happen, the physical educator needs to keep in mind the teaching strategies outlined in the following sections.

Providing Clear Explanations and Clarifying Concepts

As described in Chapter 4 of this book, the concept of an entire game or activity may not be clear to a student who is visually impaired or deafblind without specific verbal explanation, tactile exploration, and active involvement. For example, a student may not understand how home plate relates to first, second, and third base in kickball unless he or she has the opportunity to actually walk to each location to comprehend the distances between each base and where the bases are in relationship to each other. In addition, it is crucial for the student to understand the terms associated with each skill, position, and piece of equipment. For example, explanations such as the following can raise more questions than they answer: "The person who rolls the ball is the pitcher. Outfielders stand behind the bases, farther away from home plate. The team that is 'up' stands behind home base." A student who is visually impaired who has not had the opportunity to investigate those locations is left wondering, Where is home plate? What is home base? Where is "up?" The student still does not know what the purpose of the game is.

Similarly, when taking part in an activity that involves a parachute (several of which are described later in this chapter), if the student with a visual impairment or deafblindness only holds onto an individual strap or hand hold and never has the chance to feel the entire parachute, he or she may not comprehend the purpose of lifting and pulling the hand hold. When allowed to explore the parachute to understand its dimensions and given a demonstration of the way it moves, the student can be more of an active participant in any parachute game.

Important concepts such as the ones in these examples should not be taught hurriedly during a game or activity. They need to be explained purposefully, with enough time available to ensure understanding and for questions outside of the general physical education class. Learning the components of skills and games and the concepts that underlie them is important for everyone, but it is especially necessary for students who have not had experience or background in this area.

Whole-Part-Whole Instruction

Given the difficulty that students with visual impairment may have in comprehending the totality of an activity without careful explanation, the teaching approach known as whole-part-whole instruction is recommended when introducing new games and activities. In this method, the entire activity is presented first so that students understand what they are going to attempt to accomplish. Then the activity is broken down into its component parts, which are taught and practiced. Finally, the students put the parts together into the whole activity or skill.

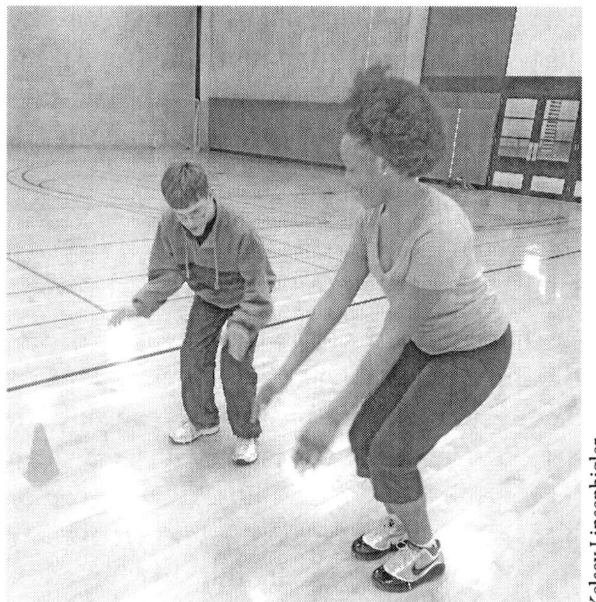

Kelsey Linsenbigler

Practicing a jump without the rope

For example, when a student is being taught jump rope, if only the jump or only the arm motion is taught, the student may never understand the overall concept of jumping rope. If the teacher demonstrates the entire skill first and then breaks it down into its components, the student will understand how the leg motion and arm motion fit together. A simple way to share the entirety of this skill is for the student with visual impairment or deafblindness to feel a classmate jumping rope (tactile modeling). The classmate may have to jump slowly and explain what he or she is doing as the student with the visual impairment feels the classmate's arms move and feels the rope at certain points in the rotation. The classmate can also say "Jump" as the student with the visual impairment jumps over the rope. Once the student understands the overall idea of jumping rope, the jump can be taught and practiced separately from the way the hands grip the rope and the way the arms swing it. After practicing each skill or each part of the activity, the student goes back to the whole activity by trying to put the parts together and jump rope. (Additional information about teaching jump rope and suggestions for adaptations are presented later in this chapter.)

Equipment

Equipment is a major consideration when setting up a physical education program for students with visual impairments. As explained in detail in Chapter 5, adaptations can be made to the size, color, weight, and texture of equipment so that it can be more easily perceived by students who are visually impaired. In addition, many pieces of equipment can be made auditory. Just a few modifications to equipment can enable students with visual impairments to become active participants in a game or activity, as in the following example:

> *When Brandon's class started a volleyball unit, Ms. Myers followed the guidelines of the AccesSports Model presented in Chapter 5, and considered the rules, boundaries, and targets or goals, including equipment. She discussed the options with Brandon, and as a result, she bought a net that had a bright pink strip on the top, they used a bright yellow trainer ball, and they added bells to the net so the sound alerted Brandon and his classmates if they hit the ball too low and into the net.*

Examples of adapted equipment are presented in the sample activities throughout this chapter. The Resources section at the back of this book provides information about companies that provide products specifically for adaptive sports or products that can be used to modify activities.

TEACHING BASIC SKILLS USING THE STEP-BY-STEP METHOD

As noted earlier, students in elementary school physical education classes learn and practice basic locomotor and object control concepts and skills and then build them into more complex skills as they progress through the grades. Students with visual impairments or deafblindness may need more specific instruction than their classmates to learn some of these skills. This section focuses on suggestions for teaching basic skills to students who are visually impaired and presents examples of how to teach specific skills, including underhand and overhand throwing, running, jumping, the standing long jump, hopping, and skipping.

Because each student and each situation are unique, how these lessons might be incorporated into a class would depend on the student with a visual impairment or deafblindness, the age of the students, the unit, the time taken by the lesson, and so forth. If possible, the student should be taught any unfamiliar basic skills before the lesson so the student can keep up with the rest of the class. The whole class might be taught a skill using the step-by-step method, and then move on once the class has grasped the concept. The student with the visual impairment may move on with the class, or, if he or she needs additional one-to-one instruction, he or she may work for a while longer with an instructor or peer tutor, as described earlier in the chapter.

Object Control Skills

Object control skills are motor skills that involve manipulating an object, such as a ball or a bat. They include basic skills, such as throwing, catching, rolling, and kicking a ball, as well as more complex skills involved in different sports and games such as bouncing, batting, dribbling, and so on. Many children may start learning these skills during the preschool years, but, as discussed in Chapter 1, children with visual impairments often miss the opportunities to learn them and need explicit instruction when they arrive in an elementary school physical education class. The most basic skills, such as throwing or kicking a ball, might be taught separately. Other skills are likely to be taught as part of a game or activity. For example, once a student knows how to kick a ball, the student can learn how to kick, trap, and dribble a soccer ball in order to play a game of soccer. In this case, a soccer ball with a bell inside or a plastic grocery bag tied around it might work best for a student with a visual impairment to learn these skills.

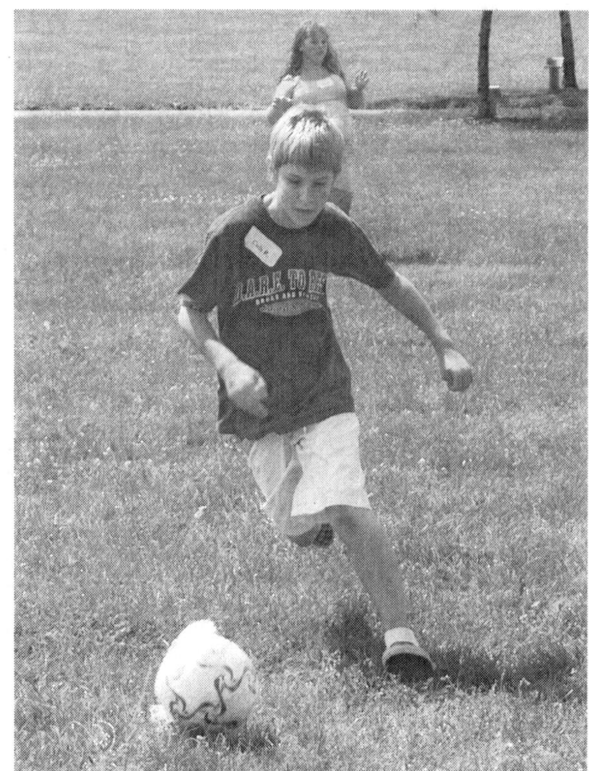

Amanda Tepfer

Tying a crinkly plastic grocery bag around a soccer ball can help a player hear the ball's location.

Basic object control skills such as throwing or kicking can be taught to students with visual impairments or deafblindness using the techniques described in Chapter 4. When introducing a student who is visually impaired or deafblind to the skills of throwing or kicking, demonstration, coupled with explanation, can be used if a student has usable vision or previous experience. As the student approximates the movements necessary, the student should be given verbal reinforcement. For example, when teaching basic kicking to a student with low vision, a ball that contrasts well with the grass or gym floor can be used. If a student has no functional vision, a ball with bells can be used, and the verbal explanation and feedback can be coupled with tactile modeling (the child feeling the movement of the instructor or a classmate), physical guidance (the teacher physically assisting the student), or both. For a student with deafblindness who is learning to kick, the ball might have both color and sound and instructions and feedback may be signed in addition to using tactile modeling and physical guidance.

Object control skills can be taught using the step-by-step procedure described in Chapter 4 and later in this chapter, in which students stand on a carpet square to help orient them and to define the range and direction of their movements. Before students can use this method to learn these skills, however, they need to learn the ready position (the teaching of which is detailed in Chapter 4) and be familiar with the terminology used to refer to body parts and positions. They also need to know which hand is their "throwing" hand and which foot is their "kicking" foot.

The skill of throwing can be introduced, following the whole-part-whole model, by allowing the student with a visual impairment to feel a classmate going through the throwing motion, along with explanation of the steps. The student with the visual impairment must feel the arm motion, hips, and step and follow through. The thrower may have to go through this several times before it is understood. Sidebar 7.3 presents the step-by-step sequences for teaching overhand and underhand throwing. When students are first learning throwing skills, it is helpful to let them start by throwing a beanbag because it is soft and easy to grasp. After the initial lessons, a softball or other type of ball can be substituted for the beanbag. Once the basic mechanics of throwing are learned, the length of the throw is based on the timing

SIDEBAR 7.3

Teaching Throwing Skills Using Step-by-Step Instruction on Carpet Squares

Step-by-Step Instruction Plan for Teaching Overhand Throwing

1. Okay, here we go. Stand on your carpet square. **(Photo A)**
2. Now, I want you to rotate—that is, turn right or left—and put the outside of your nonkicking foot toward me so you are standing sidewise to me. **(Photo B)**
3. Get into the ready position, still facing sidewise. We'll call this the sidewise ready position. **(Photo C)**
4. Keep your kicking foot planted on the back of your carpet square, and step off toward me. Point the toes of your nonkicking foot toward the front of the room.
5. Step back in sidewise ready position.
6. Step off again and point your toes forward. This time also point the fingers of your nonthrowing hand toward me. **(Photo D)**
7. Step back in sidewise ready position.
8. Step off and point toes and fingers. Step back on.
9. Step and point; step back. Step-point; step back; Step-point; step back. [Repeat until correct.]

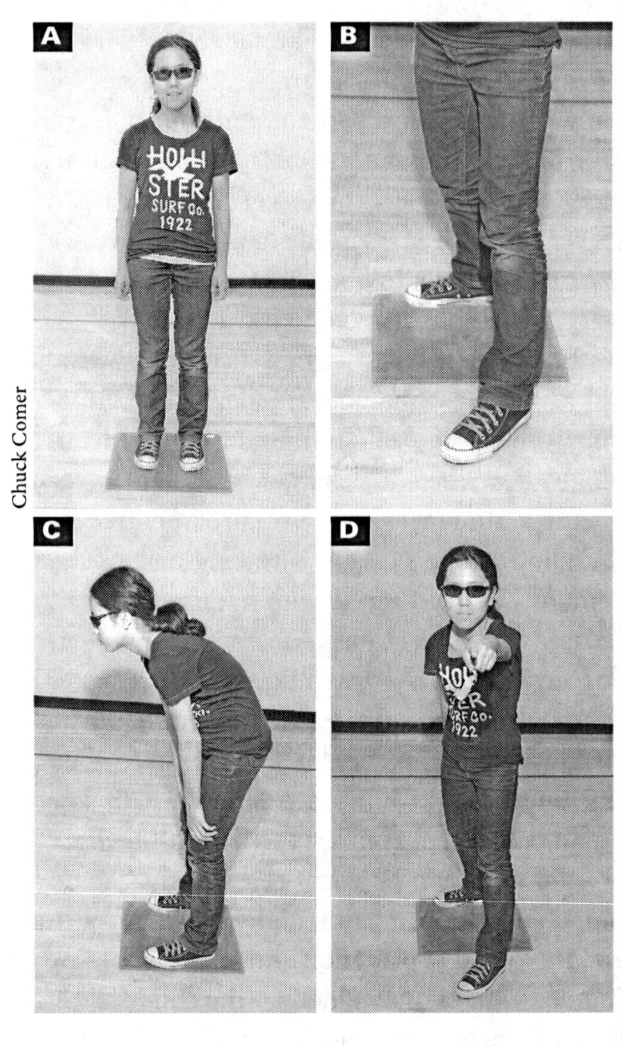

Chuck Comer

(Continued on next page)

SIDEBAR 7.3 *(continued)*

10. Now, listen before doing anything. This time when you step-point, we'll add another move. After step-point, raise your throwing hand next to your head, with your wrist and elbow bent. Then act like you are slapping me on top of the head with the palm of your throwing hand. **(Photo E)**
11. Okay, try it. Step-point, slap; back on. Step-point, slap; back on. [Repeat until correct.]
12. Listen again. This time we'll add the last step. As you slap, step off the front with your kicking foot at the same time. **(Photo F)**
13. Now, try it. Sidewise ready position. Step-point, slap-step; back on. Step-point, slap-step; back on. [Repeat until correct.]
14. It's time to throw, so get a beanbag and get in the sidewise ready position.
15. Hold the beanbag in your throwing hand where your fingers connect to your palm and then keep it there by squeezing it with your thumb and little finger. **(Photo G)**
16. This time in place of the slap, we will throw the beanbag,
17. Get into sidewise ready position.
18. Step-point, throw-step; back on. Step-point, throw-step, back on. **(Photos H, I)** [Repeat until correct.]

Substitute a softball for the beanbag and repeat if there is room and an appropriate wall to stop the ball.

Repeat until the student can consistently use the operative language to complete the skill independently.

Operative language: *Ready, step-point, throw-step.*

E
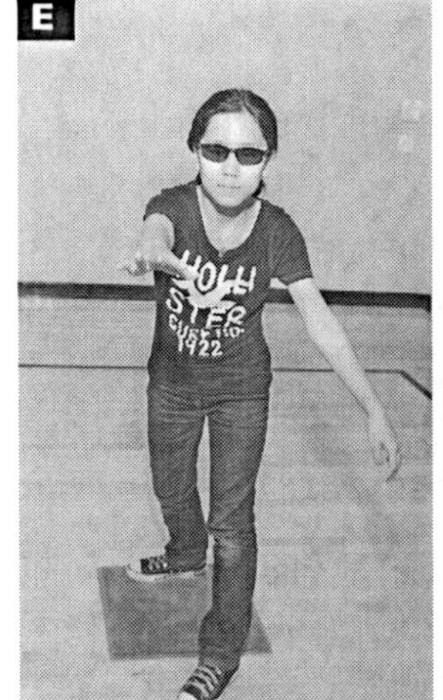

F
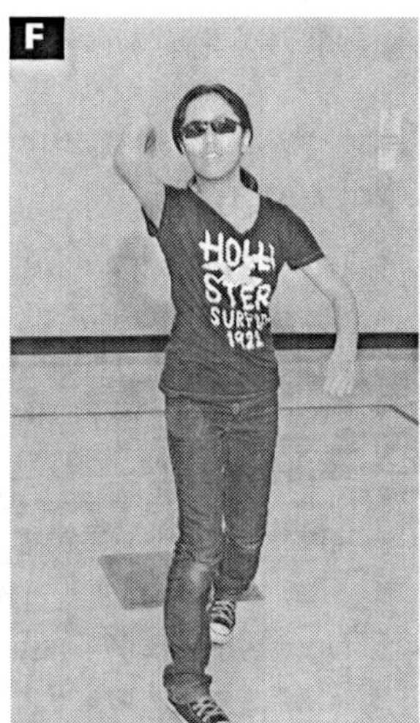

G
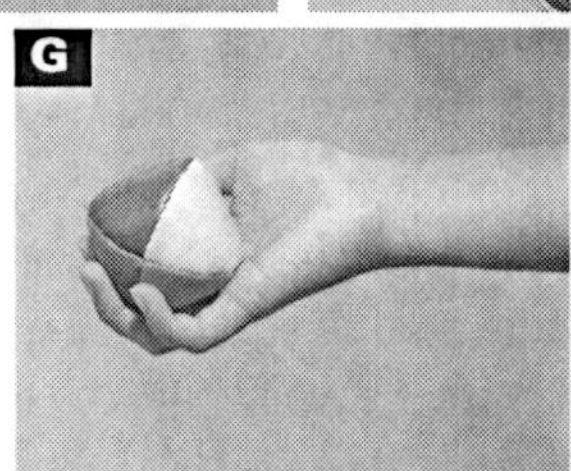

H
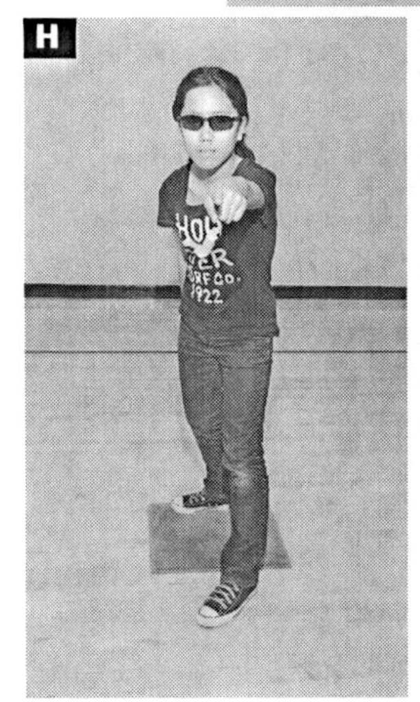

I
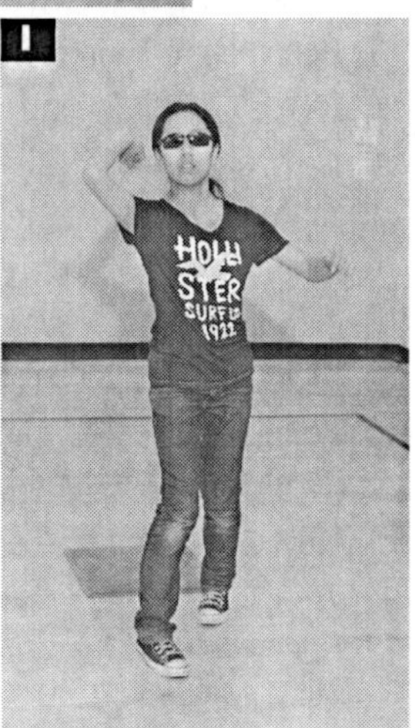

(Continued on next page)

SIDEBAR 7.3 *(continued)*

Step-by-Step Instruction for Underhand Throwing

1. Okay, here we go. Get into the ready position, but just let your hands hang by your knees **(Photo A)**
2. Step off the front with your nonkicking foot. **(Photo B)**
3. Step back on. **(Photo C)**
4. Step off and back on with the same foot.
5. Now, when I say, "Reach," reach behind you like you are trying to touch the ceiling with the back of your throwing hand. Keep your elbow straight. **(Photo D)** [Repeat until correct.]
6. This time from the reach position, when I say, "Swing," keep your elbow straight and swing your hand forward like you are going to slap the person in front of you under the bottom. **(Photo E)**
7. Reach back, swing forward, reach back, swing forward.
8. Now, show me which foot is opposite your throwing hand.
9. In the ready position, when I say, "Reach, slap-step," reach back, then step off with your opposite foot, and slap.
10. Ready, reach, step, slap. Ready, reach, step, slap. [Repeat until correct.]
11. Now, when you do the slap, step off the square with your kicking foot at the same time.
12. Ready, reach, step, slap-step. Ready, reach, step, slap-step.
13. Practice this on your own several times. Reach, step, slap-step.
14. We are going to throw the beanbag now, but first you need to hold the bag correctly. Hold it in your hand right where your fingers connect to your palm and then keep it there by squeezing it between your thumb and little finger.

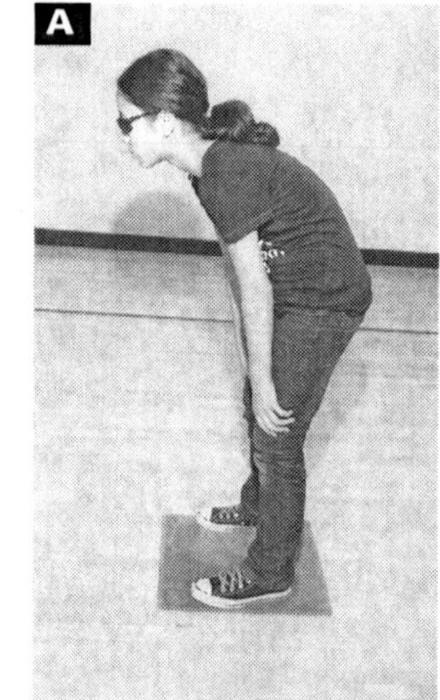
A

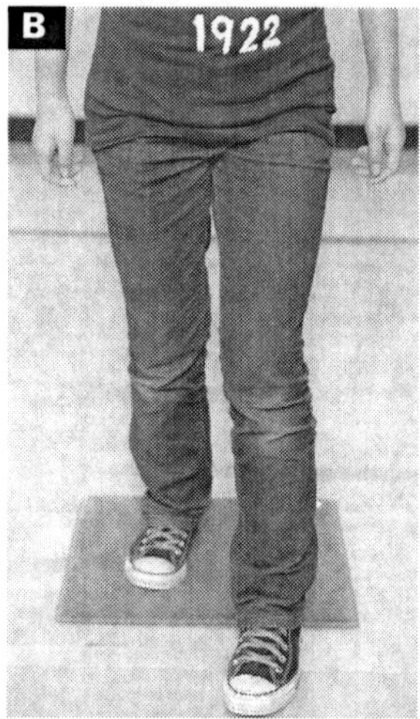

B

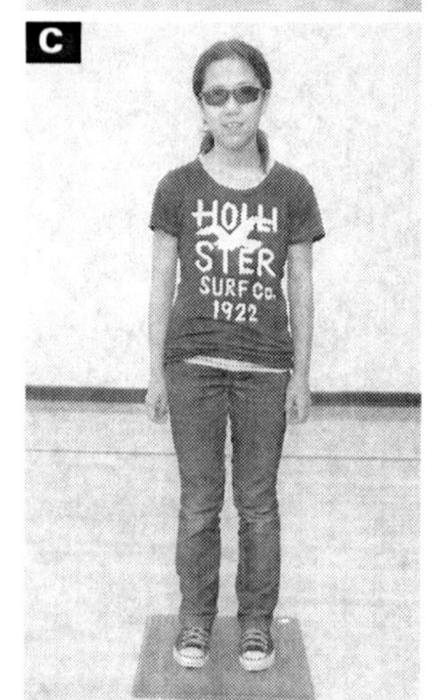

C

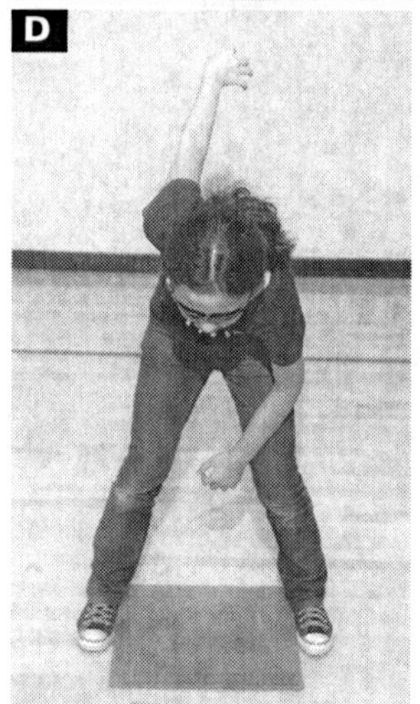
D

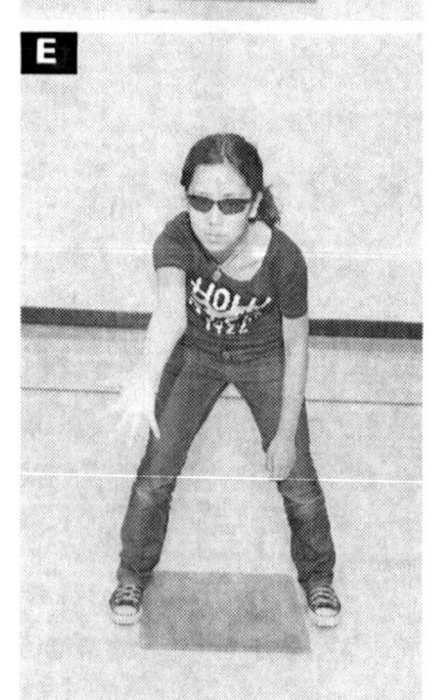
E

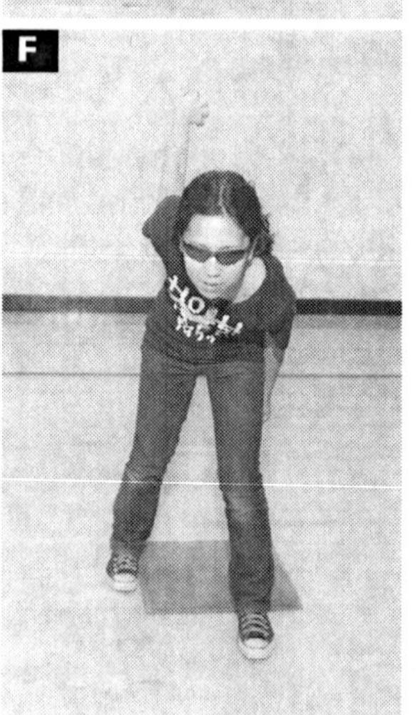
F

SIDEBAR 7.3 *(continued)*

15. This time in place of the slap, we will throw the beanbag. When I say, "Ready, reach, step, throw-step," throw the bag against the wall.
16. Here we go. Ready, reach, step, throw-step. **(Photo F, G)**
17. Great! You are doing the underhand throw!

Repeat until the student can consistently use the operative language to complete the skill independently.

Operative language: *Ready, reach, step, throw-step.*

Teacher's note: A softball, goalball, or other ball can be substituted after the initial lessons with a beanbag or bean ball. To increase throwing distance, work on coordination of the moves and on when to release the beanbag. Young children often have difficulty with the release and throw the bag straight up or down into the floor.

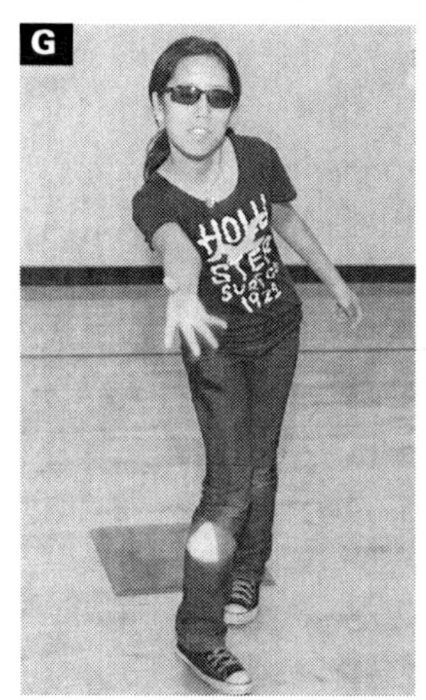
G

of the ball's release, the speed of the arm, and the speed of the body movement in the step.

Since object control skills involve manipulating an object, the teacher will also need to consider whether adapting the equipment involved would be helpful to the student who is visually impaired, as in the following example:

When Gabby, the student with deafblindness and cerebral palsy introduced at the beginning of the chapter, was 9 years old, she and her physical education teacher worked on kicking skills. At first, the teacher thought a lighter ball such as a beach ball would be better for introducing this skill. She taught Gabby using the whole-part-whole method along with physical assistance and verbal and signed feedback.

After Gabby kicked the ball twice, she stopped and asked, "Did I kick it?" The ball was apparently too light for her to know she had made contact with it. When a heavier playground ball was substituted, Gabby knew immediately when she made contact.

The teacher of students with visual impairments also suggested they place a crinkly plastic shopping bag around the ball so Gabby's classmate Federico, who is also visually impaired, could hear where the ball went after he kicked it across the room. The added weight and sound made a big difference, and Federico and Gabby were soon kicking the ball 100 percent of the time.

Teaching Basic Locomotor Skills

Locomotor skills, such as running, hopping, skipping, jumping, sliding, and galloping, propel the body in different ways. These skills may be taught individually or embedded in activities such as relay races, kickball, obstacle courses, or movement exploration. The physical education teacher decides how to introduce the locomotor skills based on the school district's physical education curriculum, previous skill level of the students, and objective of a particular curriculum unit. Good locomotor skills and the agility that results promote success in a variety of sports, fitness activities, and games. For example, the ability to slide in different directions can eventually help in defense in goalball and is beneficial in dancing.

The setting in which locomotor skills are taught to students with visual impairments needs to be planned so that the students are in an environment that is predictable and safe, both for them and for their classmates. Students with visual impairments or deafblindness can practice locomotor skills independently next to a wall or along a guide wire that they can hold on to (see Chapter 8 for more details) without worrying about safety, moving in open space, or running into others (Lieberman, 2011).

Teaching locomotor skills to students with visual impairments or deafblindness needs to be approached in a methodical and patient manner, just as with any other skill that is typically learned by watching others. The step-by-step procedure first introduced in Chapter 4 is especially helpful for teaching locomotor skills to students who lack fundamental skills and have poor body and spatial concepts. Using words as cues for the parts of a skill—such as "step-together-step" for the slide or "hop-swing, hop" for the one-legged hop—can be very helpful when teaching any locomotor skill.

The basic running technique, which is used in many sports and activities, is often the first locomotor skill taught, not only as a foundation for other skills but also to increase the self-esteem of the child. Research has shown that some children with visual impairments are self-conscious about running, are embarrassed by their running gait, and often avoid situations where they need to run (Lieberman, Robinson, & Rollheiser, 2006). Other locomotor skills should be taught according to the school's curriculum. The skip is generally the most difficult locomotor skill to learn; the leap and gallop are good prerequisites to teach before the skip is introduced.

As with teaching any skill, it is recommended that locomotor skills be taught using a whole-part-whole approach. However, because of the dynamic nature of the locomotor skills, which makes it difficult for a student who is visually impaired or deafblind to feel the whole skill while another person is performing it, it is necessary that verbal or signed explanation accompany the demonstration of the locomotor skill when the whole skill is taught.

Running

Running is one of the most basic of locomotor activities after walking, and is a component of many games, sports, and recreational activities. Running has the following components:

- Both feet are temporarily off the ground (known as the *flight phase*).
- The heel of the leading foot is placed first, then the toe.
- The arm opposite the forward leg swings forward with elbow bent.
- The back leg is bent to 90 degrees.

To present the skill of running to a student with a visual impairment, the instructor would first have the student feel the arm motion of a classmate of similar size, and then the leg motion, while giving a verbal explanation of the concepts just listed. Then the demonstrator would run while verbal explanation is again given. Once the student who has a visual impairment has a sense of how running is performed, it is his or her turn to run. Feedback and consistent cues such as "Heel-toe" and "Swing arms" should be given. The flight phase of the run is the most difficult part of the run for a child who is visually impaired, so it may take a while to comprehend and perform (Wagner & Haibach, 2012).

Many children learn to run as toddlers; however, some studies have found that children with visual impairments tend to run with a shuffling gait and little leg lift between rotations, or the full cycle of lifting each leg and putting it down to propel forward motion is limited; that is, they do not lift their back leg to 90 degrees and extend the front leg to produce a flight phase (Arnhold & McGrain, 1985; Nakamura, 1997).

In teaching running, the emphasis should be on the arm motion, lifting the front leg, and bending the back leg to 90 degrees to prepare for the next forward motion. Teaching the leg lift and back leg flexion can be done with tactile modeling and physical guidance in slow motion. To teach appropriate arm motion, some teachers have had success with a method using two 6-foot-long poles. The teacher and student each hold the opposite ends of the poles, with the teacher standing in front of the student and facing forward (away from the student). As the teacher moves his or her arms in a running motion, the poles move the student's arms in the same way. This arrangement allows the arm opposition and extension to be taught in slow motion. Then the poles can be used during an actual run to further emphasize the appropriate movement.

After students have mastered the form of running, they can run independently if they have sufficient vision, perhaps following the guidelines on a track, following a guide wire, or with a human guide using a variety of techniques. For example, they can follow a guide visually or use a version of sighted guide technique, holding onto the guide's elbow, shoulder, or hand, or hold a tether of some kind between them, such as a short rope or a towel. (Detailed information on guide-running techniques is presented in Chapter 8.)

Jumping

Jumping is a complex sequence of skills in which an individual uses leg and foot muscles to spring into the air. The simplest jump is accomplished by leaping straight up from two feet and landing in the same spot. Other jumps include the *hop,* in which the jumper leaps from one foot to the same foot; a *bound* or *step,* a jump from one foot to the other; and the *long jump,* a leap from one or both feet to both feet. The two most well-known competitive jumping events are the long jump, a contest to attain the greatest horizontal distance, and the high jump, in which competitors attempt to gain the greatest vertical height.

The standing long jump, a leap from two feet to both feet from a standing position, is generally taught as a fundamental motor skill and lends itself well to using the step-by-step method with students standing on carpet squares (see Sidebar 7.4). This skill can also be taught using the whole-part-whole method along with tactile modeling (the student feeling the demonstrator).

Many students will have already performed something that they know as the long jump, but it is highly unlikely that they have learned its parts properly. The parts of a long jump are as follows:

- Legs are bent at the knees, feet spread shoulder width.
- Straight arms reach back and up.
- Arms swing forward and legs are extended at the same time to lift the feet from the ground and propel the body up and forward.

SIDEBAR 7.4

Teaching the Standing Long Jump Using Step-by-Step Instruction on Carpet Squares

1. Okay, let's go. Stand in the ready position. **(Photo A)**
2. Step off the front of your carpet square with the foot you kick with. **(Photo B)**
3. Step back on.
4. Step off with your nonkicking foot. **(Photo C)**
5. Step back on in the ready position.
6. Jump off the front and land on both feet at once. **(Photo D)** Get back on. [Practice until the student is jumping correctly.]
7. Now, get in the ready position. Place your arms at your sides, make your elbows straight, and keep your palms at the sides of your legs. **(Photo E)**
8. Swing your straight arms behind you and up and try to reach the ceiling with the pinky fingertips of both hands. Bend your knees and look at your feet. **(Photo F)** [This has the appearance of the "set" position of swimmers on the starting blocks of a freestyle race. The back is bent parallel to the floor.]
9. Stand up. Again, ready, reach. [Practice until students attain a good reach with the face toward the feet.]
10. Stand up and shake out your arms and hands.
11. Now, ready, reach, and hold it there a second.
12. From that reaching position, keep your elbows straight and swing your arms forward with your hands open like you want to grab the person in front of you by the waist. **(Photo G)**
13. Stand up. Now, ready, reach, swing!
14. This time, as you reach back and then swing forward, follow your swing by jumping off the front of your carpet square with both feet and land on them. **(Photo H)** I'll say it this way: ready, reach, swing-jump!

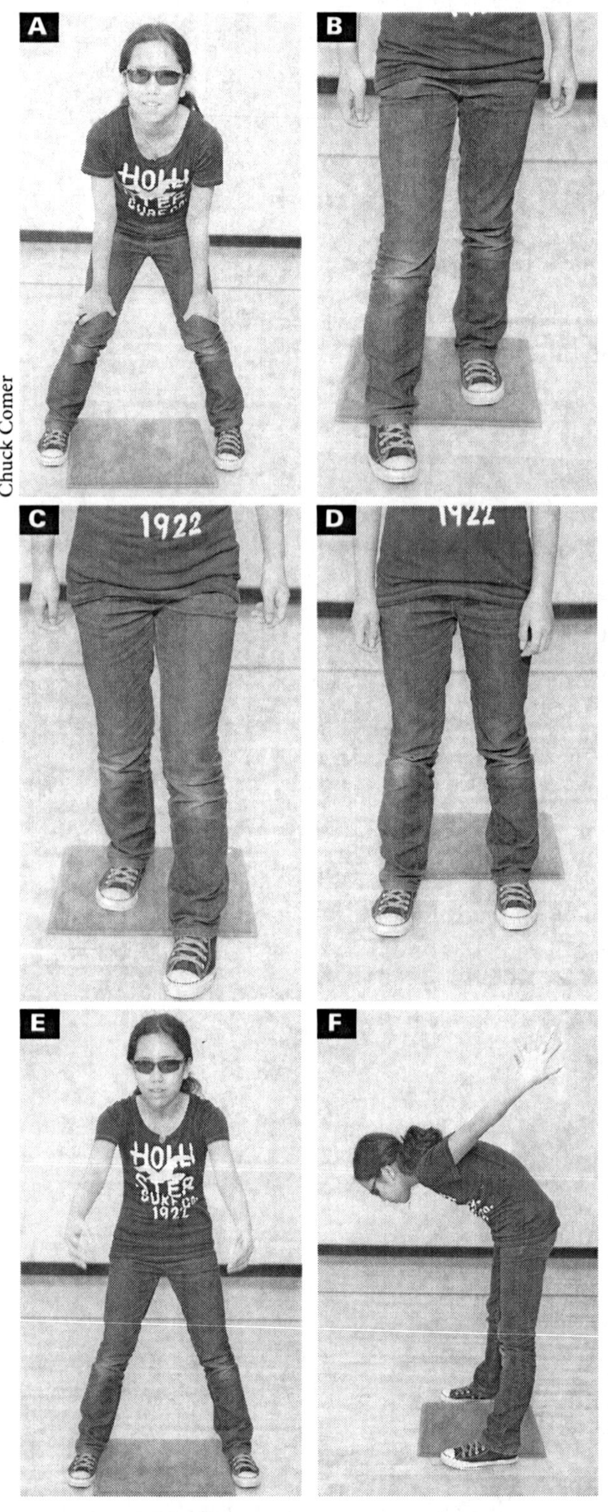

Chuck Comer

SIDEBAR 7.4 *(continued)*

15. Practice all together. Ready, reach, swing-jump. **(Photos I, J, K)**
16. Again, ready, reach, swing-jump as far as you can. You're doing a standing long jump!
17. When you jump next, I want you to land on both feet without wobbling around or falling over. We call that landing with control.
18. Ready, reach, swing-jump, control!

Repeat until the student can consistently use the operative language to complete the skill independently.

Operative language: *Ready, reach, swing-jump.*

Teacher's note: Once the basic skill is mastered, practice increasing the length of the jump.

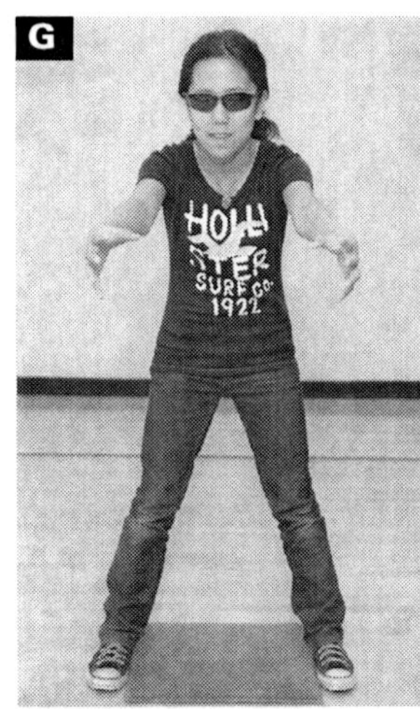

G

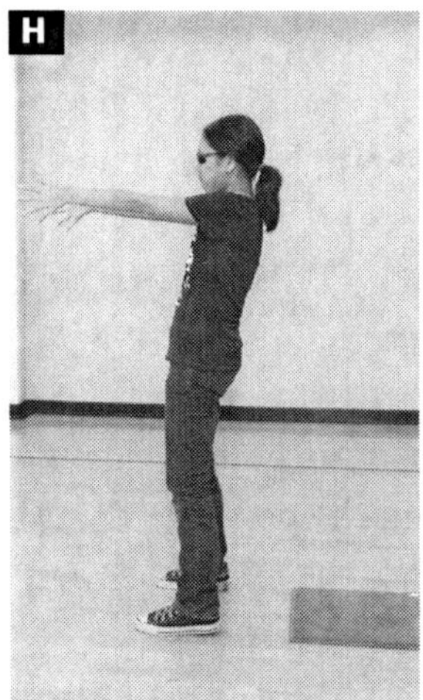

H

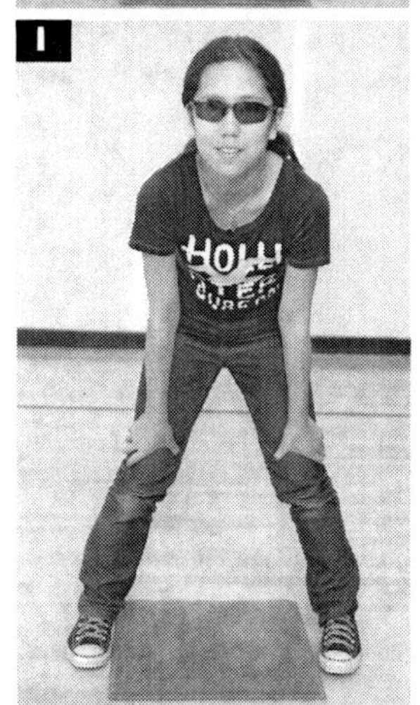

I

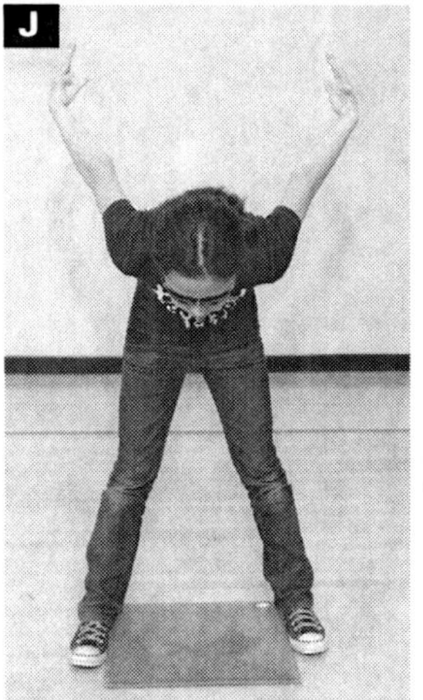

J

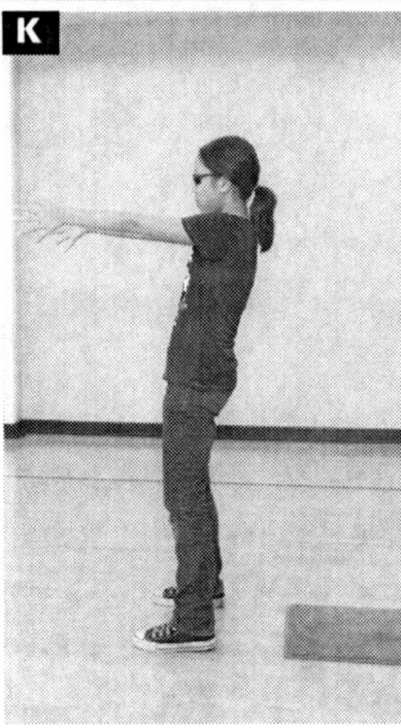

K

This skill is presented in many steps, but it is taught in four skill groups: ready, reach, swing, jump (see Sidebar 7.4). The swing and jump are eventually combined into one step. The goal is to cover as much distance as possible. The distance achieved in a standing long jump is a function of the power and speed of the reach–arm swing part of the jump—that is, the momentum gained from the force of the arm swing and the power of the leg extension. The jumper ends the jump by landing on two feet in a controlled manner.

Once the basic skill is mastered, the goal can become increasing the length of the jump, since bettering one's own best performance is a motivator for most students. Working on improving the long jump can also help teach the concept of "force" (the degree of strength with which a movement is done) to students who do not understand it by showing the way increasing the force affects the distance of the jump. To help convey the idea of force in the long jump, the word *push* or *extend* can be used to describe the action of the legs, and the word *reach* can be used for the arms. In addition, the distance jumped can be measured and shared to help the student understand how the change in mechanics and form can improve the distance jumped. Note that students may get tired after seven or eight jumps, and may need a rest before continuing to work on improving their jump.

When students have learned the standing long jump, they can progress to the running long jump. In the running jump, the basic standing jump remains the same, but occurs at the end of a short sprint. The running phase builds momentum and results in increased jumping distance. However, the addition of running adds complexity. Athletes with limited vision may have difficulty maintaining a straight trajectory during the sprint, locating the takeoff area to jump from, and landing safely in the sand pit. The running long jump is a common track and field event in middle and high school, and is discussed further in Chapter 8.

Hopping

Hopping is essentially a jump in which the jumper leaves the floor on one foot, with the other foot raised, and lands on the same foot. A hop can be done in one place or moving around a field or gymnasium. Hopping may be taught after the standing long jump (see Sidebar 7.5). Once students have learned the form for hopping, they can work on a series of three hops in a row as a final goal.

Skipping

In essence, a skip is a step followed by a hop, and then switching feet to a step and hop on the other foot, and so forth. Therefore, learning to skip needs to follow the hopping lesson. Students can be taught that a skip is a step-hop with one foot, then a step-hop with the other foot. They can learn first to skip with each foot separately, before putting both actions together to make a continuous skip (see Sidebar 7.6).

Skipping entails considerable coordination. Learning to skip helps improve agility, coordination, and leg strength.

Leaping, Galloping, and Sliding

Other basic locomotor skills include leaping, galloping, and sliding. Although these skills are not described in detail, the following

SIDEBAR 7.5

Teaching Hopping Using Step-by-Step Instruction on Carpet Squares

1. Here we go. Get into the ready position. **(Photo A)**
2. Stand on your kicking foot and lift the other foot off the ground. **(Photo B)**
3. Let's see how long you can stand like this without falling over.
4. Go back to your ready position.
5. Now, stand on your kicking foot and jump off and land on the same foot. **(Photo C)**
6. Go back to the ready position.
7. This is like a long jump, so all we have to do is add the *reach, swing-jump* arms part to the foot-to-foot hop you just did.
8. Show me a good standing long jump and say the operative words: *reach, swing-jump.* [Review long jump if needed.]
9. Now we'll do this from your kicking foot and land on the same foot.
10. Get in the ready position.
11. Ready, stand on your kicking foot. Reach, swing-hop. Reach, swing-hop. **(Photos D, E, F)**

Repeat until the student can consistently use the operative language to complete the task independently.

Operative language: *Ready, stand, reach, swing-hop.*

Teacher's note: Work on a series of three hops in a row as a final goal.

Chuck Comer

A

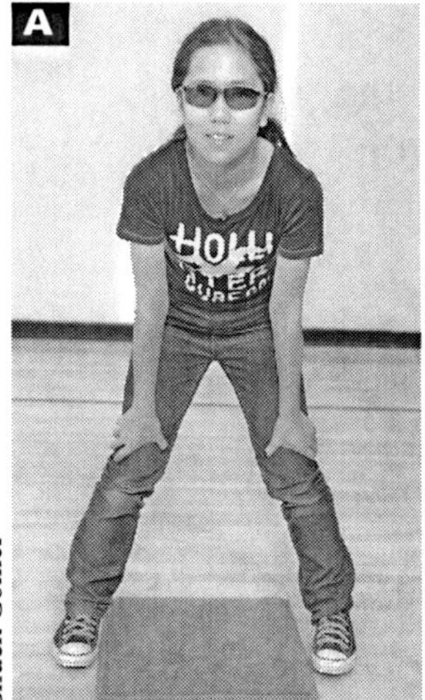

B

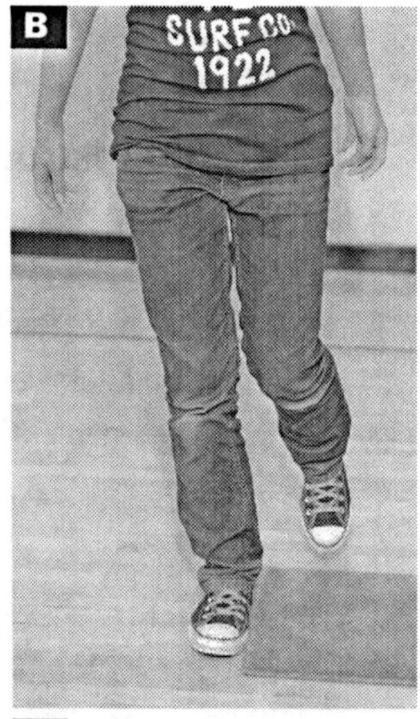

C

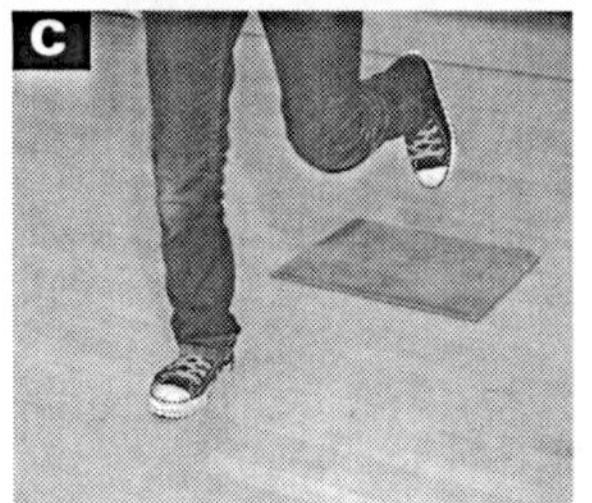

D

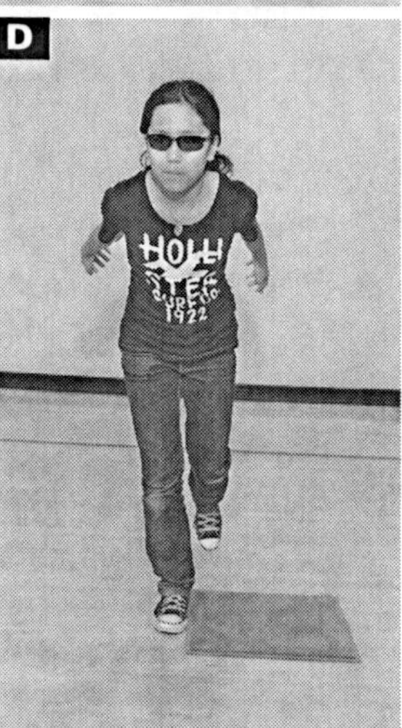

E

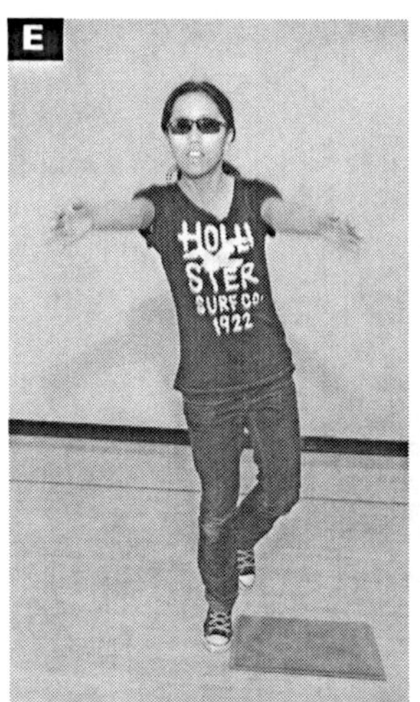

F

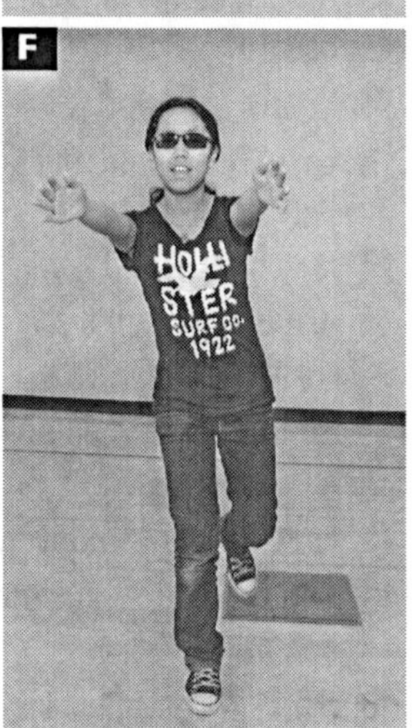

SIDEBAR 7.6

Teaching Skipping Using Step-by-Step Instruction on Carpet Squares

1. Here we go. Get in ready position. **(Photo A)**
2. Step off with the nonkicking foot. **(Photo B)**
3. Back on in ready position.
4. Step off with nonkicking foot.
5. Back on in ready position.
6. We're going to practice hopping again. What was a hop? Yes, jumping from one foot to the same foot.
7. Stand on your nonkicking foot and lift the other one.
8. Hop off the front of your carpet square. **(Photos C, D)**
9. Back on in ready position.
10. This time let's hop off with the kicking foot.
11. Lift your nonkicking foot; hop off. **(Photos E, F)**
12. Now let's put the step and hop together. Step off onto your kicking foot and then hop from it as soon as the step is made. I'll say, "Ready, step-hop." **(Photos G, H)**
13. Get in the ready position on your carpet square.
14. Ready, step-hop.
15. Let's try it again. Ready, step-hop. [Practice until correct.]
16. Now let's try it on your nonkicking foot. We'll just do the step first, then the hop, then put them together.
17. Step off onto your nonkicking foot. Ready, step. **(Photos I, J)**
18. Now let's hop with your nonkicking foot.
19. Ready position, stand on your nonkicking foot, hop off.
20. Back on, ready, nonkicking foot, hop.

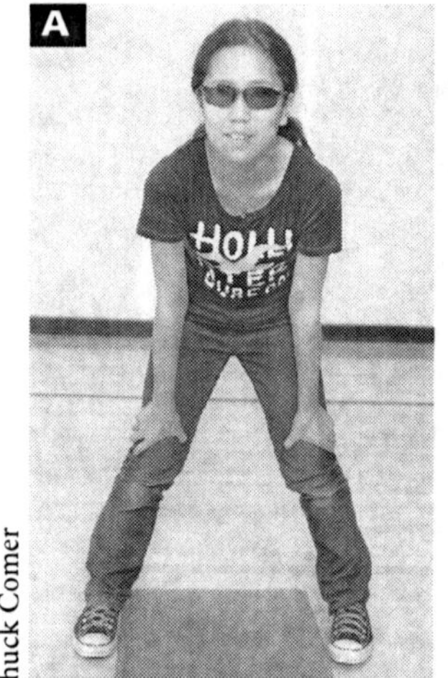

Chuck Comer

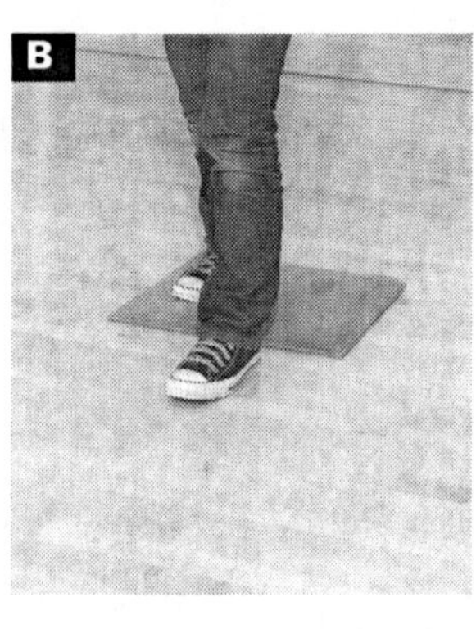

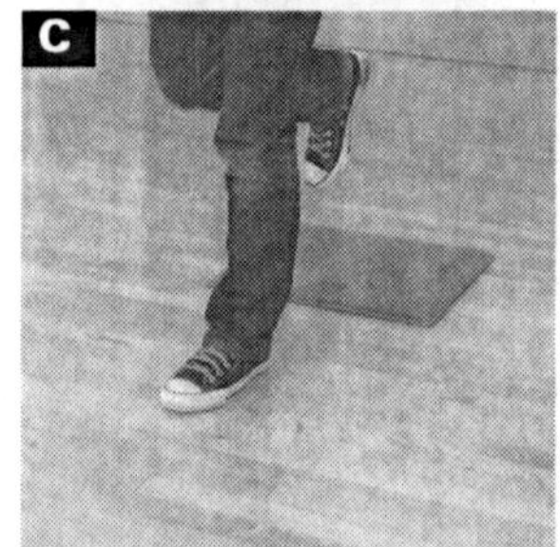

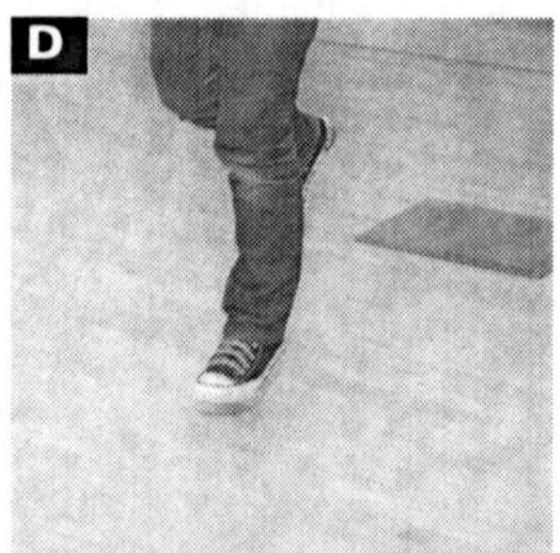

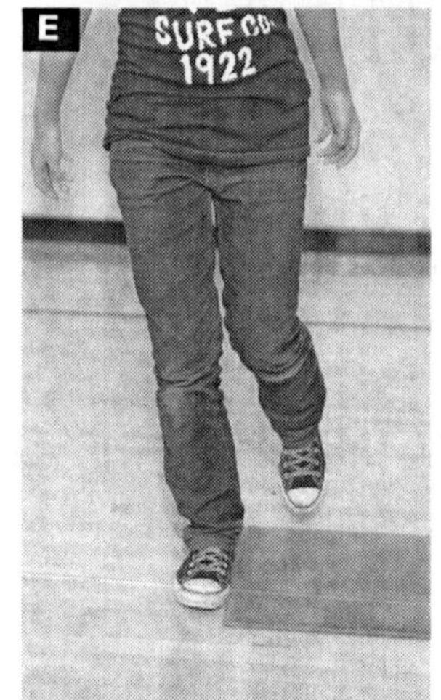

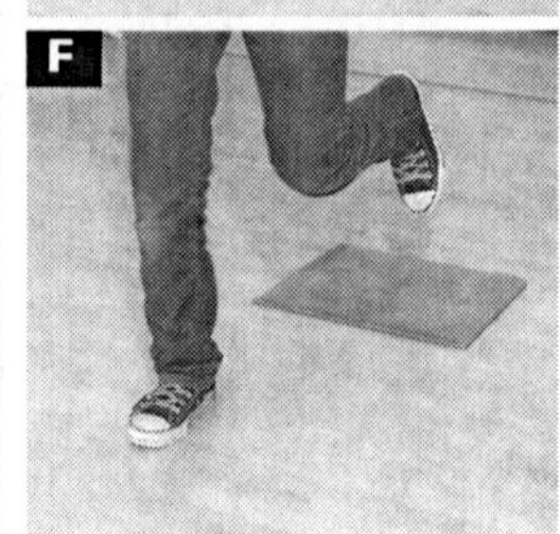

SIDEBAR 7.6 *(continued)*

21. Okay, let's try putting them together. We'll step onto your nonkicking foot, then follow with a hop on the same foot.
22. Ready position, step-hop. [Practice until correct.]
23. Now, let's put both actions together to make a skip. A skip is step-hop with one foot, then a step-hop with the other, then back to the first foot. Putting a bunch of skips together will move you clear across the gym!
24. We'll start with a step-hop with your kicking foot. Then, still going away from the carpet square, we'll switch to the nonkicking foot step-hop.
25. Ready, kicking foot step-hop, switch, step-hop.

Practice this two-step skip until students are comfortable and can use the operative language to complete the skill independently. Then continue adding as many skip steps as possible.

Operative language: *Ready, step-hop, switch, step-hop, switch, step-hop.*

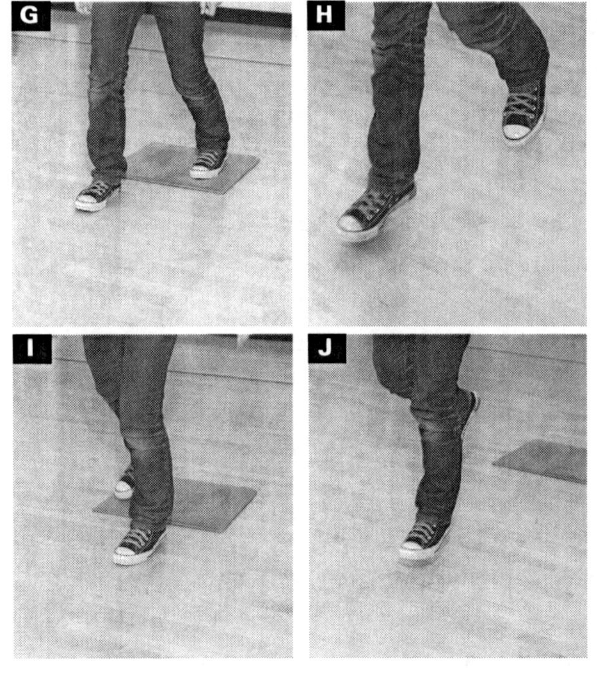

outlines of the key movements in each skill can be helpful in designing lessons to teach them:

Leap

- Take off on one foot, land on the other.
- Remain in the air for a longer period of time than in running.

Gallop

- Step forward with the lead foot, then follow by a step with the rear foot.
- The rear foot lands slightly behind the heel of the front foot.
- There are brief periods without support as the rear foot nears the lead foot.

Slide

- Step sideways with one foot.
- Move the other foot next to the lead foot.
- Keep the upper body straight.
- Transfer weight from the following foot to the lead foot.

TEACHING BASIC SPORTS SKILLS AND CONCEPTS WITH A PARACHUTE

Play parachutes have long been used in physical education and recreational settings to teach basic physical skills and concepts, as well as building cooperative skills, while adding fun to the process of learning. When a group of students lifts a parachute, the parachute catches the air, billowing and falling slowly. Students can go under or on top of the parachute, bounce objects on it, try to roll objects into the hole in the center of the parachute, and perform a variety of other activities. The parachutes used in physical education class are typically large (although they come in different sizes) and multicolored, with handles along the outside for grasping and lifting them. Large parachutes can accommodate a class of 16 to more than 20 students.

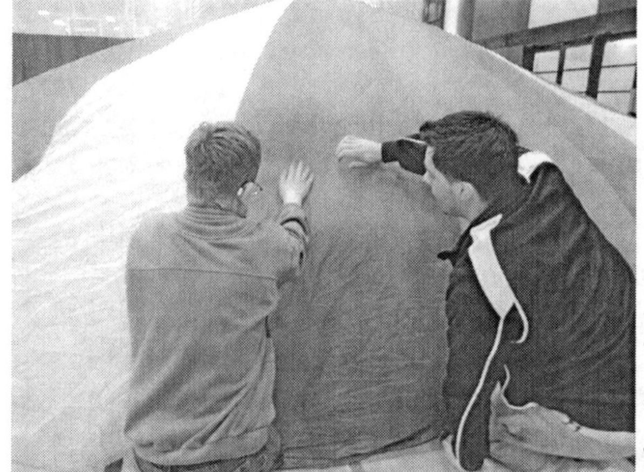
Kelsey Linsenbigler

Exploring a parachute.

Parachute activities are a different approach from step-by-step instruction using carpet squares for including a student with a visual impairment or deafblindness in an elementary classroom's skills curriculum. Physical educators have broken down instruction in basic skills and concepts into sequential lessons in much the same way that the step-by-step method does, but instead using the parachute as the learning medium.

Parachutes lend themselves to all sorts of games that can be created to build skills and sports and spatial concepts in students with visual impairments or deafblindness. The fact that the students commonly manipulate the parachute as a team also makes parachute activities ideal for skill building in inclusive learning settings, as students with visual impairments can follow the movements of the group without a lot of verbal input from teachers. In essence, the group manipulation provided by parachute activities removes the instructional communication barrier from teacher to learners with limited vision. However, as pointed out earlier in this chapter in discussing the whole-part-whole approach, it is important that students included in parachute activities understand the complete activity, not just the part of it they can see or feel in their immediate vicinity. The student with a visual impairment should first be allowed to feel and explore the whole parachute, crawl on top of it, and crawl underneath it. The student should also feel the handles and be shown how to use the handles to move the parachute up and down, left and right.

A set of simple lesson plans is presented in Appendix 7A to this chapter for using a parachute to teach the basic sports concepts of direction, level, extension, force, and time (see Chapter 1 for an explanation of these concepts) in an inclusive setting. These activities also promote cardiovascular endurance, arm strength, and flexibility. Parachute activities can be used with all different age groups to teach more advanced skills and promote fitness.

ADAPTING COMMON ELEMENTARY GAMES AND ACTIVITIES

Once students with visual impairments or deafblindness have learned basic locomotor skills and space and movement concepts, they are better able to participate in the activities of their classmates, whether in physical education class, at lunchtime, or after school. Often, common games and activities are used as elementary school physical education units, including tag, scooter activities, jump rope, parachute activities, relay races, and baseball or whiffle ball. These activities are intended to help students practice and refine their motor skills, increase their athleticism, build related skills in areas such as social interaction and team cooperation, and promote physical fitness and health. However, adaptations may still be needed for students with visual impairments to participate successfully.

When designing adaptations for a particular game for students with visual impairments or deafblindness, it is important to keep in mind the individual student's abilities and needs as well as the objective of the unit. The adaptations in the following examples are based on analysis using the AccesSports model described in Chapter 5.

Tag

Tag is an informal playground game that usually involves two or more players attempting to "tag" other players by touching them, usually with their hands. The rules of the game are flexible and may be made up by the players themselves. At the beginning, one player is "it," the individual designated to catch and tag others. The other players scatter, and "it" chases them down to tag them somewhere on the body. Once tagged, that player becomes the new "it," and the former "it" joins the other players trying to avoid being tagged. The objectives of tag are agility, coordination, fitness, spatial awareness, and turn-taking. Table 7.1 shows adaptations that can be used to include students who are visually impaired in a game of tag. The student who is visually impaired or deafblind can be "it" with the assistance of a guide or intervener. (Please note that elimination games

TABLE 7.1 Adaptations for Tag

Equipment and Goals or Targets	Boundaries	Rules
Players wear bright pinnies Students with visual impairments or deafblindness can use a swimming pool noodle (a long, narrow piece of foam) when they are "it" so they do not run into the other players "It" wears bright colors "It" wears bells	Bright cones Rope with tape over it Bright caution tape warnings placed before doors and steps	Players must walk No pushing Player with visual impairment or deafblindness can have a guide (peer tutor or intervener for a student with deafblindness) The guide can also explain what is happening in the game

in which a student who is tagged sits out are *never* recommended for students of any age or ability. Fitness activities, such as sit-ups, might be assigned as a way to earn entry back into the game, but a student should not be eliminated from a game and then sit idle during a class.)

Scooter Activities

Scooters consist of boards mounted on four wheels. Scooter games can help with the objectives of spatial awareness, movement skills, directionality, laterality, and basic game concepts. Scooters come in a wide variety of shapes and sizes. They are included in many elementary physical education curricula, and they lend themselves to a wide variety of games that are played while participants lie on their stomachs, sit, kneel, or lie on their backs while holding the handles on the scooter boards. There are entire books with scooter games, and the activity possibilities are endless. Two common scooter activities are scooter soccer and scooter tag. Table 7.2 presents some adaptations that can be used with these and other scooter games.

Scooter soccer is a game played with two teams, just like regular soccer. One team starts with the ball at center. The ball is dribbled and passed to teammates using feet. The use of hands instead of feet, or both hands and feet, can also be allowed. Other than the use of the scooter, the game can follow the same rules and play as regular soccer.

In scooter tag, two to four students are chosen to be "it." These students each have a foam ball. On the signal, the chase begins. The students who are "it" must tag another player with the ball without throwing it. If a player is

TABLE 7.2 Adaptations for Scooter Activities

The following adaptations can be used during a scooter unit for games such as scooter tag, scooter soccer, and scooter relay races. The types of scooters can vary depending on the unit and skill level of the student, the way the goals and targets are set up can be varied depending on the objective of the game or activity, the way the gym is set up can vary depending on the game or activity, and the boundaries can be modified.

Equipment and Goals or Targets	Boundaries	Rules
Square scooter Long scooter Double scooter Rope attached to the wall for students to use to pull themselves to the wall on their scooters Soccer goal Auditory sound at end of the gym for relay races Bells at end of relay Sound at end of relay race Guidewire low to floor for relay races	Bright cones Rope with tape over it Bright caution tape for warnings before doors and steps Use a wall for guidance Use guide wire low to floor	No standing on scooter No running onto scooter Relay races Scooter soccer Scooter tag

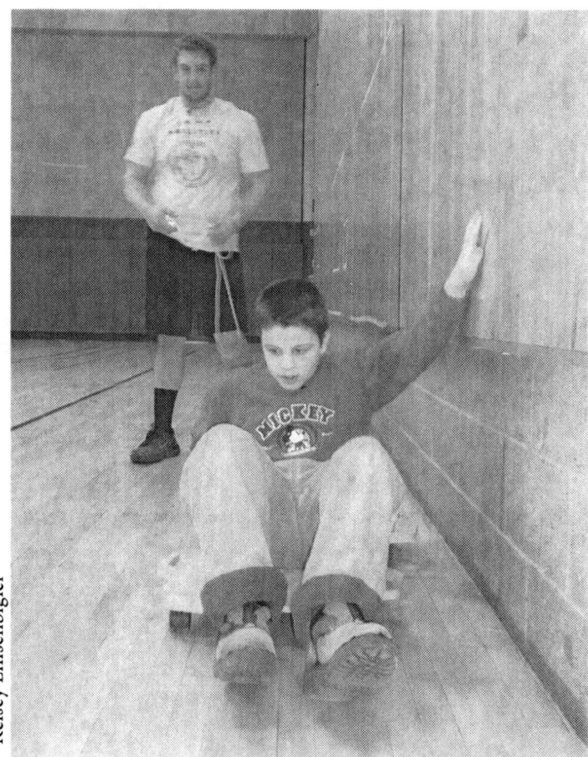

Kelsey Linsenbigler

Scooters can be used to adapt a variety of activities. This boy is using the wall of the gym to guide him as he moves on a scooter.

tagged, that player moves to a designated area (the tagged player can be asked to stand and carry the scooter for safety reasons) and perform a specified movement skill (such as push-ups, sit-ups, or any activity that the teacher wants to focus on); then the tagged player rejoins the game. Before starting, safe boundaries and rules for proper use of the scooters need to be established such as movement speed, where to place hands, and how close the scooters can get to one another. A peer tutor or intervenor can accompany students with visual impairments or deafblindness in the game so they know where they are and where they are going. Taggers should be rotated often.

Jump Rope

Like a number of other physical activities, jumping rope is a lifelong skill. Not only is it a common game for children and a competitive sport for older students and adults, but it is a part of a fitness routine for many adults, as described in Chapter 11, because it aids in agility, balance, and endurance. Jump rope can be an individual activity or a group activity, and it can be varied in many ways.

An overview of how to teach a student who is visually impaired to jump rope was offered earlier as an example of the whole-part-whole model of instruction. The parts of the skill—the grip, the arm swing, and the jump—can be demonstrated by the tactile modeling approach described earlier as well as through physical guidance, ranging from moving the student's arm through the entire swinging motion to a tap on the knee to remind the student to jump. A carpet square is too small to use to introduce jumping rope; a shock-absorbing foam mat with tapered edges is recommended instead, such as the one that comes in the APH jump rope kit (see the Resources section) that defines a safe space in which to jump and helps give students a sense of where they are in space when they jump (Lieberman, Schedlin, & Pierce, 2009).

The student can practice the arm motion first without the jump rope and then by swinging the rope overhead and forward, allowing it to hit the ground in front, and walking forward over it, one leg at a time. Students who use wheelchairs can roll their chair over the rope, or students with limited use of the legs can roll their body over the rope. For students who are able, jumping over the rope can then be practiced in the following sequence of increasingly difficult steps (Lieberman, Schedlin, & Pierce, 2009):

- Step over a low rope (1 to 2 inches high) tied to a chair or held by two people.
- Jump over a rope tied between chairs or held by two people at a height of 6 inches.
- Jump over a swinging low rope at a height of 1 inch with verbal direction or assistance.
- Swing the jump rope with both hands forward over the head and let the rope fall to the ground; then walk over the rope one foot at a time.
- Swing the jump rope with both hands over the head and let the rope fall to the ground and run with one foot in front of the other consecutive times.
- Jump rope with two feet at a time over the rope.
- Jump rope with two feet at a time over the rope at a faster pace.
- Jump rope with two feet at once swinging the rope backward. Jump rope for a specific number of times or for a specific length of time.

A variety of adaptations to the physical environment, such as the following, can be used to adapt jump rope for students who are visually impaired (Lieberman, Schedlin, & Pierce, 2009). These are summarized in Table 7.3 along with suggested adaptations to the rules.

- Jump ropes may be made of different materials, such as plastic, that a student may find easier to turn, and may have different handles or grips that are more or less comfortable.
- Beaded or brightly colored jump ropes can be used for greater visibility.
- A rope can be threaded through a section of a hula-hoop, which can be hung at the rope's center; this makes the rope heavier, and it can be easier to hear the hoop hitting the floor.
- The jump rope can be cut in half, so that the two ends are separated and the rope does not hit the ground under the feet when it is turned. Doing this allows the student to practice only the arm motion and then add

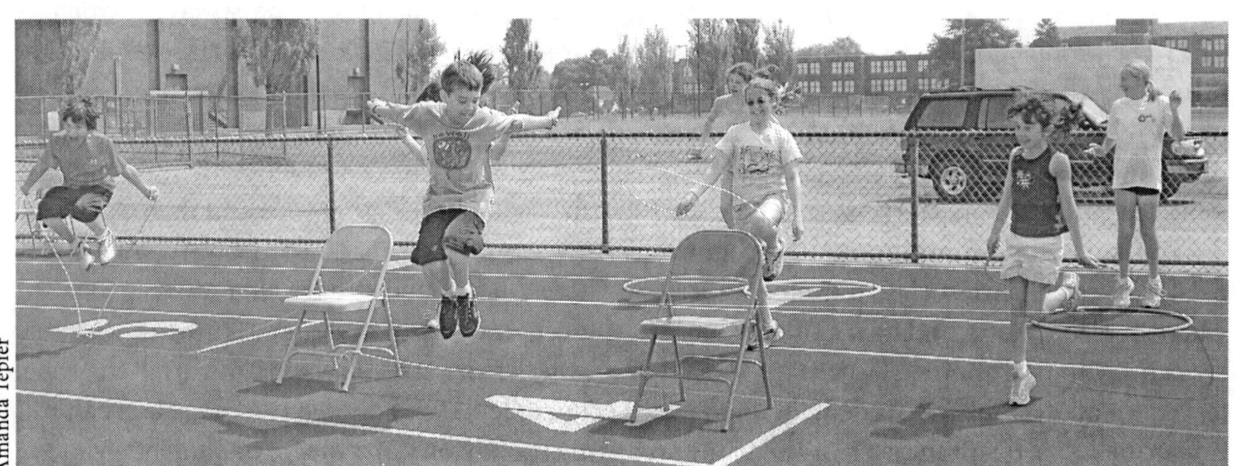
Amanda Tepfer

Practicing jump rope in a variety of ways: jumping over a rope tied to a chair, jumping in and out of hula hoops, running over the rope, and jumping with both feet over the rope.

TABLE 7.3 Adaptations for Jump Rope

Equipment and Goals or Targets	Boundaries	Rules
Beaded rope Plastic rope Cloth rope Bells on rope Hula hoop rope Jump rope cut in half Ropeless jump rope Bright tape wrapped over the rope	Bright caution tape Bright cones Warnings placed before doors Correct space ensured Floor mats used to help with orientation	Walk over rope Jump over 6-inch-high rope with tape over it Jump at own pace Use guidance of a peer Use arms only Use legs only Use music to set the beat Jump with partners Encourage everyone to take a turn jumping with blindfolds

the jump without worrying about timing or height of the jump or becoming tangled in the rope.

- A "ropeless" jump rope can be used that also allows the arm motion to be practiced without worrying about tripping; these devices consist of handles with short sections of rope and may digitally monitor the number of jumps.
- A mat can be used to set the boundaries of the jumping area so the student does not move too far when jumping.
- Music can be used to keep the beat for jumping.

In addition to individual jumping, with some additional adaptations, students who are visually impaired can participate in group jumping and games. The child with the visual impairment can be a rope turner. When he or she jumps, verbal and musical cues can assist with the cadence of the rope. The cue may be as simple as "Up, up, up" when the rope must be swung upward, or it can be more constant such as "Up, down, up, down."

In addition, instead of "running in" while the rope is turning, the student can be allowed to start by standing next to the rope, with it resting on his or her ankle. A count of "1, 2, 3, and over" is used to signal when the rope is turned to assist with timing.

Relay Races

A relay race is a race between two or more teams, in which each team member participates in only part of the race and is then relieved by another member of the team. Usually, each team stands in a line, while a racer goes to a designated point and returns to tag the next racer at the head of the line, who cannot start until he or she is tagged. The goal of relay races is to improve the locomotor skills of agility, speed, coordination, directionality, and laterality. Races can be done cooperatively or competitively and can be held inside or outside. Students can race individually or in pairs, and teams can be of any size, although it is important that they not become too large, as allowing students to spend too much time standing around defeats the purpose of the activity.

Students with visual impairments can participate in relay races by being paired with a classmate or paraeducator, if they have one, or

TABLE 7.4 Adaptations for Relay Races

Equipment and Goals or Targets	Boundaries	Rules
Scooters Carpet squares	Ropes Run next to wall Verbal cues Tactile lines placed on floor to guide runners Guide wire Bells Radio Bright cone at turning point Sound/music at turning point Peers yelling at turning point Loud bell to ring at turning point	Students must move on scooters Students must move on carpet squares Use trained peer tutor Ensure partner is trained and knows how to guide appropriately Use tactile cues Shorten distance Increase distance

by having them run along a wall or guidewire. Students who are deafblind can be paired with a trained peer tutor or their intervener. It is preferable to use peer tutors as guides rather than professionals, when possible, as it provides more age-appropriate social interaction. Visual or audible markings at the designated turning point or end point can also help guide runners. Table 7.4 suggests some specific adaptations that enable students with visual impairments or deafblindness to participate in relay races.

Baseball and Whiffle Ball

A variety of different kinds of balls, bats, and batting tees can be used to adapt baseball and its variations to enable students with visual impairments or deafblindness to play, as illustrated in Table 7.5. The bases and base path can also be adapted. In addition to adapting a regular game of baseball or whiffle ball for a student who is visually impaired, the entire class can be introduced to beep baseball, a game developed specifically to be played by individuals who are blind or blindfolded. Beep baseball is described in detail in Chapter 9. Again, if a student is deafblind, then the student can be paired with a trained classmate, or the intervener or paraeducator if the student has one. It is important to make sure that the details of the game are explained to students who are blind or deafblind, as this game can be boring if a student is in the outfield or in line to bat and does not know what is going on.

MOTIVATING STUDENTS

Regardless of whether students have a disability or not, how they are introduced to physical activity and sports is a strong determinant of their motivation to continue participating into adulthood. Including students with visual impairments or deafblindness in physical education and other games and sports activities with their classmates is a crucial part of that process (Ponchillia, Strause, & Ponchillia, 2002). It is also important to examine the factors in the way physical activity is presented that might increase students' motivation to continue being physically active.

One model of motivation that has been applied to physical activity indicates that motiva-

TABLE 7.5 Adaptations for Baseball or Whiffle Ball

Equipment and Goals or Targets	Boundaries	Rules
Plastic bat	Yellow ribbon on fence	Pre-teaching skills before unit begins
Batting tee	Bright bases	Physical assistance
Whiffle ball with bells inside	Auditory bases	Verbal assistance
Softball	Different textures on path	Bat off tee
Ball on string	Guide wire to bases	Bat from a string
Beep baseball		Run with trained peer
Bright Nerf ball		Describe what is happening in the game
Large bat		Provide assistance in the field with locating the ball and knowing where to throw it
Bright bat		
Light bat		

tion is linked to the need for activities that satisfy innate psychological needs for autonomy, competence, and relatedness (Kilpatrick, Hebert, & Jacobsen, 2002). *Autonomy* is the perception of self-control or the ability to make choices for oneself; *competence* is an internal knowledge that one has the skills to accomplish one's goals; and *relatedness* is the inner sense of the ability to get along in the social world.

Thus, students with visual impairments or deafblindness can be motivated to participate in physical activity in an elementary physical activity curriculum by making sure that the experience encourages autonomy, promotes success that fosters feelings of competence, and stimulates the development of social relationships. The ultimate goal is for students to be intrinsically motivated to participate in physical activity—that is, to enjoy physical activity for its own sake—rather than by external rewards or punishments, which tend to undermine autonomy and therefore ultimately undermine motivation as well (Kilpatrick, Bartholomew, & Riemer, 2003; Kilpatrick, Hebert, & Jacobsen, 2002).

The following recommendations are intended to foster an increased adherence to an active life by making physical activity an intrinsically motivating activity (Agran, Hong, & Blankenship, 2007; Kilpatrick, Hebert, & Jacobsen, 2002):

- Give positive feedback. Positive feedback should be given as the main form of feedback, but minimal instructional or corrective feedback is expected and appropriate.
- Promote specific goals. Base goals on task mastery, not on competition, comparisons, or outperforming others. Task mastery tends to eliminate outside pressures from competition that are beyond the student's control. Measure progress by measuring growth in each student, not among students.
- Promote moderately difficult goals rather than hard-to-achieve ones. More attainable goals are more likely to promote success and foster a feeling of competence and mastery. Err on the side of less difficult, rather than more difficult.
- Provide choice of activities. Providing choices promotes autonomy, while forcing participation in a single activity leads to perceptions of coercion.

- Provide a rationale for activities. Giving the rationale for the activity also promotes autonomy, and not doing so causes perceptions of being controlled.
- Promote the development of social relationships. An increased sense of satisfaction and belonging contribute to developing a sense of relatedness to others.
- Give rewards sparingly and carefully. Rewards have the potential to undermine autonomy and motivation, because the reward itself may come to be the goal, as opposed to the love for physical activity and movement. Giving rewards is appropriate, however, under many circumstances, such as temporarily motivating a new behavior that is not intrinsically appealing until the behavior itself becomes more desirable.

CONCLUSION

Using the strategies outlined in this chapter—along with some time, energy, patience, and creative thinking on the part of teachers, specialists, parents, and other caregivers—students with visual impairments or deafblindness can be active and full participants in the activities of their elementary school physical education class. In addition, students will be learning and practicing many of the skills in the core areas of the expanded core curriculum, discussed in Chapter 3, such as O&M skills and concepts, recreation and leisure skills, social interaction skills, self-determination and independence skills, and sensory efficiency skills (Sapp & Hatlen, 2010).

Students who are introduced to physical activity early on and who are included in the physical education curriculum throughout their years in elementary school are getting the tools to be safe and successful in physical activities and the opportunity to develop a love of activity that can continue into adolescence and adulthood. They will most likely be ready to participate in the more advanced games and sports taught in junior high and high school and perhaps move on to competitive athletic events, as discussed in the next chapter.

APPENDIX 7A

Lesson Plans for Using Parachute Activities to Teach Sports Concepts

Site: Gymnasium or large room
Materials: 12-foot parachute and audible ball
Objectives: The objective of these activities is to develop and improve the understanding of the concepts of direction, level, time, extension, and force in an inclusive setting. Students will also work on cardiovascular endurance, arm strength, and flexibility.

ACTIVITY 1: WAVES

When this activity is done correctly, the parachute simulates the motion of waves in the ocean or a pool.

1. Spread the parachute out flat on the ground.
2. Have students squat down next to it and grasp it with both hands, fingers up and thumbs down.
3. Have students use small hand movements to *slowly* lift the edge of the parachute and put it back on the ground.
4. Have students use small hand movements to *moderately* lift the edge of the parachute and put it back on the ground.
5. Have students use small hand movements to *quickly* lift the edge of the parachute and put it back on the ground.
6. Have students repeat these movements until they master the concepts of slow, moderate, and quick.
7. Test the mastery of these concepts by giving random commands until they are consistently performed accurately.

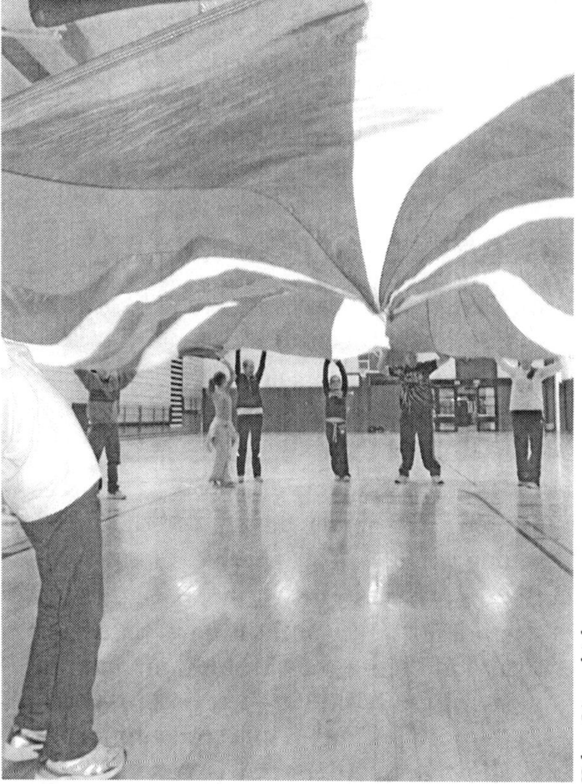
Kelsey Linsenbigler

Making waves with a parachute.

ACTIVITY 2: LEVEL WAVES

1. Have students spread the parachute out flat on the ground.
2. Have students squat down next to it and grasp it with both hands, fingers up and thumbs down.
3. Have students use small hand movements to quickly lift the edge of the parachute up to their ankles and put it back on the ground.
4. Have students use small hand movements to quickly lift the edge of the parachute up to their waists and put it back on the ground.
5. Have students use small hand movements to quickly lift the edge of the parachute up over their heads and put it back on the ground.
6. Repeat these movements but replace the words *ankles* with *low level, waist* with *medium level,* and *above their heads* with *high level* until mastered.
7. Test the mastery of these concepts by giving random commands until consistently performed accurately.

ACTIVITY 3: SEE-SAW PULL

1. Have the students spread the parachute out flat on the ground.
2. Have the students begin the activity by sitting around the parachute, so that it is in front of them.
3. Have the students grasp the parachute using two hands, fingers and thumbs down.
4. From the sitting position, have the students *slowly* pull the parachute back and forth in a see-saw motion, making sure to fully extend their bodies when they are pulling. A cue could be "arms above head."
5. From the sitting position, have the students *moderately* pull the parachute back and forth in a see-saw motion, making sure to somewhat extend their bodies when they are pulling.
6. From the sitting position, have the students *quickly* pull the parachute back and forth in a see-saw motion, making sure they do not extend their bodies when they are pulling.
7. Randomly give the commands for slow and big extension, moderate and some extension, and fast and no extension.
8. Test the mastery of these concepts by giving random commands until consistently performed accurately.

ACTIVITY 4: CHUTE LIFT

1. Have the students lay the parachute out flat on the ground.
2. While standing, have the students bend down and grasp the parachute with both hands, fingers and thumbs down.
3. Have the students lift the parachute to midlevel (waist), then raise it back and forth between high level and midlevel softly, "like butterfly wings."
4. Briefly note the soft sounds and breezes that are created by the parachute. The teacher may say, "Feel the breeze from the movement of the parachute. What does it sound like?"
5. Have the students lift the parachute to midlevel (waists), then raise it back and forth between high level and midlevel really fast, "like hummingbird wings."
6. Briefly note the loud snapping sounds and wind that are created by the parachute. The teacher may say, "Feel the breeze from the snap of the parachute. What does it sound like?"
7. With the teacher counting cadence by saying, "Up, down, up," so that all children work as a team, have the students lift the parachute to midlevel (waists), then raise it back and forth

between high level and midlevel softly with the teacher's commands.

8. With the teacher counting cadence by saying, "Up, down, up," and so forth, have the students lift the parachute to midlevel (waists), then raise it back and forth between high level and midlevel fast with the teacher's commands.
9. Have the students describe the sound of teamwork compared to no teamwork. If the students do not work as a team, the parachute will flap and snap loudly, as it will not be moving smoothly up and down.

ACTIVITY 5: MUSHROOM

The students piled up under the parachute create a lumpy shape that looks like a mushroom.

1. Have the students lay out the parachute flat on the ground.
2. From a standing position, have the students bend down and grasp the parachute with both hands, fingers and thumbs down.
3. Have the students lift the parachute up over their heads at high level and quickly bring the parachute down, tightly behind them.
4. Have the students lift the parachute up over their heads at high level and quickly bring the parachute down in front of them to low level (below knees), and then tightly behind them.
5. Have students alternate bringing the parachute down in front of the body and in back of the body randomly until the mushroom shape is achieved consistently.

ACTIVITY 6: ONE-HAND RUN

1. Have the students lay the parachute out flat on the ground.
2. Mark the left hands of all the students with a washable tattoo or tactile marker such as a wrist band of their choice.
3. From a standing position, have the students bend down and grasp the parachute with their tattooed hand, extending the other hand and arm away from the parachute.
4. While still holding on, have the students quickly walk forward around in a circle.
5. Then have the students stop and change hands with the opposite hand holding the parachute and the opposite hand and arm extended.
6. Have the students quickly walk forward around in a circle.
7. Have the students quickly walk, then give random direction and hand changes until they make the hand and direction exchanges quickly and efficiently.

Teacher's note: Many games can be made of this direction activity, including changing direction after each 10 steps, changing the speed of walking from slow like a turtle to fast like a rabbit, walking backward, and so forth.

ACTIVITY 7: PUNCHING BAG (JUST FOR FUN)

1. Have the students lay the parachute out flat on the ground.
2. While standing, have the students bend down and grasp the parachute with both hands, fingers and thumbs down.
3. Have the students raise the parachute over their heads to high level, take three steps in, quickly lower the parachute to the floor, and kneel.
4. Without leaving their kneeling position, have the students "punch" the air out of the parachute until it is flat.
5. Repeat as a fun break at any time during the lesson.

ACTIVITY 8: BALL ROLL

1. Have the students lay the parachute out flat on the ground.

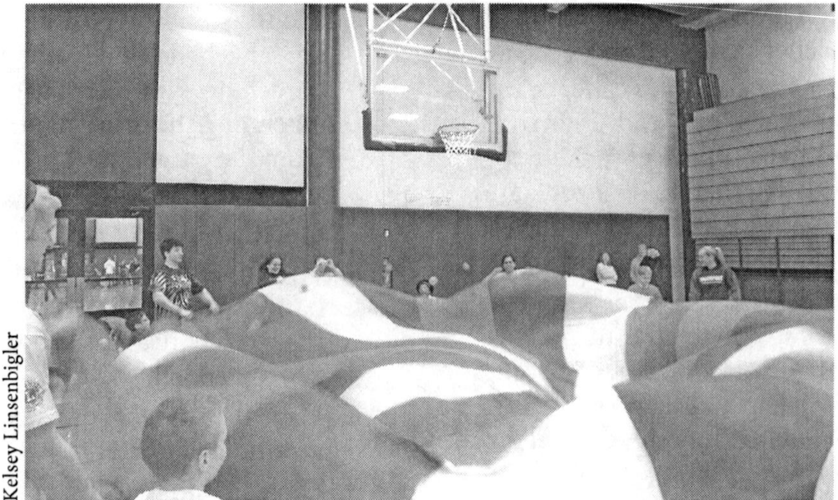
Kelsey Linsenbigler

An activity with a parachute and balls.

2. While standing, have the students bend down and grasp the parachute with both hands, fingers up and thumbs down.
3. From the standing position, have the students manipulate an adapted ball containing bells or a beeper on the parachute to try to roll the ball into the hole in the center.
4. While trying to get the ball into the center of the parachute, have the students use whatever skills necessary, focusing on level, extension, and force.
5. Have the students talk about how they got the ball in the hole, encouraging them to use terms related to level, extension, and force.

Physical Education and Sports Activities in Middle School, High School, and Adulthood

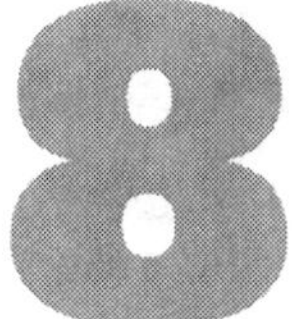

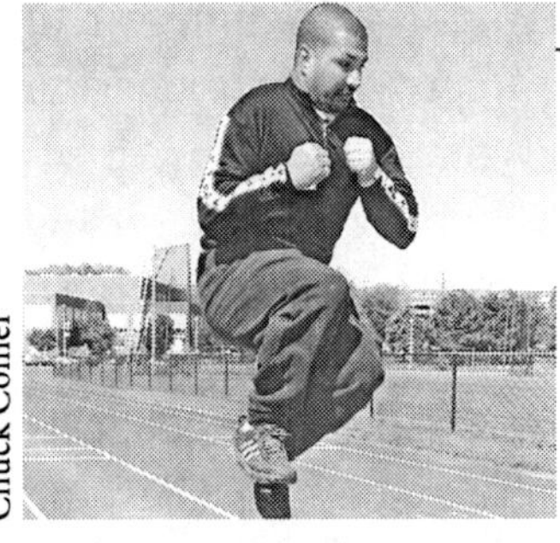

Chuck Comer

IN THIS CHAPTER

- **Physical Education in Middle School and High School**
- **Sports Activities for Adolescents and Adults**

Jamalia, a freshman at a small county high school of some 350 students, loved to swim and had spent much of her childhood summers in the water. However, she felt that her severe visual impairment prevented her from participating in her school's sports programs. But then her teacher of students with visual impairments found out about a device made out of a modified lawn sprinkler that would let her know when she was approaching the end wall of the swimming pool. Jamalia obtained one of the devices and practiced swimming laps in a friend's swimming pool all summer between her freshman and sophomore years. After this experience, she was convinced that she could compete on her school's swimming team, so she reported for swimming tryouts in the fall.

The swimming coach was reluctant at first, but Jamalia's newfound confidence convinced him to give her a chance to try out. After Jamalia made the team, the coach contacted the United States Association of Blind Athletes for assistance with other adaptations, and he soon became one of Jamalia's strongest advocates. She swam in all the school meets that year and won two third-place finishes in league meets in the backstroke event.

As students make the transition from elementary school to middle school and then to high school, the nature of their physical education classes changes in response to the physical, social, and cognitive developmental changes they are undergoing during this time in their lives. The primary purpose of physical education programming in elementary school is to equip students with basic physical skills, such as running, jumping, throwing, and kicking (Rink, 2009). As children move into middle school, however, the focus changes to generalizing the use of these basic skills to modified or simplified game situations, while in high school students learn the aspects of functioning in complex game settings (Rink, 2009). Older high school students differ little from adults in their ability to play complex games, so they are generally treated as adults during their later years in physical education. Because of this, the high school curriculum is frequently based on students' choice rather than on the prescribed curricula that are used in elementary and middle schools (Rink, 2009).

This chapter discusses the continuum of physical education programming from middle school to high school and the implications of such programming for the physical education of students with visual impairments or deafblindness. Then it describes a variety of sports and other activities commonly included in such programs, with specific information about how these activities can be made accessible to students with visual impairments or deafblindness. Chapter 9 will address sports developed specifically for individuals with visual impairments, and making recreational and fitness activities accessible is covered in Chapters 10 and 11, respectively.

As described in Part 1 of this book, participation of youths and adults with visual impairments or deafblindness in sports activities in general tends to be quite limited (Ponchillia, Armbruster, & Wiebold, 2005), and sports media coverage of games played by competitors with disabilities that might spark interest in these activities is rare. To provide information needed to encourage young people with visual impairments to become more physically active and to become involved in recreational and competitive sports, this chapter includes detailed information on a wide range of sports activities, including information on adapting each activity and on competitive opportunities for athletes with visual impairments or deafblindness. Because young people with visual impairments have few sports heroes with whom they can identify and whom they can emulate, short profiles of successful athletes with visual impairments or deafblindness are presented for each sport, to provide role models that teachers and parents can share with children.

PHYSICAL EDUCATION IN MIDDLE SCHOOL AND HIGH SCHOOL

The content of physical education programming in middle school and high school varies significantly, largely because the two groups of students are so different developmentally in terms of their cognitive, social, emotional, and physical development. Middle school children are experiencing rapid growth spurts and accompanying coordination issues, the emotional ups and downs of puberty, and the desire to be like the others in their age group. In comparison, high school students are physically and emotionally more like adults and are beginning to break away from their reliance on peer groups, becoming more individualistic (Rink, 2009). Consequently, the middle school curriculum is generally designed to take that expected developmental growth into consideration, while the high school curriculum is usually not. In addition, because many high schools offer physical education classes in only one or two of their four years, it is impractical to offer a sequenced curriculum for high school physical education.

The physical education content standards developed by the National Association of School Physical Educators (NASPE, 2004; see Chapter 3) serve as building blocks for the development of physical education curricula across the United States. Although the standards apply to all grade levels, the way that the standards are implemented differs from elementary to middle and high school. Sidebar 8.1 provides an example of how the standards would be applied in the middle school curriculum, as suggested by Rink (2009), who has provided guidance to help physical educators convert the standards into objectives and content frameworks for the delivery of sound physical education in public schools and provided much of the material for this discussion.

SIDEBAR 8.1

Emphases of the NASPE National Standards in Middle School Physical Education

The following list shows how the NASPE standards might be applied to a middle school physical education curriculum:

Standard 1: Demonstrates Competency in Motor Skills and Movement Patterns to Perform a Variety of Physical Activities

By the end of middle school students should be able to

- achieve mature forms of basic skills
- participate with skill and achieve competence in the basic skills in a variety of sport, dance, gymnastics, and outdoor activities
- use skills and tactics successfully in modified games or activities of increasing complexity

Middle school programs should develop students' basic skills in an activity to a level of competence, meaning that they should be able to demonstrate good form and consistency in the use of the form.

By the end of middle school, students should be using skills in modified gamelike situations, such as playing 3 against 3 in basketball or 7 against 7 in soccer. Changing the game space and number of players need to be modified when making modified gamelike conditions. By the end of middle school, students should know and be able to execute the basic tactics of both invasion and net activities.

Standard 2: Demonstrates Understanding of Movement Concepts, Principles, Strategies, and Tactics as They Apply to the Learning and Performance of Physical Activities

By the end of middle school, students should have the cognitive expectation that they can

(Continued on next page)

SIDEBAR 8.1 *(continued)*

- identify critical elements of sport-specific games and activities that characterize good performance
- identify basic tactics of both invasion and net activities and how to use them effectively in modified game situations
- know the basic principles of conditioning for a sport or an activity
- identify principles of good practice
- use information from the disciplines as well as feedback from others to improve performance

Standard 3: Participates Regularly in Physical Activity

Students need to be able to take what they learn in the physical education classroom and apply it to what they do outside of the class. Emphasis in this area is to

- understand the importance of being physically active on a daily basis
- participate in physical activity on a daily basis
- understand their own interests and abilities in the area of physical activity
- make lifestyle choices to be physically active

Middle school students have many opportunities to choose to participate in structured or unstructured activities, which makes the middle school years an ideal time developmentally to help these students choose wisely in terms of the amount of physical activity they engage in on a daily basis. Students need to know where and when they can participate outside of the class in all of the activities that are taught in the curriculum. Also, helping students understand where their interests may lie ought to be a part of every program.

Standard 4: Achieves and Maintains a Health-Enhancing Level of Physical Fitness

Students at the middle school age level should

- be able to set personal fitness goals and assess the extent to which they have achieved those personal goals
- have the skills to assess their own cardiovascular endurance
- identify the relationship between regular participation in physical activity and fitness
- meet the standard for fitness identified for their age group
- identify the health-related benefits of physical activity
- be comfortable with identifying and using the components of fitness to talk about their own fitness status and to identify what they can do to improve or maintain their own personal fitness levels

Standard 5: Exhibits Responsible Personal and Social Behavior That Respects Self and Others in Physical Activity Settings

Experiences in physical education class should be positive ones. The intent of this standard is to help students act in responsible ways. Students should

- interact with others in a positive way regardless of skill level, gender, or status within the group
- accept responsibility for conducting themselves in a safe and productive manner in class
- work independently
- demonstrate respect for self and others

Standard 6: Values Physical Activity for Health, Enjoyment, Challenge, Self-Expression, and/or Social Interaction

Middle school programs that provide students with an opportunity to experience all of the benefits from physical activity include a wide variety of different kinds of activities and are taught so that students can achieve enough skill and depth with these experiences to realize these benefits. Learning for this standard involves helping students to

- value physical activity for the positive personal effects of that activity

SIDEBAR 8.1 *(continued)*

- identify different positive effects of participation in different kinds of physical activity
- use movement to express feeling
- identify personal likes and dislikes of physical activity in terms of their personal effects and in terms of the kinds of activities that are personally attractive

Sources: Adapted, with permission, from J. E. Rink, "Foundations of the Middle School Curriculum," in J. E. Rink, *Designing the Physical Education Curriculum: Promoting Active Lifestyles* (New York: McGraw-Hill, 2009); National Association for Sport and Physical Education, *Appropriate Instructional Practice Guidelines for Middle School Physical Education.* (Reston, VA: NASPE, 2001).

The Middle School Curriculum

As already noted, physical education in middle school focuses on teaching students to use the basic skills learned in elementary school in practical, simplified sports and game settings. The transition from practicing basic skills to sports skills—for example, from underhand throwing to bowling, kicking to soccer passing, or jumping to long jumping—is made during this period. Middle school students begin learning skills in simplified conditions, and teachers gradually add complexity to the conditions. The middle school program should develop students' basic skills in an activity to a level of competence, and the skills and concepts should increase in complexity from grade 6 through grade 8.

Middle school student programs ought to include a variety of movement forms, such as aquatics, team sports, dual sports, individual sports, outdoor pursuits, self-defense, dance, and gymnastics (NASPE, 2009) and not rely only on team sports. By the end of middle school, students should have learned to control both their own movements and the objects used in the activities and to understand the major tactics of so-called invasion games (ones in which the aim is to invade the territory of the other side in order to score, such as basketball or soccer) as well as net games (such as badminton; pickleball, a pre-tennis game using a whiffleball; and tennis). However, middle school students need not play under full game conditions. Teachers can modify the rules of the game to simplify them, much in the same fashion that activities are modified to make them simpler for students with visual impairments or deafblindness (as explained in Chapter 5). Such modifications might include reducing the number of players—for example, playing a 3-against-3 game of basketball—or simplifying scoring by, for instance, awarding points for hitting the rim of the basket and eliminating penalties or other rules that continuously stop play. The specific sports and activities covered in middle and high school programs are similar, but the complexity of the skills taught and the game conditions are not.

The High School Curriculum

The high school physical education curriculum, as already mentioned, is frequently offered in one or two years and is usually not sequential, and students commonly choose their own activities in it. Many high school curricula also emphasize participation in physical activity programs outside the classroom and attempt to establish lifelong patterns of exercise and other health-promoting behaviors. Sidebar 8.2

SIDEBAR 8.2

Sample High School Physical Education Curriculum, Expressed as Goals and Learning Objectives

The following sample curriculum gives goals and objectives showing how the NASPE national standards can be applied to physical education in high school:

Standard 1: Demonstrates Competency in Motor Skills and Movement Patterns to Perform a Variety of Physical Activities

Goal

- Be competent in three different activities in two different movement forms

Specific Objective

1. Demonstrate competence in three different activities from two of the following:
   - **a.** Team sports—basketball, volleyball, lacrosse, soccer, field hockey
   - **b.** Individual/dual sports—gymnastics, bowling, archery, tennis
   - **c.** Outdoor pursuits—canoeing, backpacking, kayaking, wall climbing
   - **d.** Fitness and training—weightlifting, jogging, aerobic dance
   - **e.** Dance—line and folk dance, modern, African
   - **f.** Martial arts—yoga, tae kwon do, karate

Standard 2: Demonstrates Understanding of Movement Concepts, Principles, Strategies, and Tactics as They Apply to the Learning and Performance of Physical Activities

Goals

- Know why physical activity is important
- Use both a training and an activity approach to maintain or improve fitness
- Design a personal activity plan to improve health-related fitness based on scientifically based knowledge
- Use discipline- and activity-specific knowledge to improve performance and learning

Specific Objectives

1. Can describe the benefits of participation in physical activity
2. Can plan a program to improve fitness using a training-and-activity approach
3. Can identify the safety, rules, and tactics of the activities chosen for competence development
4. Can describe one principle of learning and one principle of biomechanics that would improve performance in each activity taken

Standard 3: Participates Regularly in Physical Activity

Goals

- Understand the relationship between physical activity and a healthy lifestyle through the lifespan
- Possess the skills, knowledge, and disposition to maintain a high level of physical activity independently
- Participate regularly in physical activity
- Identify community resources for participation in physical activity

Specific Objectives

1. Can identify the major sources of physical activity and community resources for people of different ages
2. Participates for at least nine weeks in a structured physical activity outside of school
3. Participates at least three times a week in moderate to vigorous physical activity outside of a physical education class

SIDEBAR 8.2 (*continued*)

Standard 4: Achieves and Maintains a Health-Enhancing Level of Physical Fitness

Goals

- Independently apply training principles to maintain or improve a level of fitness
- Assess personal fitness status
- Meet the health-related fitness standards as defined by Fitnessgram
- Achieve personal fitness goals after a period of training

Specific Objectives

1. Meet the health-related fitness standards as defined by Fitnessgram.
2. Independently apply training principles to diagnose, set goals, and establish a personal fitness program to maintain or improve levels of fitness

Standard 5: Exhibits Responsible Personal and Social Behavior That Respects Self and Others in Physical Activity Settings

Goals

- Positively influence the behavior of others in physical activity settings
- Develop a personal philosophy of participation that is inclusive of others of different ages, ability, gender, race, ethnicity, socioeconomic status, and culture
- Hold themselves personally responsible for safe practices, settling conflicts in a positive way and establishing rules, procedures, and etiquette in physical activity settings

Specific Objectives

1. Be inclusive in their relationships with others in physical activity settings.
2. Know how to be an independent and responsible participant in a wide variety of physical activity settings

Standard 6: Values Physical Activity for Health, Enjoyment, Challenge, Self-Expression, and/or Social Interaction

Goals

- Can identify the potential values of different kind of activities
- Can identify the activities that provide personal pleasure and why they provide pleasure
- Is willing to learn new activities

Specific Objectives

1. Can identify the potential values of different kinds of activities
2. Can identify the activities that provide personal pleasure and why they provide pleasure
3. Demonstrates a willingness to learn new activities by their selection of activities in the program

Source: Reprinted with permission from J. E. Rink, *Designing the Physical Education Curriculum: Promoting Active Lifestyles*, Box 10.4, "Goals Translated into Specific Objectives for Meadowbrook High School" (New York: McGraw Hill, 2009).

contains a typical example of a high school program written with learning objectives.

Effects of the Physical Education Curriculum on Students with Visual Impairments or Deafblindness

The degree of access that students with visual impairments or deafblindness have to physical education activities is affected by the differing contents of the curricula in middle and high school. In particular, access to the middle school curriculum can be somewhat more restrictive than in most high schools, depending on the skill of the physical education teacher in adapting activities, because the middle school curriculum requires students to participate in fast-moving invasion sports (in which the objective is to enter or "invade" the opponents' territory to score points) and net activities. These activities require the visual tracking of objects, such as basketballs, baseballs, and whiffle balls, which can be extremely difficult for students with visual impairments or deafblindness. In high school, however, students with low vision or no vision often have a choice of curricular activities and can select activities that are more appropriate for their visual ability or can be more easily modified for them.

In addition, team and invasion sports have been deemphasized in physical education classes in recent years (Rink, 2009), and the national content standards describe a broad view of physical education, well beyond just sports activities. Therefore, participation in sports activities, whether in physical education class or outside the school curriculum, has increasingly become the student's choice. It should be kept in mind, however, that allowing students to choose their own activities may also limit the range of experiences for some students with visual impairments or deafblindness who may avoid certain activities that they mistakenly consider too difficult or impossible, either because those students may not have adjusted to their disabilities in terms of sports participation or because they simply lack sufficient experience with physical skills to know their own potential.

As discussed in Chapter 1, this kind of self-imposed limitation and the other limitations related to visual impairment and deafblindness discussed in that chapter can decrease students' access to physical activity and physical education classes. In contrast, students with visual impairments or deafblindness who have had previous experience in school physical education classes or in summer sports education camps are more likely to participate in future sports activities (Ponchillia, Strause, & Ponchillia, 2002; Ponchillia, Armbruster, & Wiebold, 2005). Moreover, anecdotal evidence, such as the experience of Christopher, whose story is introduced in Chapter 1 and who is profiled later in this chapter as a wrestling role model, indicates that participation in sports can have profound positive consequences for some individuals with visual impairment or deafblindness.

The aim of this chapter, therefore, is to facilitate such choices and make the option of participating in sports activities in school, as well as outside of it, more easily available to students with visual impairments or deafblindness. The remainder of this chapter provides educators, parents and other family members and caretakers, and other advocates with the information necessary to successfully implement sports programs for adolescents and adults with visual impairments or deafblindness and thus increase the possibility that they will continue such activities throughout their lives.

SPORTS ACTIVITIES FOR ADOLESCENTS AND ADULTS

People with visual impairments or deafblindness participate in virtually every sport of consequence and at every level: in back yards or sandlots, at the local "Y" or community parks, on intramural or interscholastic teams, on exclusive club teams, on intercollegiate teams, on international teams of athletes with disabilities, and on the U.S. Olympic team. Given the wide range of sports played by these individuals, priority has been given in this chapter to covering those most commonly played by adolescents and adults with visual impairments or deafblindness and that are common in the middle and high school curricula. Most of the activities presented here are also sponsored by the United States Association of Blind Athletes (USABA) and the authors' summer sports camps. The USABA is a membership organization composed of athletes with visual impairments and their supporters that provides sports education, promotes involvement of its members in mainstream competitions, and provides them with competitive opportunities. The organization also works with the U.S. Paralympic committee and the International Blind Sports Foundation (IBSA) to select athletes with visual impairments or deafblindness to represent the United States in international events, including the Paralympic Games, held in conjunction with the Olympics. (These organizations and the international competitions they sponsor are described further in Chapter 12, and the Resources section at the back of this book provides contact information for these and many other sports-related organizations that serve people with visual impairments and deafblindness.) The USABA and the IBSA recognize a system of classification for athletes with visual impairments based on their visual abilities (see Sidebar 8.3). It should be noted that the B4 category for athletes who are visually impaired but not legally blind is recognized only by the USABA and thus is not encountered in the international competitions discussed in this chapter.

The sports activities described in this chapter include individual track, cross-country, and field events; individual aquatic events; wrestling; judo; rowing; tandem bicycling; and dragon boating. The sections on each of these activities contain a description of the activity, a brief history, the adaptations required by people with visual impairments or deafblindness to participate, the competitive options for individuals who are visually impaired or deafblind and their rules, and tips for teachers or coaches about how best to present the activity. (Readers will also find descriptions of each sport, the rules for competition, and training tips and other information on the website of the USABA, www.usaba.org. Another resource for adaptations to sports as well as recreation activities is *The Encyclopedia of Sports and Recreation for People with Visual Impairments* [Liebs, in press].) This detailed information presented on sports activities is best understood in the context of the model of sports adaptation presented in Chapter 5. The adaptations for each activity

SIDEBAR 8.3

Vision Classification for Official Sports Competition

The International Blind Sports Federation (IBSA) and the United States Association of Blind Athletes (USABA) hold competitions in various sporting events for people who are legally blind or deafblind. To ensure fairness in the competitions, athletes compete in specific classifications or divisions based on the amount of vision an athlete has, so that athletes compete only against those with similar degrees of vision, that is, those who have no functional vision generally do not compete against those with any degree of vision. The last category, B4, is a relatively new one and was implemented to support participation among athletes who have visual impairments but are not legally blind. It is used only in USABA events.

IBSA Visual Classifications

Class B1. No light perception in either eye up to light perception, but inability to recognize the shape of a hand at any distance or in any direction

Class B2. From ability to recognize the shape of a hand up to visual acuity of 20/600 and/or a visual field of less than 5 degrees in the better eye with the best practical eye correction

Class B3. From visual acuity above 20/600 and up to visual acuity of 20/200 and/or a visual field of less than 20 degrees and more than 5 degrees in the better eye with the best practical eye correction

USABA Classification for Low Vision

Class B4. From visual acuity above 20/200 and up to visual acuity of 20/70 and a visual field larger than 20 degrees in the better eye with the best practical eye correction

Source: United States Association of Blind Athletes, *Visual Classifications*, retrieved 4/3/12 from http://usaba.org/index.php/membership/visual-classifications/.

described here are based on the AccesSports system, and the adaptations for each event can be classified according to whether they modify the targets or goals, the boundaries, or the rules of the activity. Adaptations used in a particular competitive event are also highly dependent on the athlete's competitive vision classification.

The descriptions and adaptations for each sport are presented as if the athletes are participating in a competitive event. This was done to ensure coverage of the most complex situation under which adaptations might have to be used. Most individuals who will ultimately use the adaptations are likely to be participating in a school class or an informal personal practice session or setting. Regardless of the complexity of the situation, the same adaptations generally apply.

Athletics or Track and Field

Description

Athletics is the term used internationally for what are often known in the United States as track events or track and field. Athletics is one of the oldest known sporting events, dating back to the original Greek Olympiad. According to the International Association of Athletics Federations, the world governing body for track and field, the activities included under the rubric of athletics are track and field events, cross-country racing, road running, race walking, and mountain walking (International Association of Athletics Federations, n.d.).

Track events are held on standard tracks of 400 meters in length and include the following:

- *Fast-paced sprints* (100 and 200 meters).
- *Hurdle races:* Sprint races in which competitors must pass over a series of hurdles (low obstacles) before crossing the finish line.
- *Middle distance races:* 400 and 800 meters.
- *Distance races:* 1,500, 3,000, and 5,000 meters.
- *Cross-country racing:* A form of distance running that takes place over natural terrain, such as golf courses or parks, rather than on the paved oval tracks used in track meets.
- *Road races:* A form of long-distance race conducted on roadways that are closed to traffic on the day of the event. The marathon is the best-known road race.
- *Relay races:* Races of varying distances in which teams of four runners compete by passing a baton—a smooth, hollow, one-piece tube—sequentially from one runner to the next after each runner completes one-quarter of the race distance.

The field events found in track meets at the middle and high school levels include the following throwing and jumping events and the pole vault:

Throwing Events

- *Shot put:* A throwing event in which a heavy metal ball, called the shot, is propelled by pushing the ball at an approximately 45-degree angle by forcefully extending the arm, waist, and leg joints, while simultaneously stepping quickly from the back to the front of a raised circle
- *Discus:* A throwing event in which a discus, a heavy disk of wood or hard rubber, is propelled from under the palm of the hand at an approximately 45-degree angle, with force created by the competitor first crouching at the back of a raised ring, rapidly spinning, and then allowing the discus to fly out of the hand near the front of the circle and travel as far as possible while the competitor stays within the throwing ring.

Jumping Events

- *Long jump:* An event in which a competitor attempts to jump a greater horizontal distance than other competitors by first taking a fast running approach and then leaping from a takeoff board into a sand-filled pit
- *High jump:* An event in which a competitor attempts to jump over a horizontal bar at a greater height than other competitors by first taking running steps, leaping over the bar head first and face up, with the body horizontal to the bar, and then landing on a cushion
- *Pole vault:* An event in which a competitor uses a pole to vault over a horizontal bar at a greater height than that vaulted by other competitors by first taking running steps, planting the end of the flexible vaulting pole, leaping and pushing off with the pole over the bar feet first, and then landing safely on a cushion

Adolescents and adults with visual impairments are in general capable of involvement in all these sports, with the possible exception of hurdle races and the pole vault. Many are members of their local clubs or school track and field or cross-country teams or simply participate as individuals in classrooms, or in open running events (Ponchillia, Strause, & Ponchillia, 2002). In addition, track and field is the most popular among the sports offered by the USABA (Ponchillia et al., 2002). The thousands of children who have participated in these events at the authors' summer camps also attest to the popularity of the events and to the ease with which children with visual impairments or deafblindness can participate. Access to participation and competition for people with visual impairments is probably better than in most other sports, because there are countless open meets available in communities nationwide. Also, the adaptations required for competition in inclusive or open events are simple, affect rules minimally, and are routinely accepted by meet officials. As already noted, the only track and field events that do not yet lend themselves well to any available adaptation and therefore rarely include anyone with a visual impairment are hurdle races and the pole vault. The specific adaptations for track and field events are presented in the following discussion.

Adaptations

Running Adaptations

There are several adaptations that will enable an individual with a visual impairment or deafblindness to participate in running or race walking events. The adaptations described in this section are aimed primarily at running competitively, while those used in more recreational or fitness settings will be covered in Chapters 10 and 11. The adaptive technique depends on the type of event and the runner's degree of vision and hearing. Most notably, runners in the B1 and B2 visual categories (see Sidebar 8.3) are permitted to use guide runners, while those with the highest level of vision (B3 and B4 in USABA events) are not, nor are they allowed to use any other modifications. The distance being run in a specific event affects the method of guiding used. Fast-paced sprint races require far more specific interaction between guide and athlete and more practice than distance races. While these techniques can be useful in practice, not all of them are permitted in formal competitions.

Guide Runner. A runner with vision may run with a runner in the B1 or B2 category, serving as a guide runner. Guide runners can be used in all running events by athletes in those categories. Generally, runner and guide are assigned two track lanes and hold opposite ends of a rope tether, and the guide runs slightly ahead until nearly the end of the race, where the guide must drop behind the runner the

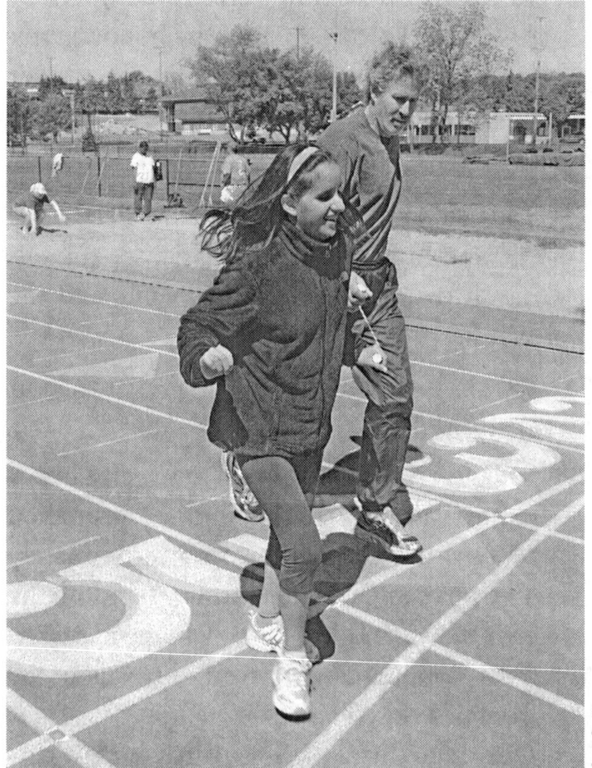

Chuck Comer

A student and instructor running with a tether. The guide must let the runner go first when crossing the finish line.

moment before they reach the finish line. The tether is usually a short rope that is knotted at each end, so that it can be held between and at the base of two fingers. The tether should not be wrapped around fingers or wrist, since a fall with the rope in such a position could injure a joint. The tether allows both the runner and the guide to swing their arms freely, which is not possible when the runner holds the guide's arm.

When individuals are first learning to run with guides, they start by walking, then jogging, and then running together on a track or other smooth running surface. Some people prefer a longer tether, to allow a more natural arm swing, while some prefer a more rigid plastic pole; others may hold the elbow, shoulder, or hand of the guide. The guide needs to serve as a sort of play-by-play announcer, informing runners about the conditions of the track, their position in the race, and when they are attempting to pass slower runners. In road races or other off-track areas, it is the guide's responsibility to inform the runner about such matters as upcoming hills, turns, curbs, and uneven footing. For runners who are deafblind, communication while running may need to be limited to essential information related to distance covered and safety, with other information conveyed before or after the run. In a race, guides must be faster than runners so that runners can perform at their best and guides can focus on the complexities of maneuvering among the other competitors.

Considerable practice is required for both the runner and the guide to coordinate starts coming out of starting blocks. Runners who are deafblind and thus cannot hear the report of the starter's pistol require some adaptation to indicate the start of a race. For a middle- or long-distance race, guides usually indicate the start by tugging on the guide rope at the instant the starter's pistol is heard. Because a sprint race can be won or lost at the start, however, a separate person will generally be used to tap a sprinter who is deafblind on the back at the time of each of the three starter's commands: Mark, set, go.

Runners who have enough vision can use a guide and even follow the guide visually, but only B2 athletes are permitted this modification in sanctioned races. In this case, guides often wear bright orange shirts or other easily identifiable garb and position themselves in the runner's best visual spot to make following easier.

Visual Adaptations. Although it is not permitted in sanctioned races, runners with sufficient vision can sometimes be assisted in other races or in practice runs by increasing lane visibility by using chalk or white tape to broaden certain lane markers. Runners with sufficient vision can also use the inside lane of a track so that they may visually follow the curb or grass line. They can also hold their heads down and perhaps orient on the lane markers. During competitive distance races, runners with functional vision might also use a competitor who has a similar pace as a kind of guide runner by following the competitor closely through the traffic of the race and then sprinting ahead just before the finish line.

Sprints

Calling. Calling is a technique that allows runners to run sprint distances in a straight line independently by having a caller who serves as a target toward which they run by constantly announcing their lane position. This technique is generally used in practice only; it is no longer allowed in continental, world, or Paralympic competition. In brief, the caller stands in the same lane as the runner, just before the finish line, and helps the runner line up correctly by yelling, "Point at me, here, here, here!" During the sprint, the caller repeatedly yells the runner's lane number: "Four! Four! Four!" to keep the runner aligned. More details about calling appear in Chapter 11.

Guide Wires. A wire or rope can be strung along a track lane and followed by B1 or B2 athletes. In the past, multiple wires served as lane markers for several competitors running simultaneously. This practice has generally been supplanted in competition by guide runners, since competitors generally achieve faster times with guides. The use of guide wires in running for fitness is described in Chapter 11.

Cross-Country Running

Since a cross-country race takes place on a course with variable and unpredictable terrain, runners with visual impairments should have the opportunity to preview and practice on the course prior to the race. When runners use guides, guides must also be prepared to describe the running surface that they are approaching, such as, "We're about to begin a gradual downhill. At the bottom, the ground gets very bumpy for a few steps, so I'll count down 3, 2, and we'll be there on 1. Ready, here we go, 3, 2, 1." For independent runners depending on their limited but functional vision, key spots such as course turns can be marked with ribbons, colorful plastic bags, or highly visible traffic cones. Runners also need to be aware of the need for additional ankle support, given the unpredictable running surface.

ROLE MODEL

MARATHON RUNNER

Steve Gokey

In 2008, Steve Gokey was unique among the 17,000 runners signed up to take the starting signal in the Chevron Houston Marathon. He was the only person without sight in the 26.2-mile event. "I love running; I love sports," says Gokey, 55, who works as a switchboard operator for the Modesto, California, police department. "It's recreation, but very competitive for me." He has run nearly two dozen marathons, including four times in the Boston Marathon. "It never gets old," Gokey said. "Finishing, and the idea of finishing and getting my medal and wearing my medal for a week, it never gets old." Gokey was born blind, making his disability different from those who had sight and lost it later in life, he said. "I've been fortunate," he said. "It's not a big deal. It's an inconvenience at times but I've adjusted pretty well with it. I don't have any fear with it." He trains at home on a treadmill. "There are days I don't like to train," he said. "It does take a certain amount of discipline."

In a marathon, a team of four guides each take a segment of the race to guide him around the course. He links to his guides by using two 5-foot-long PVC pipes, the kind used in plumbing. "They hold on one end and I hold on the other," he said. "The pipe balances me. It feels like the treadmill. It's probably psychological but it works out." His guide may tell him his location on the course, or if there's a turn coming or a change in the surface like a railroad track crossing.

Relay Races

A formal relay race takes place on either the straightaways or curves of a circular track, and the baton must be passed to the next runner within a specified exchange zone. Runners in a relay race use the same adaptations as in other running events, but the baton exchange may also require adaptation. In sanctioned races, the exchange may be made from guide runner to guide runner, from guide to a runner, or from runner to runner. The most efficient exchange, and therefore the one most used in competition, is from guide to guide. However, if a runner-to-runner exchange is used, the following technique is effective:

- In a modified handoff, the waiting runner yells the name of the approaching runner at short intervals. The waiting runner holds his or her arm straight out at his or her side, instead of behind, as in a traditional relay race, but with the palm still facing toward the baton carrier. The approaching runner yells "Go, go, go!" as he or she approaches the waiting teammate, and the waiting teammate begins to run. The approaching runner places the baton on top of the waiting teammate's extended arm and slides the baton down along the forearm and into the waiting hand as the two team members run a few steps together.
- The batons can be made more visible with bright tape.
- Runners can wear a bright glove on the hand that will receive the baton.

The modified handoff takes a good deal of practice to be efficient.

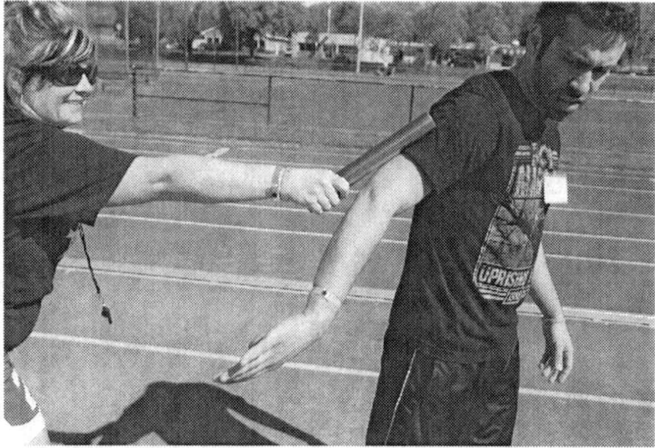

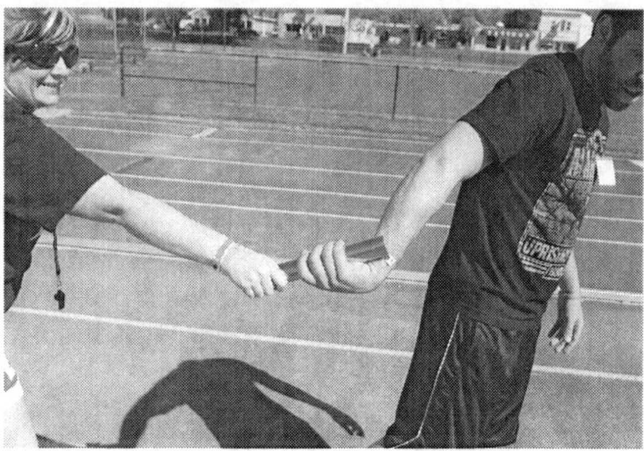

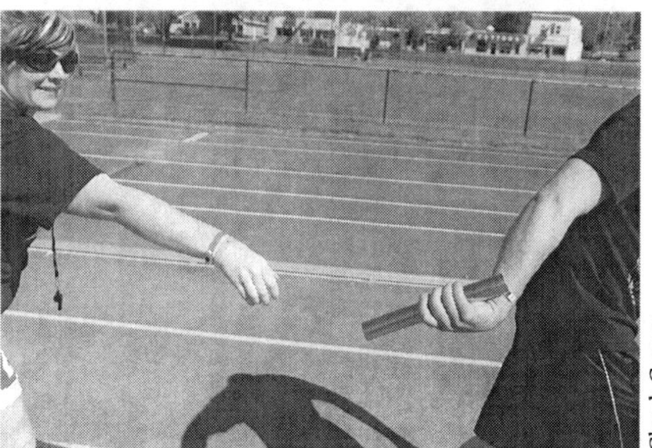

Chuck Comer

Sports camp staff members demonstrate the modified baton exchange used in relay races, in which the runner slides the baton down the extended arm of the waiting team member.

Adaptations for Field Events

Shot Put

In competitions the shot-putter is required to stay within a circle while putting, and the shot must land within the legal throwing area. The adaptations for this sport therefore mainly involve marking the throwing circle visually or with tactile materials to help the athlete maintain orientation to the boundaries. However, the standard shot put circle has a "box" or raised area in the front portion that can serve this purpose. A caller can also be used to help orient the shot-putter to the boundaries of the

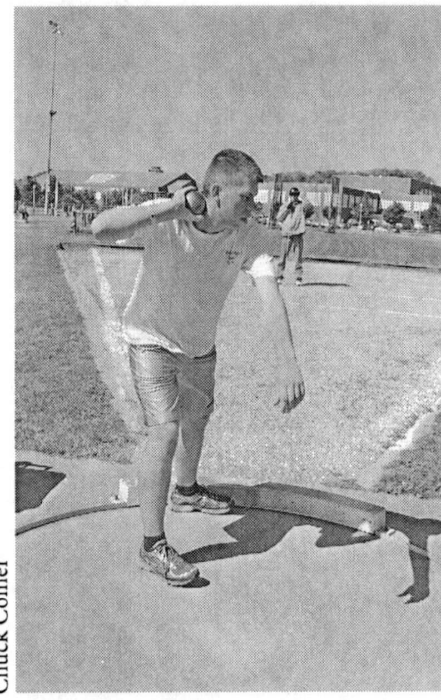
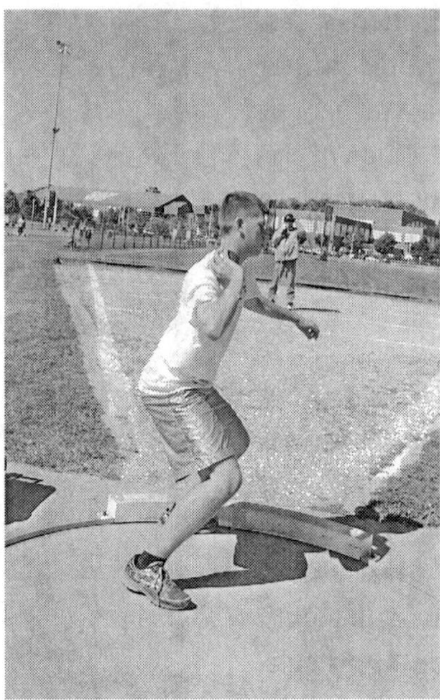
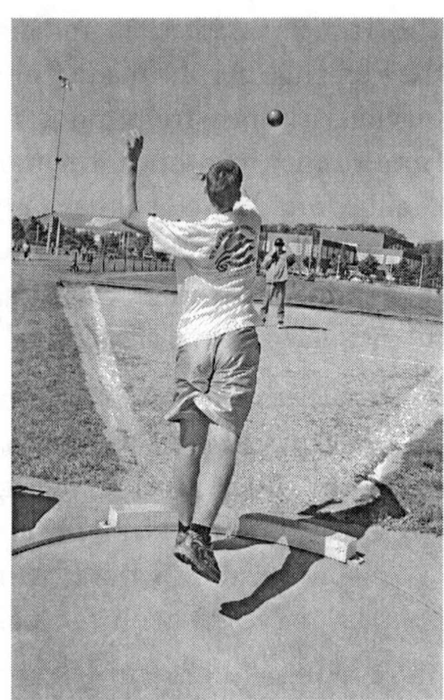

Chuck Comer

Releasing the shot put. The raised area in the front of the shot put circle and the caller standing in the field orient the athlete to the direction in which the shot should be released.

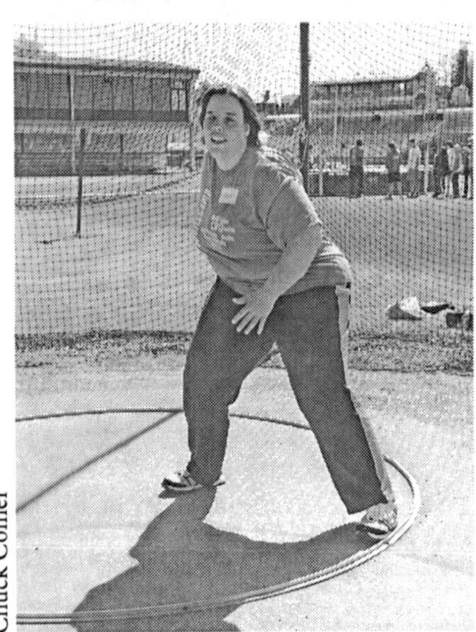
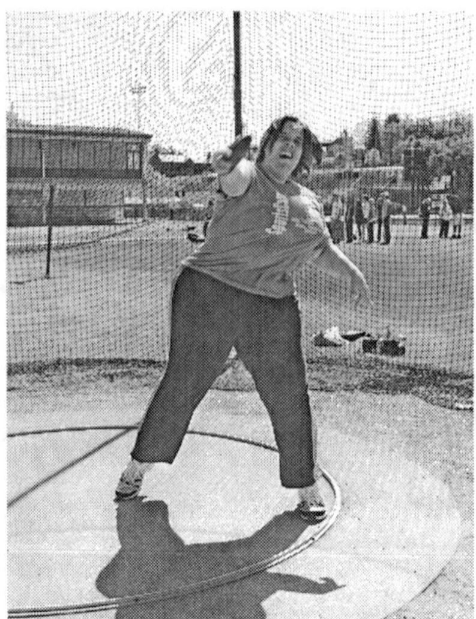
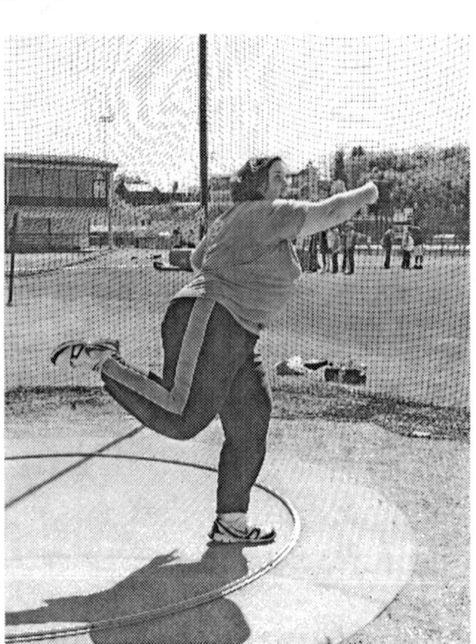

Chuck Comer

A sports camp staff member demonstrates the discus throw.

circle and throwing area by standing in the throwing area and giving a verbal command.

Discus Throwing

As with the shot put, the throw in the discus event is made from within a fixed circle and must land within throwing boundaries. Again, the main adaptations are orienting the thrower to the boundaries of the circle and its front and back.

Long Jumping

The setup for the long jump is described in Chapter 4, and Chapter 7 includes a detailed

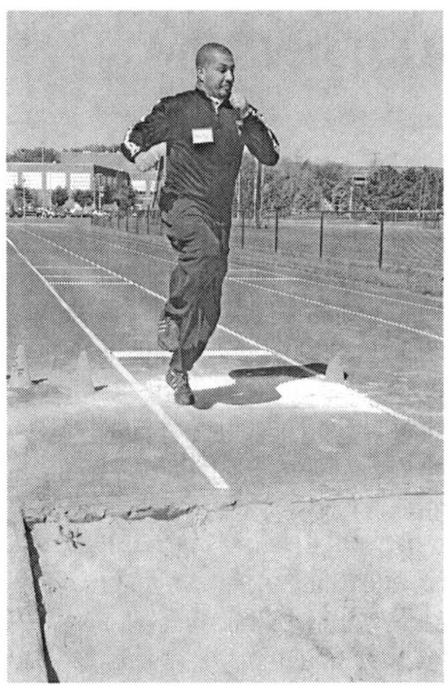
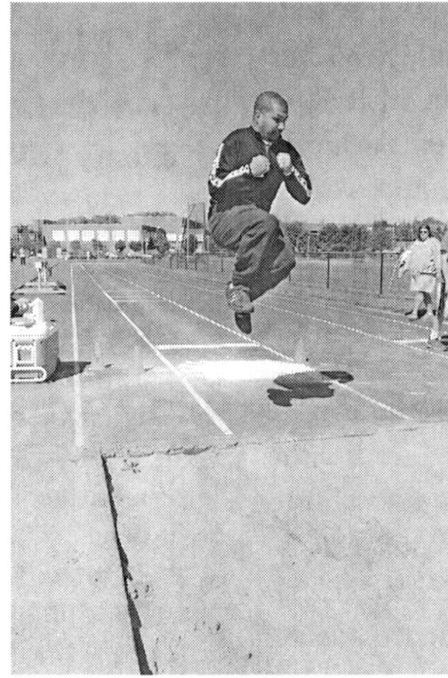
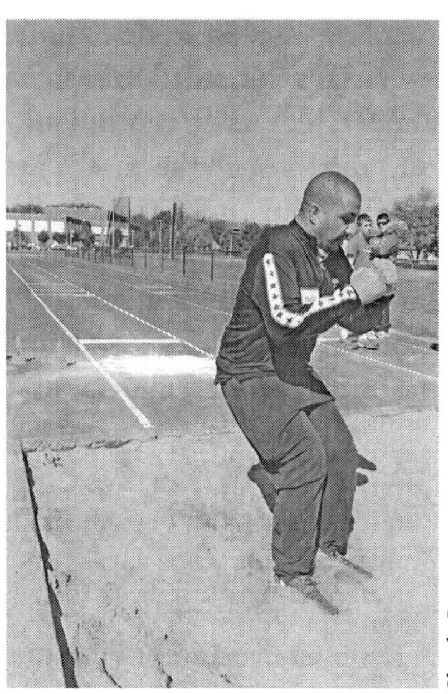

Chuck Comer

A sports camp staff member demonstrates the long jump.

description of how to provide instruction in the basics of this skill. The major difficulties for competitors with visual impairments in long jumping are staying on the running approach, stepping on the board properly, and landing safely in the pit. The most independent and efficient adaptation for B1 athletes is using a caller. The jumper begins on the runway at a distance that allows for a 3-step approach, and the caller faces the jumper at the end of the sand pit. The caller yells "Here" and asks the jumper to point directly at him or her to verify the jumper's alignment. If the jumper points straight at the caller, then the caller yells through cupped hands, "Okay—ready—Go! Go! Go! Go!" The caller also uses an abort command ("Stop!") if the jumper begins to veer off the runway.

The standard takeoff board can be replaced for B1 athletes in sanctioned events by a modified board made with a light dusting of talcum powder on a 3-foot section of runway about 3 feet before the edge of the pit. The jump distance is then measured from the jumper's footprint in the powder, rather than from the front edge of the board as is customary.

Teaching a new jumper when and where to jump is accomplished virtually the same way as it is with sighted jumpers, that is, by having the jumper count steps. It is not usually done by telling the jumper when to jump by giving a command. The teaching sequence begins with a standing long jump, moves to a 3-step approach, and increases in steps until the jumper attains a safe approach with a maximum jump distance. Each time jumpers begin a new series of jumps following a significant break, they start by reestablishing their "steps." Jumpers using a 3-step approach place their heels in the middle of the takeoff board (or powder board), take three large steps away from the pit, turn around and face it, and place a marker in the grass to designate where they should begin their running approach. They then begin to run with the foot they will jump from and run across the board and through the landing pit.

A coach watches to determine if the jumper's toe strikes the board near its middle. If so, the jumper repeats the technique, but instead of running through the pit, the jumper leaps from the board to attain the longest jump possible. If the toe is short of or past the board on the run through, adjustments are made to lengthen or shorten the approach length until the toe strikes the board correctly and consistently.

Deafblind jumpers can use a guide rope stretched alongside the runway, across the takeoff board, and over the sand landing pit to maintain a straight approach during a running long jump. A knot can be added to the rope one step before the jumping board to alert the jumper to the upcoming jump point. Also, step counting can be practiced in the same fashion as that used by B1 athletes.

The takeoff board can be made more visible for individuals with functional vision by placing stripes on it using black or brightly colored 2-inch vinyl tape. Also, the runway can be marked on both sides with 2 to 4 inches of brightly contrasting tape. (If tape does not stick to the runway, it can be tacked down with small nails with large heads.)

ROLE MODEL

LONG JUMP

Elexis Gillette

Elexis Gillette, a B1 athlete, attended a summer sports education camp for athletes with visual impairments as a high school freshman in the early 2000s. He was introduced to the long jump at the track and field introduction clinic, and it was immediately obvious to the coaches that Elexis was a fine athlete who had outstanding potential as a long jumper. The following year, the athlete's O&M instructor encouraged him to join his high school track team. He did, and it has been nothing but success for Gillette since that time. First, Elexis became captain of his school track team and competed successfully against sighted athletes in open meets. His successes there led him on to national track competitions at USABA-sanctioned meets, where he eventually qualified for the Paralympics and other international events. He has gone on to achieve international acclaim by winning silver medals in long jump at the Athens, Beijing, and London Paralympics. He broke the 21-foot mark in two Paralympics, and his 2004 performance established a new American record for B1 athletes. He hopes to eventually break the 22-foot mark.

High Jumping

The major challenge in high jumping for athletes with visual impairments or deafblindness is locating the crossbar. Raised marks can be placed on the runway at the point where the jumper starts running. The jumper must then repeatedly practice the direction of approach and the number of steps to take before jumping. The jumper can be oriented to the direction of the run up—the approach to the jump—by hanging a beeper or other sound source on the bar or one on each of the crossbar standards. As in the long jump, athletes with deafblindness can follow a guide rope stretched from their starting point, under the bar, and over the landing pad to orient them to the location of the bar. Likewise, a knot placed in the rope one step before the jumping point can be used to alert the jumper of where to begin the jump. Step counting can accomplish this as well. Athletes generally start jumping first without a crossbar and gradually work up to using one.

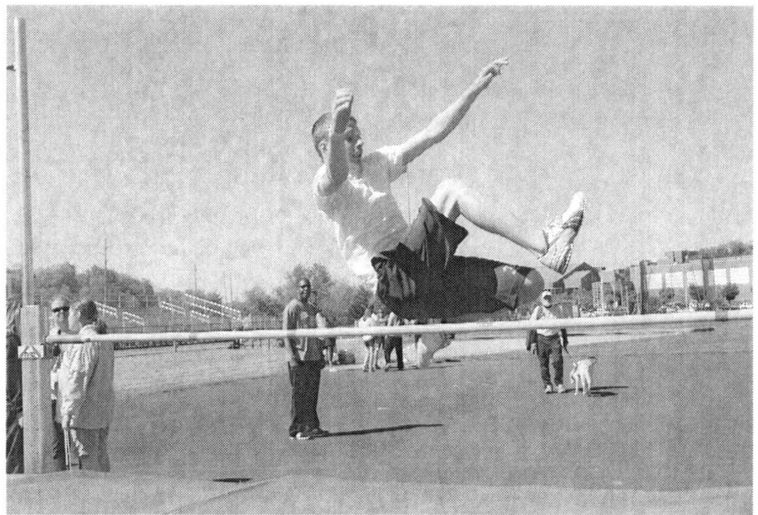

Chuck Comer

Practicing the high jump.

The high jump crossbar is generally striped black and white, but it can be made even more visible for athletes with low vision by hanging strips of 2-inch black or bright orange tape across its length. The bar is much more easily seen if the tape hangs down about a foot. Bright markers on the runway can also aid jumpers with low vision in their approaches.

Aquatics or Swimming

Description

Swimming, like athletics, is a sport that is relatively easily accessible to individuals with visual impairments or deafblindness and that offers a wide range of opportunities for participation. Many students with visual impairments participate in swimming for recreational purposes, and many compete on intramural, interscholastic, or club teams. This section focuses primarily on swim racing, while swimming for recreational or fitness purposes is covered in Chapters 10 and 11, respectively.

Swim racing has been a major sport for people with visual impairments or deafblindness, as evidenced by its inclusion in the first Paralympic Games in 1960. Its popularity is most likely related to the relative ease with which it can be adapted to meet the needs of swimmers with little or no vision.

Swim racing includes four swimming stroke classes or types:

- backstroke
- breast stroke
- butterfly stroke
- freestyle or front crawl stroke

Competitors in freestyle races are able to use any stroke, but they must use only that stroke during the entire race. Since the front crawl stroke is the fastest stroke, however, it is usually used in freestyle events.

The following are the swimming events included in the Paralympic Games:

- 50-meter freestyle
- 100-meter freestyle
- 400-meter freestyle
- 100-meter backstroke
- 100-meter breaststroke
- 100-meter butterfly
- 200-meter individual medley
- 4×100-meter freestyle relay
- 4×100-meter medley relay

Men and women compete separately in official swim meets. Much as in track and field, individuals compete in events ranging from sprints (50 meters), to middle distance (100-meter), through distance (400-meter) races. Also, swimmers can compete in individual medleys, which combine all four swimming strokes in one race or in freestyle or medley relays.

The USABA and the U.S. Paralympic Committee promote this sport nationally and internationally for competitors with visual impairments. In addition, USA Swimming, the national governing body for swimming in the United States (see the Resources section), encourages athletes with visual impairments to compete in local swim meets.

At the international level, swimmers compete in one of three classifications based on the IBSA categories: S11 (the same as B1, which includes swimmers with the most vision loss who must wear darkened goggles unless they have prosthetic eyes); S12 (the same as B2); and S13 (the same as B3). Youths 17 years of age or younger are divided into age groups, 15 and younger and 16 and over, and are further segregated by gender. Complete swim racing rules are available on the International Paralympic Committee website (http://www.ipc-swimming.org/Rules_Regulations), which includes modifications to USA Swimming rules.

ROLE MODEL

SWIMMING

Trischa Zorn

Trischa Zorn was an alternate to the 1980 U.S. Olympic swim team, missing a spot by just 1/100th of a second. However, Zorn went on to compete for the United States in her sport in the Paralympics, becoming the most decorated athlete in the history of the games. She won an outstanding 55 medals (41 gold, 9 silver, and 5 bronze), along with eight world records (50-meter backstroke, 100-meter backstroke, 200-meter backstroke, 200-meter individual medley, 400-meter individual medley, 200-meter breaststroke, 4x50-meter medley relay, and 4x50-meter free relay). She is a four-time All-American and was the first athlete with a visual impairment to earn a Division I athletic scholarship. In 2012, she was inducted into the Paralympic Hall of Fame. Zorn has become so well known that there is a question about her in the popular board game Trivial Pursuit!

Adaptations

The major adaptations required for swim races are the following:

- modifying the race starting position
- alerting swimmers when they are approaching the end of the pool during the multiple laps of a race or at the race's end
- keeping swimmers swimming straight within the boundaries of a swimming lane

Swimmers with visual impairments or deafblindness need to be properly oriented when starting the race to make sure they begin swimming in a straight line within their own lane. In addition, swimmers with deafblindness may have difficulty hearing the starting gun. Starting straight is usually accomplished by having the swimmer place his or her toes over the pool or starting platform edge, reaching down to use hands to make sure that toes are perpendicular with edge, and mentally projecting a point in the water 20 feet away at which to dive. When a swimmer is learning this procedure, the imaginary point can be reinforced by having a teacher in the water to give the diver an auditory or visual clue. As is the case with sprint races, competitors with deafblindness can be alerted to the start of the race by having their coach tap them at each of the starter's commands, "Mark, set, go," if they cannot hear the starter's gun or feel its vibrations.

Maintaining a straight-line path during a race is accomplished by practicing, particularly focusing on correcting a veer from the path after contacting the floats or rope of the lane markers. Practice primarily involves ways to keep from getting entangled in the lane marker ropes. After swimmers have made contact with a lane marker, they need to keep their swim kick low under water, turn their head away from the rope, and extend their stroke laterally across the head and away from the rope. Teachers and coaches should also be aware that swimmers tend to overcorrect, which can take them into the rope on the opposite side.

Alerting swimmers at the right moment that they are approaching the end of the lane is crucial, as crashing into a wall when swimming all-out during a race can cause serious injury. Although sighted swimmers may see the wall as they approach it, there are two standard methods of indicating that the wall is near: (a) the symbols painted on the pool floor, aimed at swimmers using crawl, breast, or butterfly strokes, and (b) the pennant-like flags that hang from a cable suspended across the pool just above the water's surface that can be seen when swimming the backstroke.

Alerting the swimmer with a visual impairment that he or she is approaching the end of the pool can be done in several ways. The most common method is "tapping" the swimmer. The tapstick is a pole approximately 5 feet long, usually bamboo, with a tennis ball attached at one end. The tapper must strike the swimmer firmly between the shoulder blades when the swimmer is about 3 feet from the end of the lane. Races with one or more turns require two tappers.

Another method of alerting swimmers when they are approaching the wall is using an easily constructed device that sprays water on the swimmers' backs when they are a specified distance from the wall (Scheib & Ponchillia, 1999). One version of this device, known as the Aqualert, is a modified lawn sprinkler that attaches to a water spigot and continually projects a spray onto the water of a single lane. A second version, known as the Aqualert II, is a more highly engineered device consisting of a long spray boom that is attached to the backstroke flag cable and projects an easily detected continuous fine spray down onto swimmers' backs as they pass. A study of the Aqualert II found that, although the system requires a short learning period, research participants preferred it to the tapstick, primarily because it gives consistent,

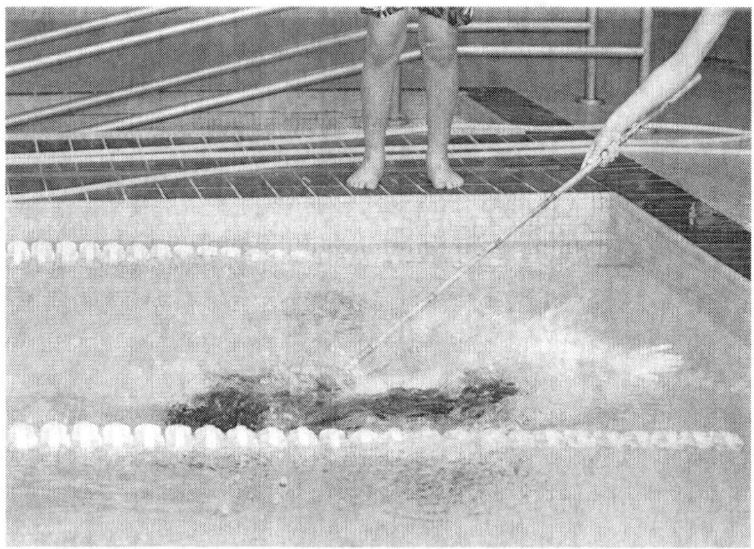

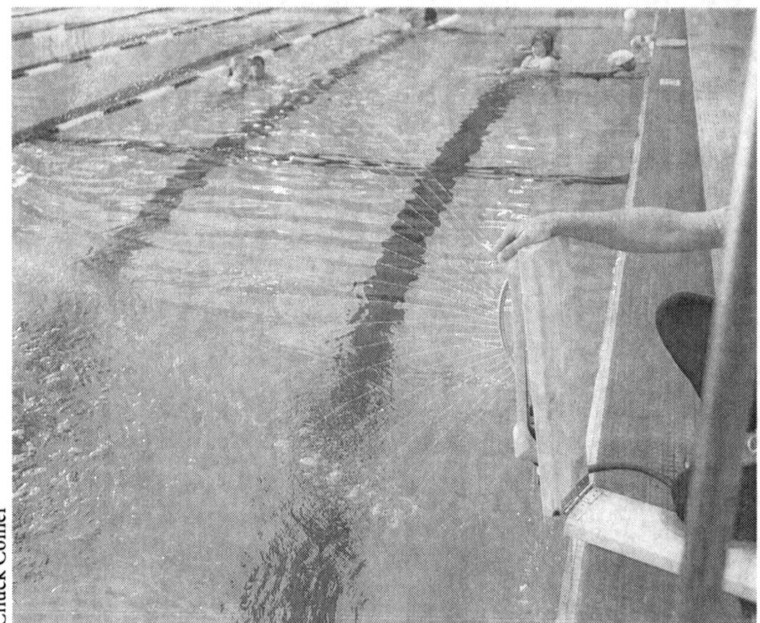

Chuck Comer

Two methods of alerting swimmers when they are approaching the end of the pool: a tap stick (top) and a modified lawn sprinkler (bottom), known as the Aqualert.

reliable feedback and, unlike the tapstick, can be used independently (Scheib & Ponchillia, 1999).

Additional modifications to the rules of swimming competitions sanctioned by USA Swimming are as follows:

- having the coach tap a swimmer to indicate a turn or the finish line
- speaking to swimmers if they drift into the wrong lane
- hanging strips of ribbon low enough for the swimmers to touch them as they

stroke, lowering the backstroke flags, using bubbling devices, or showering water from the backstroke flags

- giving swimmers the option of starting the race from the diving blocks, the pool edge, or in the water
- having the coach give an athlete who is deafblind a tactile starting signal
- having the coach or another swimmer start a relay participant with a nonverbal signal such as touching
- giving B1 swimmers leeway in the requirement that both hands must touch the wall simultaneously and on the same level for breaststroke and butterfly

Teaching Tips

Teachers or coaches working with swimmers who are visually impaired or deafblind need to be aware that the noisy and reflective pool environment can be frustrating to some swimmers, particularly those with little vision, as, under high levels of noise, they are essentially deafblind. The following suggestions are designed to increase communication and promote instruction in aquatic activities:

- Provide orientation to the pool and environment to help the swimmer organize and plan pool entries and exits.
- Have the teacher wear a thin synthetic black shirt and running tights to make his or her leg or arm actions more visible underwater.
- Teach new skill concepts on the pool deck for ease of instruction and positioning.
- Use sign language with swimmers who are deafblind during instruction. A flotation device may be used to free hands for signing when teaching in the deep end of the pool.
- Be sensitive to issues of touching and provide appropriate substitutes for touching the teacher, such as having parents or caregivers model positions or movements.
- Offer a running commentary to describe what others are doing, using students' names frequently.
- Use lane lines during lap swim and stroke practice to provide tactile boundaries for staying within a lane.
- Use auditory signals to orient swimmers to the proper direction, for example, placing a radio near the deep end (however, the signal may not work well under conditions of high noise).
- Place raised block or braille numbers on the wall next to the corresponding depth markers so swimmers can find the appropriate height independently by trailing down the wall, and get into the pool at the depth they desire.
- Have participants bring a magnet to place on their lockers, if braille labels are not available, so they can locate their lockers independently. The magnet can easily be removed when they are finished. (Lepore, Gayle, & Stevens, 2007)

In addition, it is important to maintain safety precautions in a pool environment, such as the following:

- Provide a spotter for participants to give verbal feedback to swimmers in case the swimmers become disoriented.
- Inform swimmers of any hazards in the environment.
- Be aware that swimmers with certain eye conditions must avoid bumping their head or eyes (see Chapter 5).

- If the pool is shared, provide a somewhat segregated environment and use a sighted spotter to intercept balls and kickboards and to prevent other swimmers from bumping into swimmers with limited vision.
- Have sighted spotters provide cues for swimmers who want to jump or dive.

Wrestling

Description

Wrestling is one of the world's oldest sports activities. Competing wrestlers having been depicted in ancient cave drawings traced back some 15,000 years (Rousseau, 2012). In the most common form of wrestling in the United States, competitors attempt to defeat one another by a "fall," that is, by pinning the opponent's shoulders to the mat for a period of 1 second. However, if neither wrestler can complete a fall during a match, the winner is determined by points. Points are awarded as follows:

- 2 points for a *takedown* (bringing the opponent from standing to the mat)
- 1 point for an *escape* (getting out of the grasp of an opponent)
- 2 points for a *reversal* (moving from being in the grasp of an opponent to having the opponent in one's grasp or under control)
- 2 or 3 points for a near fall (exposing an opponent's back to the mat but not attaining a pin)

This point system is used in college wrestling, also known as folkstyle or scholastic wrestling. It is the most common style in the United States and is familiar to the thousands of parents who have watched their elementary, middle, or senior high school children take part in Saturday wrestling meets. Two other styles, freestyle and Greco-Roman wrestling, are also practiced in the United States. Greco-Roman wrestling differs the most from folkstyle wrestling in that Greco-Roman prohibits the use of the legs and all holds must be applied above the waist. Freestyle and folkstyle are nearly identical, except a fall is more difficult to obtain in folkstyle because the shoulders must be held to the mat for 1 full second, whereas freestyle falls occur when the shoulders simply touch the mat.

> **ROLE MODEL**
>
> WRESTLING
>
> ***James Mastro***
>
> Jim Mastro is among the best wrestlers with a visual impairment to have ever stepped onto a mat. Jim, a Bemidji State University physical education professor, lost his vision as a teenager, and then became a dominant wrestler in high school and college. He was selected as an alternate on the U.S. Olympic Team, a three-time medal winner at the National AAU Wrestling Championships, a National Intercollegiate Champion in Greco-Roman wrestling, and a gold medalist at three different Paralympic Games. After wrestling was dropped from the Paralympic Games, Dr. Mastro switched sports and became a dominant judo competitor.

Adaptations and Competitive Options

Wrestling is a sport for everyone, regardless of their gender, size, or age. Although it has generally been a male-dominated sport, opportunities are now widespread for girls as well. Unlike in many other sports, small participants are not at a disadvantage, because they compete only against those within their own weight class.

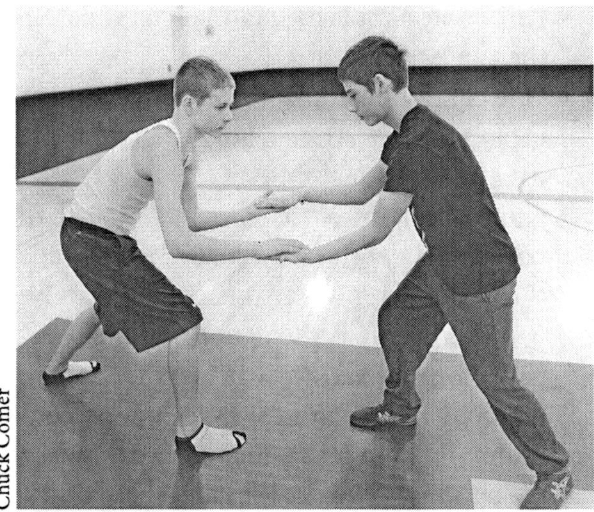

Chuck Comer

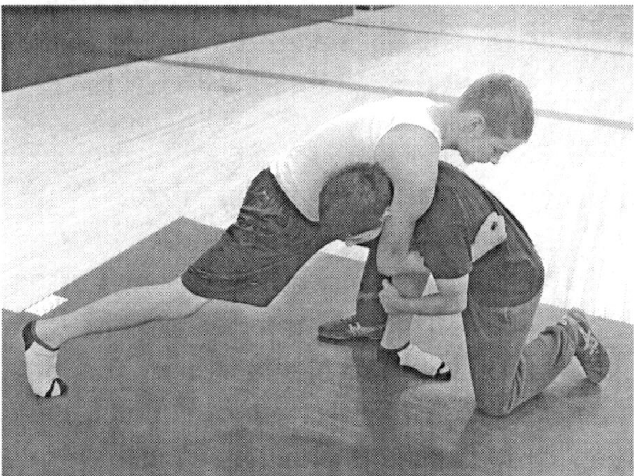

The only adaptation required for wrestling competition is that the athletes must maintain constant contact when standing, by touching fingertips; one hand up and one hand down.

Wrestling is as available to athletes with visual impairments or deafblindness as it is to others, because it requires only a single simple adaptation that has been readily accepted throughout all levels of wrestling competition. As described by the USABA (http://usaba.org/index.php/sports/sports-adaptations/), the adaptation requires the wrestlers to maintain physical contact while standing as well as when on the mat. In the standing position, the opponents touch hands, one hand with fingers up and the other with fingers down. Wrestling is sponsored by the USABA nationally, but it is not sanctioned internationally by IBSA, nor is it a Paralympic sport at this time. However, wrestling in school meets is quite common for athletes with visual impairments.

Teaching Tips

Wrestling lends itself to hands-on instruction by its very nature. In most cases, it is preferable to teach wrestling movement skills by tactile modeling or physical guidance rather than relying on verbal descriptions. It is natural to teach a move, such as single-leg takedown, by executing the takedown move on the student. Although in most other instructional situations, physical guidance, especially using force, is usually the method of last resort, in wrestling it is expected of a sparring partner or teacher. As is always the case when using physical contact, a discussion of the technique with the wrestler first is advised.

Teachers and coaches should also keep in mind that although most students with visual impairments will learn and exhibit wrestling skills in much the same fashion as other students, some with limited physical skills or physical education concepts may have difficulties in early lessons (see Chapter 1). Since wrestlers are attempting to take down or pin one another, they use a great deal of speed and force. Students with limited understanding of or experience with force and speed are often shocked by the force and aggressive actions used by their opponents. As a consequence, such students often want to quit or drop out of the introductory wrestling clinics at the sports camps. At least two approaches have been used to address this problem. One approach is to discuss concepts of force and speed with students before they ever engage in physical contact. A second approach is that the student's initial opponent is a teacher or coach who increases both force and speed gradually until the student can understand and cope with those experiences.

Judo

Description

Modern judo was developed by Jigoro Kano in Japan in 1882 and became an Olympic sport at the 1964 games in Tokyo (Olympic Studies Center, 2011). It was first included in the Paralympics at Seoul, Korea, in 1988. The number of competitors grew to 60 by the 2004 Athens games, and 132 athletes competed at the 2008 games in Beijing. Judo is a grappling sport somewhat akin to freestyle wrestling in that the primary objective is to pin an opponent. However, judo differs markedly from wrestling because judo uses throws, joint locks, and strangles to win a match.

Scoring of judo matches is also somewhat similar to wrestling, but judo uses traditional Japanese language in its scoring system, as well as in conducting the matches. Therefore, the objective of judo is to score an *ippon* (one full point). Once such a score is achieved, the competition ends. An ippon can be scored in one of the following ways:

- One contestant executes a skillful throwing technique which results in the opponent being thrown largely on the back with considerable force or speed.
- One contestant maintains a pin for 25 seconds.
- One contestant cannot continue and gives up.
- One contestant is disqualified for violating the rules.
- One contestant applies an effective armbar or an effective stranglehold (this does not usually apply to children).
- One contestant earns two *waza-ari* (half points). A waza-ari can be earned by (a) a throwing technique that is not quite an ippon (for example, the opponent lands only partly on the back or with less force than required for ippon); (b) holding one contestant in a pin for 20 seconds; or (c) when the opponent violates the rules three times.
- If the time runs out with neither contestant scoring an ippon, the referee awards the win to the contestant who has the next highest score.

Judo is relatively popular in the United States, but most people know little about the traditional terminology it uses or how a match is conducted. The Judo Information Site website (www.judoinfo.com/competition.htm) provides an excellent description of much basic information, including the following:

- The competition uniform is usually referred to as a *gi* (pronounced "gee," with a hard "g" sound). It is made of heavy material, so it can be used to throw opponents.
- A match is termed a *shiai.*
- Contestants bow to one another initially.
- The match begins with the referee's command *"hajime"* (begin).

Adaptations and Competitive Options

Judo is a sport that demands a physical and strategic performance, testing the skills of strength, touch, balance, and sensitivity. Because it began initially as a martial art aimed at developing agility, self-confidence, self-

ROLE MODEL

JUDO

Andre Watson

Andre Watson is 5'10" and weighs 195 pounds. He was born in 1976 in Philadelphia, earned a doctorate in clinical psychology at Widener University, and is now a practicing psychologist. Dr. Watson competed in judo for only three years before he had earned medals at both the 2005 IBSA Pan Am Games and the 2005 World Cup. Watson initially became interested in judo because of his previous experience with wrestling. He said, "Judo gave me an opportunity to reconnect with that side of me that I really loved in wrestling."

discipline, and independence, it is an ideal activity for promoting these skills in students with visual impairments or deafblindness or in building confidence in individuals who have a newly acquired vision loss.

Judo for competitors with visual impairments or deafblindness, like athletics and swimming, is governed by IBSA and by the U.S. Paralympic Committee in the United States. Both organizations have similar rules, which are based on adaptations to the current rules of the International Judo Federation. Each athlete with a visual impairment is unique, and competitors may need varying degrees of assistance depending on their visual acuity, experience, age, and so forth. However, unlike most other sports, competitors in all three vision classifications compete in one open class. Competition is also divided into gender and weight classifications, as it is in most other sports.

Adaptations of judo rules require action by both coaches and referees (IBSA, n.d., "Judo Rules"; Ohlenkamp, 2000). The adaptations re-

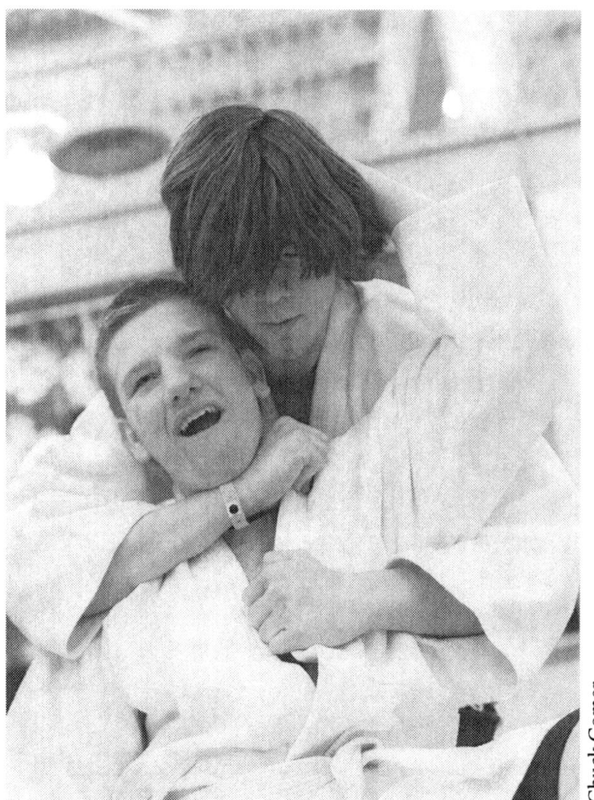

Chuck Comer

Practicing a judo move.

late primarily to the start and finish of the match and the communication of the referee's scoring:

- A coach or assistant guides competitors to their side of the mat when called.
- A corner judge then guides competitors to their starting mark.
- After the judges are seated, the referee announces the beginning of the match and the competitors bow to each other. The referee claps once with arms outstretched in front. The competitors then advance and engage in *kumi kata* (gripping each other's gi). This starting position is used to permit the competitors to grip each other freely. Until hajime (begin) is called, the referee

should ensure that the competitors do not step away or change their foot positions.

- When the competitors have their feet even or parallel with each other, the referee announces "Hajime" to begin.
- Each time the competitors separate during a match, the same procedures are used to resume competition.
- All referee hand signals used during the match must also be spoken simultaneously.
- Referees may take the opportunity during a break in the action to verbally inform the contestants of the score and time remaining.
- At the end of the match, the corner judge again provides whatever assistance is needed to help competitors exit the mat.

The rules also call for the danger zone, a 1-meter-wide area that surrounds the competition mat, to be distinguishable by touch or by having the referee call "Mat" when necessary to ensure safety and to prevent the unintentional rule violation of entering the danger zone. In addition, specific hand signs are designated that can be made on the body for the referees to use with competitors who are deafblind, in order to signal when to begin, when to pause, the score, and so forth.

Teaching Tips

Teaching judo to students with visual impairments uses the same methodologies as was previously described for wrestling. Like wrestling, judo is a sport of quick and complex movements, making it difficult to teach in the usual way of modeling a move and then having the student observe it with either limited vision or touch. Instead, it is easier and more effective to have the teacher or coach show the student the move by actually using it on the learner. Because judo competitors or even those learning judo become accustomed to "reading" their opponent's movements in order to determine what move to use to counter it, they respond well to learning through physical guidance. Students who are deafblind need to have instructions signed to them in their preferred mode of communication. Since it would be difficult to spell out each judo term, it is important to agree on specific signs and for the interpreter or intervener to use them consistently. As with any new skill, repetition is important until the student understands the skill. Sidebar 8.4 provides some additional coaching tips for working with judo students who are visually impaired (Ohlenkamp, 2000).

As was also discussed with regard to wrestling, teachers and coaches need to assess each student's understanding of the concepts of force and speed. If students show little willingness to quickly pursue a foe, they may be shocked by the speed and force used by other students who have a good understanding of these concepts. Remediation of the problem requires teaching these concepts. (See the previous section on Teaching Tips under Wrestling for teaching suggestions.)

Tandem Cycling

Description

Tandems are bicycles designed to carry more than one person. The term *tandem* does not refer to the number of people carried on the bicycle, however; rather, it is derived from the arrangement of the seats, one behind the other (bikefortwo.com). (A bike with two riders side-by-side is called a sociable, surrey bike, or duo bike.) Tandem bikes have been around nearly as

SIDEBAR 8.4

Suggestions for Working with Judo Students with Visual Impairments

The following are some suggestions for judo instructors working with students with visual impairments. When teaching judo to a student with deafblindness, refer to the communication suggestions in Chapter 4.

- Use verbal descriptions to supplement demonstrations. Be as exact and descriptive as possible. When describing an action or intended result, avoid using phrases such as "like this," "Put this hand here," or "Move it this way." Terms that rely on visual cues will provide no information to a student with a visual impairment, and such terms can be confusing. Clearly specify which body parts are involved in the technique (right or left, inside or outside).
- Do not disrupt the class to have a student with a visual impairment or blindness feel the position of the instructor. Feel free to use the student as a partner in the demonstration, but try not to single out the student in a way that delays the rest of the class and makes the student with the impairment feel self-conscious.
- Deal with the student with a visual impairment as an individual. Learn how much vision the student has, and do not make assumptions about the student's abilities or skill level. There are uncoordinated students who are blind just as there are highly athletic students; there are slow and fast learners; there are weaknesses and there are strengths to take advantage of. Address individual needs, but do not treat a student with a visual impairment as if that student has a handicap.
- For students who could benefit from it, begin with an orientation to the room and mat area. Allow the student with the visual impairment to become aware of his or her surroundings through exploration and verbal descriptions, noting any potential hazards, to allow the student to be as self-sufficient as possible.
- During instruction or training, provide audible cues so that students can determine their location in the room without sight. Do not allow students with visual impairments to drift off the mats or into danger, but avoid grabbing or pulling them to direct them, unless necessary for safety. Offer to guide them if you think they may need assistance. Rely on verbal instructions to respect the dignity of the individual.
- Challenge a student with a visual impairment like any other student. Expect full participation and maximum effort.
- Fully integrate students with visual impairments or deafblindness into regular judo classes whenever possible, but permit opportunities for competition and training with other students with visual impairments as well. Educate all the students on the special competition rules for athletes with visual impairments.
- Listen to your students and let them tell you if they need assistance. Feel free to ask what you could do to help.
- Avoid teaching based on stereotypes. Although some athletes with visual impairments may be good at mat work, it is a myth that they like mat work. Athletes with visual impairments can do foot sweeps, they can excel in *ukemi* or *kata*, and they can be effective in all other aspects of judo.
- Athletes with visual impairments do not want others to look at them with sympathy. Likewise, they do not want to feel as if what they do is inspiring. It does not take special courage for an individual with a visual impairment to pursue judo. Such athletes would like the same opportunity to participate as anyone else without carrying along any baggage or special responsibilities. All students of judo are courageous and inspiring, and all of them overcome great difficulties and personal handicaps.

Source: Adapted with permission from N. Ohlenkamp, "Coaching Judo for Blind Athletes" (2000), retrieved 7/4/12 from www.judoinfo.com/vicoach.htm.

long as the bicycle itself, having been invented in Great Britain by Dan Albone and Arthur James Wilson in 1886 (Griffin, 2011). Tandem cycling was popular during the early 1900s, dropped off significantly after World War II, and has regained some of its popularity since then. Assuming factors not related to the bicycle itself are equal, such as the skill of the riders, wind direction, and the like, tandems generally outperform single bicycles in races, because they have twice the power, their wind resistance is about the same, and the drive train friction is not much greater than that of a one-seater.

One of the reasons for the tandem's recent revival is that it has become a high-tech machine that performs at the same level as one-seater racing bikes. The performance level is, in part, as a result of the high tech innovations developed by Bill McReady, a bicycle technician working in the 1950s (Griffin, 2011). However, it also seems likely that the inclusion of tandem racing in the Paralympic and IBSA World Games has spurred bicycle engineers' interest in developing faster tandems.

Tandem cycling differs from the other sports activities discussed in this chapter, in that it is not truly an adapted sport. That is, although communication between the two riders needs to be coordinated, tandem cycling does not require true adaptation or modifications to make it accessible to people with visual impairments or deafblindness. Rather, the sport is simply carried out with one person on the back seat of the bicycle who has a visual impairment and one on the front seat who does not.

Tandem cycling is also a sport that is both competitive and recreational; people use it to exercise and enjoy the scenery in such events as the Annual Great Bicycle Ride Across Iowa, in which thousands participate (www.ragbrai.com), to tour beautiful places, or to ride a nearby bike path on a quiet evening. For more information on recreational tandem cycling, see Chapter 10.

Cycling is a perfect sport to get people with visual impairments and people with vision together, working as a team toward a common goal. The rider in the front seat, known as the captain or pilot, steers. The rider with a visual impairment pedals from the rear seat and is referred to as the "stoker" or "co-pilot."

Tandem cycling became a Paralympic sport in Seoul in 1988 (www.paralympic.org/sport/para-cycling), at which time road racing was introduced for athletes with visual impairments. Events are gender specific or include both genders in mixed teams; they are offered as road races, taking place along existing roadways or as track events, held on long, circular tracks or on highly banked velodromes.

The Paralympic cycling events include the following:

- men's road races over distances ranging from 100 to 135 kilometers, among circuits of 5 or 10 kilometers, or in races between two towns
- women's road race events over shorter distances (between 50 and 70 kilometers)
- "mixed" road racing—a man and a woman together—over distances ranging from 60 to 85 kilometers
- time trial races for individuals or teams of three tandems for men

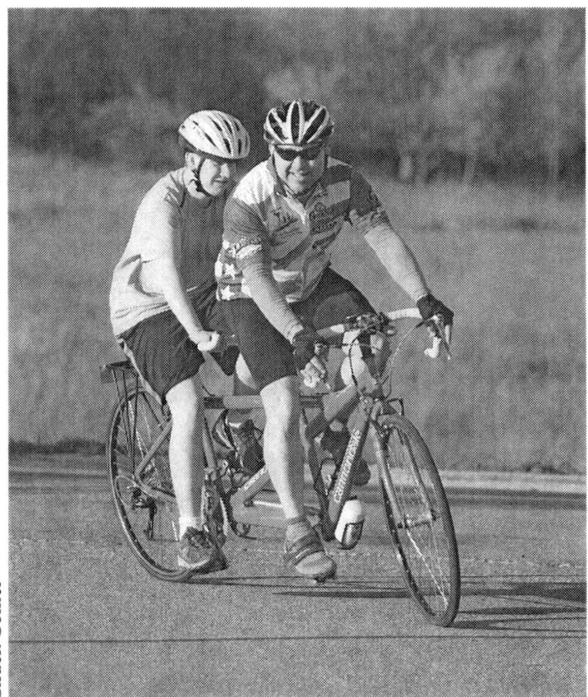
Chuck Comer

Success in tandem cycling relies on communication between captain and stoker.

ROLE MODEL

PARALYMPIC CYCLING CHAMPION
Karissa Whitsell

One of the top cyclists with a visual impairment in the world, Karissa Whitsell won four medals as a tandem bike racer with sighted partner Katie Compton at the 2004 Paralympics in Athens. She and Mackenzie Woodring also won gold, silver, and bronze medals at the 2008 Beijing Games. But Whitsell also likes the freedom of riding solo, with another rider alongside on another bike to point out potential hazards. Vision loss from macular degeneration leaves her with only blurred peripheral vision, but that has never slowed her down. She ran road races with her father when she was 3. Named female athlete of the year by USABA in 2004, the Eugene, Oregon, resident has her sights set on earning more gold medals and breaking her personal records at future summer Paralympic Games.

- indoor competitions in velodromes
- sprint, an event in which two tandems compete over a distance of 1,000 meters
- individual pursuit, over 4,000 meters for men and 3,000 meters for women and mixed teams
- 1-kilometer time trial in mixed races and 500-meter time trial for women

Rules and Competitive Options

As already noted, there are no special adaptations required for tandem cycling competitions. The rules for tandem cycling competition primarily apply to the pilot and are intended to prevent the team member with a disability from recruiting a pilot who has elite cycling status and gaining unfair advantage. Therefore, anyone who is an active elite rider cannot be a captain in an official tandem race. Elite riders can be either amateur or professional riders. Amateur cyclists can ride as pilots if they have not been selected by their national federation to participate in international competitions sponsored by the International Cycling Union (UCI, the international governing body for bicycle racing), for at least three years. Also, in order to qualify as a pilot, a former professional cyclist must have stopped cycling under his or her professional permit for three years and none of the cyclist's earnings can have come from cycling races for the last three years. In addition, the minimum age for taking part in official IBSA competitions is 16. The events take place for B1, B2, and B3 categories together.

Teaching Tips

Teaching Learners with Previous Cycling Experience

If would-be riders with visual impairments have had cycling experience, their skills should be assessed, but there is generally no need to reteach riding skills. Rather, a communication system must be established between the captain and the stoker to avoid injury and to increase the team's efficiency. Sidebar 8.5 outlines the steps for introducing an experienced cyclist to tandem riding and provides communication tips for captains of tandem bicycles.

SIDEBAR 8.5

Steps for Introducing Tandem Cycling to an Experienced Cyclist

Communication between captain and stoker when riding a tandem bicycle is the key to efficiency and safety. The following steps can be used to introduce a rider who is visually impaired to the tandem bicycle, the riding techniques, and the communication used:

- Allow the stoker to inspect the bike and its parts, pointing out any parts that were missed in that initial look.
- Explain mounting, pedaling, balance, and dismounting techniques before attempting them on the bicycle.
- Roll the bike forward and turn the pedal cranks until both front and back pedals are up on the right side.
- Both riders stand on the left side of the bike.
- Both riders step over the crossbar and place the right foot lightly on the up pedal, keeping weight on the left foot.
- When ready, the captain gives the command, "Mount," and both riders take one firm downward pedal stroke together, stop pedaling, and sit down to get balanced on the bike. When the bike is stabilized and the left feet are placed in the pedals, the riders continue pedaling. For riders with deafblindness, these instructions must be communicated with a tactile signal on the hand or arm.
- Both riders pedal as much forward as down; too much down stroking makes the bike wobble, especially if pedals are matched in rotation.
- Both riders lean slightly into, not away from, turns.
- The captain alerts the stoker when he or she wants to slow down or stop.
- The captain alerts the stoker when he or she needs stronger pedaling help, such as on a hill or to speed up to avoid a traffic problem.
- When the captain wants to stop, he or she tells the stoker, "Slowing to stop. Prepare to dismount." At the moment the bike reaches the point of complete stop, the captain gives the dismount command, so the stoker can dismount as the bike stops. Mistiming here can result in the stoker dismounting while the bike is still moving and could result in an injury from being hit in the calves by the pedals. Again, these instructions must be communicated tactilely with a rider who is deafblind to ensure cooperation and safety.

Note that the stoker cannot tell the difference between the pilot's slowing down deliberately and slowing because they are climbing a steep hill. The stoker may therefore misunderstand why the bike is slowing and, for example, pedal harder while the captain is trying to slow to stop at a busy intersection, or stop pedaling on a steep upgrade, thinking the captain is coming to a stop. To avoid such misunderstandings, it is important for the captain to use clear communication, such as, "Coming to an intersection" or "We're starting a steep climb."

Teaching Learners Who Have Never Ridden

Learners with visual impairments or deafblindness who have never ridden a bicycle can start by learning on a stationary bike and then progressing to riding the tandem. Learners can be enrolled in a stationary bike spinning class, or the instructor can work directly with the learner using a stationary bike, starting with the following steps:

- Introduce the parts of the stationary bike.
- Make sure that learners who are deafblind know the terms and signs for the various parts and how they work together.
- Teach pedaling, including stroke rhythm, pedaling frequency and rhythm, and forward stroking using a metronome and/or music.
- Build the learner's stamina in preparation for riding.

Once a spinning class has been completed, students have only to learn the bike's parts and functions, controlling balance on the bike, and communicating with the captain. As with experienced cyclists, start by introducing the tandem bicycle's parts and their functions, allowing the student to investigate each. Even though stokers do not normally operate the gearshift or brake mechanisms on a tandem cycle, they should understand where they are on the bike and how they affect riding performance. Some parts in particular, such as the toe clips and the relationship between the front and back sets of pedals, are important for understanding the roles of the stoker and captain.

A captain with a stoker who is riding for the first time needs to be an experienced rider to provide the stability that novice stokers usually lack, and the riding environment should be free of traffic. If the captain is new to riding a tandem, he or she should ride the bike alone at first in order to get accustomed to the longer wheelbase and maneuvering requirements.

The steps for the initial rides are similar to those for more experienced riders, as are the communication requirements. The captain may need to pay more attention to some of the following details with a beginning rider:

- To mount the bike, the captain gets on first and holds the bike steady with both brakes set, while keeping a wide leg stance.
- After the stoker gets on, the captain should communicate where the pedals are positioned for starting the ride. The right pedal should be just forward of straight up. If the pedals are out of position, the stoker pedals backward until the pedals are in starting position. (It is sometimes advantageous to remove toe clips with new riders with visual impairments, because it may be difficult to place the feet into the clips at first.)
- With the captain still holding the bike upright, when the stoker is in both pedals, the stoker announces, "Ready," or signs or gestures if the stoker is deafblind.
- Both riders begin with one good push with the right foot, pause for the captain to get his or her left foot in pedal, glide until the bike is stable, and then begin pedaling.
- To stop and dismount, the captain announces, "We're stopping, but keep your feet in the pedals," and then the captain brings the bike to a gradual stop and braces the bike with brakes locked and a wide stance.
- After the captain announces, "Okay, dismount right [or left]," the stoker gets off and stands away from the bike so the captain does not kick the stoker while dismounting.

- Agreed-on physical gestures must be used to convey signals for stopping and dismounting to the stoker who is deafblind to ensure a smooth and safe stop.

Rowing

Description

Rowing competition among organized crews is one of the oldest and most traditional sports. Races between oared galleys were held in ancient Egypt and Rome. In the United States, the National Association of Amateur Oarsmen was established in 1872 and renamed the United States Rowing Association in 1882. US Rowing, as it is commonly called, is recognized by the United States Olympic Committee as the national governing body for the sport (www.usrowing.org).

Rowing, like tandem cycling, requires no substantive adaptations. An individual with a visual impairment who had rowing experience before losing vision or who has had substantial training in rowing can simply participate on a rowing team with sighted teammates after an adequate practice period.

Rowing has two forms. In crew or sweep-oar racing, two, four, or eight crew members sit facing the stern of the boat, each rower pulling one oar. The vessel is steered by a team member called the *coxswain,* who sits in the stern of the boat, facing the crew, and does not row. The job of the coxswain is to steer the boat, decide tactics, and establish and maintain the speed and rhythm of the strokes of the rowers.

The other form of rowing, in which no coxswain is used, is called sculling, or scull racing. It is performed by an individual, by a pair, or by a team of four rowers with each rower facing the stern and pulling on a pair of oars.

The boats, referred to as shells, vary in length. These long, slim craft may weigh as little as 14 pounds. The shells contain seats that slide back and forth to accommodate body movement while rowing and shoes, called footboards, to hold the rowers' feet in place. The oars are affixed to the shell by oarlocks and are usually about 12 feet long, with blades of 24 to 36 inches in length and 6 inches in width. The stroke begins with placing the oar in the water and ends when the oar has reemerged and is poised to begin another cycle. The stroke may be broken down into four parts: the recovery, catch, drive, and release. Power for the stroke is supplied by the driving of the rower's legs and the force of the pull through the shoulders and back, which is made possible by the sliding seat. This entire sequence of rhythmic, balanced movements is repeated from 32 to 40 times per minute, depending on conditions. (See also the discussion of indoor rowing machines for fitness in Chapter 11.)

Rules and Competitive Options

The sport of adaptive on-water rowing is growing in popularity around the world, and in 2003, the International Rowing Federation (FISA; www.worldrowing.com) adopted an adaptive rowing classification system. There are three types of events for rowers with disabilities that are based on type of disability and number of team members (Gilbert, 2007). These include the following:

- legs-trunk-arms mixed-gender four with coxswain, 1,000 meters with sliding seats
- trunk-arms double scull 1,000 meters with fixed seats
- men's and women's single sculls, 1,000 meters, arms only, with fixed seats

FISA is the sole world governing body for rowing. The sport is practiced by athletes in 24 countries. Races are held over 1,000 meters for all four events. FISA introduced adaptive rowing on a world championship level at its 2002 World Rowing Championships in Seville, Spain. The number of participating countries has grown from 7 the first year to 16 in 2007 (Gilbert, 2007). The first Paralympic rowing competition was held in Beijing in 2008. The vision classifications used by FISA are identical to the IBSA classifications described earlier in the chapter (see Sidebar 8.3).

ROLE MODEL

ROWING

Jamie Dean

James (Jamie) Dean is a former Sports Education Camp athlete who after early success in goalball at the youth national level went on to win a spot on the Wake Forest University rowing team. Like Jim Mastro, he lost his vision as a result of retinitis pigmentosa. He was a Fletcher Scholar in the Graduate Law School at Wake Forest and has been a rower on the U.S. Rowing Team three times. He has won the Adaptive Four with Coxswain competition at the 2007 U.S. Rowing National Championships, competed internationally in the FISA World Championships in 2006 and 2007, and was on the silver medal–winning U.S. team in the 2008 Beijing Paralympic Games. After the silver medal finish, Jamie said: "When we began our push to the finish, we completely caught the competition by surprise. . . . The last 20 strokes of our race were the sweetest I've ever taken. The boat was absolutely flying, with adrenaline and excitement taking over where the muscles were tempted by fatigue to fail."

Teaching Tips

As in all teaching situations that include equipment, it is essential to allow learners to investigate the boat and oars, including all of their integral parts. In the case of very lightweight boat shells, it is also important to teach participants how to get in and out of the boat. In addition, since this sport relies on the exact timing of strokes and the commands of the coxswain, learners must know the language of communication.

If the participant has never rowed with either a single or double oar, that skill also needs to be taught before trying it on the water. As with tandem cycling, the essential stroke can be taught on an indoor trainer. There are several rowing machines that will suffice, but the product known as the Concept2 rowing machine is especially good for this purpose, because the company offers a free download of Erg Chatter, software that makes the device accessible to rowers who are blind. In addition, Concept 2 has begun to promote stationary rowing competitions among people with visual impairments (Concept2, n.d). For learners who are deafblind, inspecting the boat on land using touch and practicing the stroke on the rowing machine and in the actual boat on land may be beneficial. In addition, as with any other sport, the signs for the parts of the boat, oars, and rowing concepts also need to be taught.

The rhythm of rowing is learned through hearing and "feel." Aerial Gilbert (personal communication, November, 2007) explains this as follows:

> Rowing is a sport that requires the rowers to row backwards, keep their focus in the boat, and not be looking around. The ideal rower is the one that is focused on what she

> is feeling and hearing: feeling the movement of one's body moving forward and backward, the power and application, and hearing the oars turning in the oarlocks. She is also hearing the seats of the rowers behind and or in front moving up the slide, and of course listening to the coxswain's commands. A drill that is used regularly to get the rowers to feel the movement of the boat is to have all the rowers close their eyes for a part of the training session. The longer this is done, the more effective it is.

Gilbert reports that in rowing, oars are used in either the square position (oar blade facing backward in the same direction as the rower) or feathered, that is, with the edge of the blade facing backward. In order to know when the oar is feathered, Gilbert notes that placing a notch on the handle or taping a coin to correspond with the position of the blade edge is helpful in making sure the broad side of the oar is kept in the water during a stroke.

Explaining the role of the coxswain is an important part of teaching about crew races. The coxswain's functions include the following:

- to be in command of the boat
- to steer the boat
- to coach the crew
- to let rowers know if they are catching the stroke late or early
- to let rowers know if they need to change their stroke in order to be in sync with the others
- to provide motivation and encouragement to the crew
- to inform the crew where they are relative to other crews and the finish line
- to make any necessary tactical decisions
- to keep the boat and rowers safe at all times

Consequently, understanding communications from the coxswain is an essential part of rowing.

Given the importance of communication in this sport, working with a rower who is deafblind would require a good knowledge of the techniques for communication with people who are deafblind discussed in Chapter 4. As far as is known, there are no deafblind rowers competing in international rowing, so the adaptations suggested here for interpreting the coxswain's commands are based more on knowledge of the sport and of deafblindness than on experience. However, the rowing rhythm would most likely be sensed by a rower with deafblindness and learned with practice. In addition, the coxswain's call could be communicated by thumping the boat's hull with a foot as the call is made. Communication might also be facilitated by placing the rower who is deafblind in the seat nearest the coxswain where a prearranged set of tactile signals could then be transmitted to the rower, either by thumping the hull, tapping the individual, or using a remote electronic device placed on the rower's skin. For example, a touch on the left shoulder could mean slow down your stroke, and a touch on the right shoulder, speed it up.

Dragon Boating

Description

Although it is not taught in high school and has a limited number of competitive opportunities at present, dragon boating, or dragon boat racing, has been included in this chapter because, like rowing, it is easily accessible to people with visual impairments or deafblindness and it appears to have significant potential for growth. The use of dragon boats is believed to have begun some 2,500 years ago in South Central China (Barker, 1996). The custom of dragon boating supposedly began after similar boats were used in an attempt to save a Chinese scholar from drowning one day near the summer solstice. The sport has been practiced continuously in China since that time. The Hong Kong Tourism Bureau helped move dragon boat racing into the modern era by donating teak dragon boats to countries around the world. In 1986, the Hong Kong Pavilion at Expo '86 donated four teak dragon boats to the city of Vancouver, British Columbia, Canada. Community leaders in Vancouver quickly saw the potential in creating a multicultural event that would bring together the Chinese and non-Chinese citizens for a fun event and festival, giving birth to the Canadian International Dragon Boat Festival, now known as the Alcan Dragon Boat Festival.

The original boats were loaned or rented to Toronto, Victoria, Seattle, and Los Angeles and quickly helped spread the seeds for modern dragon boat racing throughout North America. Taiwanese-style dragon boats have also been donated to sister cities in North America to help found the Portland Kaohsiung Dragon Boat races in Portland, Oregon. Today there are clubs, teams, and festivals all around the United States. Major dragon boating events are still held around the time of the summer solstice.

Modern dragon boat racing is governed by the International Dragon Boating Federation (IDBF). The IDBF has organized the World Nations Dragon Boat Racing Championships for representative national or territorial teams every two years since 1995, but dragon boating is not yet an Olympic sport. The IDBF recognizes two types of racing: *sport racing,* the more formal IDBF-sanctioned races, and *festival racing,* more traditional and informal types of races, which use varying rules. Sport racing distances are typically 250 meters, 500 meters, 1,000 meters, and 2,000 meters and are held under formal rules of racing. A festival race is typically a sprint event of several hundred meters; 500 meters is a standard distance in many international festival races.

The dragon boat team is made up of a caller (coach) who stands in the front and calls the

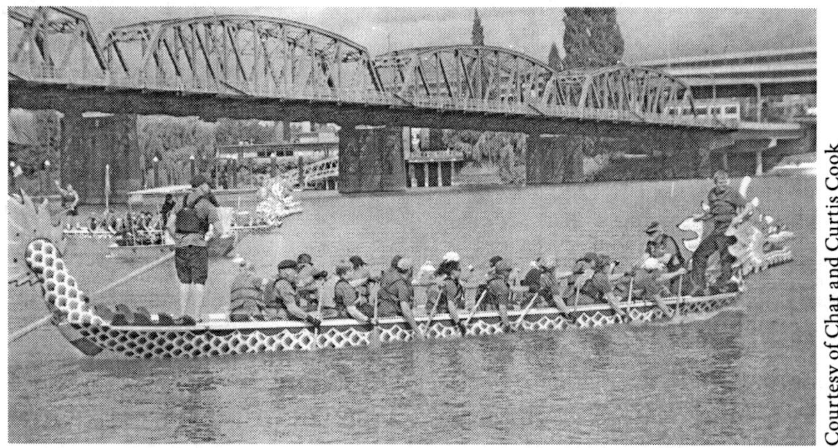

Courtesy of Char and Curtis Cook

The Lethally Blind dragon boat team racing in the Rose Festival Regatta in Portland, Oregon, in June 2012. Of the 21 team members, 15 were blind.

ROLE MODELS

DRAGON BOATERS

Bonnie Cooper and Char Cook

Bonnie Cooper is a 50-year-old single mother from Portland, Oregon, who is deafblind as a result of Usher syndrome. She works for an equipment manufacturer, bending, shaping, and welding metal parts and shipping the finished products. Through the Oregon State Commission for the Blind, she was introduced to a dragon boat paddling team named Blind Ambition, in which she honed her skills. She then joined the Portland-based 150-member Wasabi Paddling Club. Bonnie competed for and won a spot on the U. S. Masters Women's Team B, which competed in Berlin, Germany, at the International Dragon Boat Federation World Dragon Boat Racing Championships. Whatever Bonnie does, she gives it 100 percent. She is very dedicated in her workouts on the boat. She paddles with her team three times a week, for a total of three to four hours per week.

Char Cook, like Bonnie Cooper, took up dragon boating after the age of 50 years, after she had become a grandmother,. Char lost her center vision to retinitis pigmentosa, a progressive retinal disease, when she was a child. Her version of becoming a paddler follows:

> I hated it at the beginning, but I stayed with it because I had committed to the group. At the end of the first two-month practice time and after those first races, I quit and was glad for it. But I had made a couple of good friends on the first boat, and they insisted that I keep trying, so I did. After months and months of practicing three days a week in all weather conditions, I fell in love with the sport.
>
> Some folks like my friend Bonnie are naturals. They do it well from the beginning; they have a good stroke and their timing is perfect. Then there are the folks like me. It was difficult for me to learn the stroke. My timing had issues which didn't get resolved right away, and my fitness level was in the basement. But I liked it, so I kept on practicing. That's been almost six years ago, and I am passionate about the sport now. I often bring groups of newly blinded adults down to the dock to experience paddling. I also bring groups of kids from the school for the blind down to paddle. They love it immediately. It's a real team sport and no accommodations are needed. It's just, get fit, get instruction, and practice your guts out.
>
> In 2005 I tried out for Team USA. The World Dragon Boat Games were being held in Berlin, Germany. I made it, and Bonnie Cooper and I were the first blind paddlers to ever race at the world level. . . . The sport is a happening one and is one that can fully embrace the person who is blind or visually impaired!

race, a tiller who stands in the back and steers the boat, and 20 paddlers (Charlene Cook, personal communication, October 28, 2007). The paddlers sit side by side on bench seats. The paddles are similar to canoe paddles, but are somewhat shorter and have a T-shaped handle grip. As is the case in rowing, timing of paddle strokes among the 20 team members is crucial to success.

Rules and Competitive Options

As is the case with crew or scull rowing, there are no adaptations or special rules governing competitors with visual impairments or deafblindness. In fact, there are no competitive opportunities outside of traditional IDBF-sanctioned events. Competitors with visual impairments are rare and are simply part of sighted teams. The sport is covered in this chapter be-

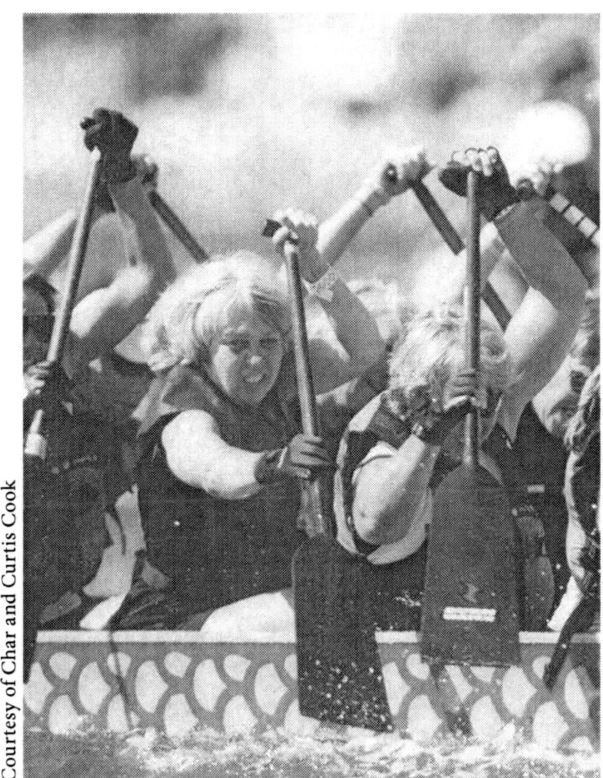
Courtesy of Char and Curtis Cook

Char Cook, member of Team USA in the 2005 Dragon Boat World Games.

cause it appears to have outstanding potential for growth among people who are blind, are deafblind, or have low vision. It appears that there are presently at least three teams of paddlers with blindness or deafblindness active in North America: in Vancouver, British Columbia, the British Columbia Blind Sports and Recreation Association; the Houston, Texas, Lighthouse for the Blind team, Blind Fury; and Blind Ambition PDX in Portland, Oregon, which bills itself as the first blind dragon boat team in America to compete equally with 80 other teams (see the Resources section for more information on these teams). The sport's greatest potential appears to be for individual paddlers with visual impairments to become part of an existing team. The Portland team includes a woman who is deafblind who qualified for and competed on the USA team in the IDBF world championships.

For suggestions on teaching the sport of dragon boat racing to individuals with visual impairments, see the teaching tips in the section on rowing, as the sports are similar.

CONCLUSION

As the wide variety of sports and competitive events highlighted in this chapter demonstrates, the opportunities for sports participation among students and adults with blindness, deafblindness, or low vision are virtually limitless. The sports activities described in this chapter have been mastered by many athletes with visual impairment or deafblindness, as illustrated by the role models included in each activity section.

Virtually every sports activity can be modified and made accessible to some degree by using the AccesSports Model described in Chapter 5. In addition, the adaptations required to play many sports not described in this chapter have already been developed, and the information is available from sources such as organizations and websites devoted to those sports (see the Resources section of this book for contact information for many of these organizations). Additional mainstream sports that are played by people with visual impairments or deafblindness include Alpine skiing, cricket, golf, gymnastics, lawn bowling, Nordic skiing, powerlifting, soccer, and waterskiing. Some of these sports that are considered more often in a recreational category or those not routinely taught in high school physical education curricula are discussed in Chapter 10. Competitive sports designed specifically for individuals with visual impairments are described in the next chapter.

9 Organized Sports for Children and Adults with Visual Impairments

GOALBALL AND BEEP BASEBALL

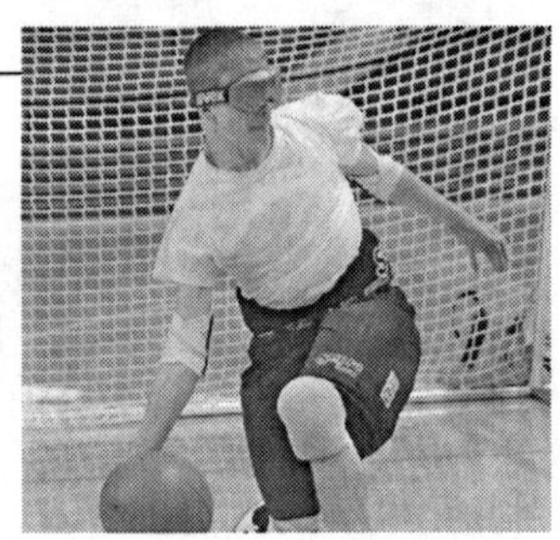

Chuck Comer

IN THIS CHAPTER

- **Goalball**
- **Beep Baseball**
- **The Eyeshade and Low Vision**
- **Adaptations for Students with Deafblindness**

James and Dorian, two adolescent boys who are completely blind as a result of retinoblastoma, a hereditary retinal cancer, both signed up for a local goalball program at the beginning of the school year. Unlike most children with this condition, who have vision for some part of their early childhood years, Dorian had had no vision since birth because his eyes had to be removed within a few days of being born, while James did not totally lose his vision until he was nearly 10 years old. Before that time, James had had sufficient vision to see the motor movements of his peers and learned basic physical concepts and skills by watching them play, while Dorian did not.

After a few practice sessions in the goalball program, it was apparent to the coaches that the two boys had highly different skills and conceptual knowledge. James, having seen veteran players demonstrate blocking, dove on his side hard at 90 degrees to the trajectory of the ball with both arms extended, and the ball hit him in the chest before it could pass him. When he stopped the ball, his body was nearly parallel with the goal line.

Dorian, although he had received verbal instructions and a tactile demonstration of blocking, had difficulty with the conceptual aspect of the skill. When a softly thrown ball approached him from his right front, he did not dive toward it. Instead, he dropped from his hands and knees to his right hip in a sitting motion, and while continuing to face forward reached toward the passing ball with a half-hearted movement of his right hand. Also, he reacted long after the ball had already passed him. These behaviors indicated that Dorian's concepts of extension, time, and rate were not well developed. He simply did not realize how far and how quickly he had to extend his arms and body to reach the ball before it passed him and became a goal for his opponents.

During the next several weeks, the coach started to lay the groundwork for teaching Dorian sports concepts.

■

Neil is a 45-year-old former basketball player and coach who lost most of his vision as a result of diabetic retinopathy. During his rehabilitation program, Neil learned to play goalball and became involved with a local goalball club. He played the game a few times recreationally, but, other diabetic complications prevented him from playing competitively. However, Neil soon became highly interested in coaching goalball, first becoming the assistant coach and then head coach of the local club team for two seasons. He moved on to coach the state youth goalball team, and after two years and a great deal of hard work and effort, he was named head coach for the USA goalball team. Neil's innovative style and dogged dedication led the USA team to their first medal finishes in many years in the Paralympics and World Games. ■

The sports described in the previous chapter developed over the years primarily as activities for children and adults with a full complement of vision, and were then adapted for people with visual impairments or deafblindness. A few sports activities, however, are specifically identified with blindness. The most well-known of these games are goalball and beep baseball. Goalball, as its name implies, is a goal sport, but it is one that was originally invented specifically to be played by people with blindness. Although beep baseball is technically an adapted version of baseball, its numerous adaptations make it easily identifiable as a sport specific to people with no vision or whose vision has been totally blocked by an eyeshade or occluder. A version of beep kickball has also recently been developed. These specialized games might also be played by an entire class of sighted students while blindfolded to help them understand the skills of the student with a visual impairment and to learn more about using their own senses of hearing and touch.

As has been stressed throughout this book, physical activity, and particularly participating in group activities such as sports, has positive effects on participants that go beyond the immediate benefits for health and fitness. For young people with visual impairments, the opportunity to play a sport designed specifically for their abilities not only teaches physical and conceptual skills but also boosts self-confidence and self-esteem; provides a venue for learning social skills, cooperation, and discipline; and promotes pride in their self-identity. Goalball, beep baseball, and beep kickball also offer the benefits that come from playing any team sport, such as learning to depend on other team members, working together until the team becomes a single unit, and winning or losing as a team.

Based on pre-camp interviews at the authors' sports camps, it appears that both goalball and beep baseball have a high level of name recognition among students with visual impairments, but most of those students interviewed had little knowledge of the specifics of the games, as did the campers' teachers and parents or other caretakers. This chapter aims to remedy this knowledge deficit by providing detailed descriptions of these two sports and sufficient information to enable teachers, parents and other family members or caretakers, students, or other interested persons to implement teaching units in physical education classes or to initiate local goalball or beep baseball programs. The information in this chapter is derived from the national organizations that sponsor goalball (the United States Association of Blind Athletes) and beep baseball (National Beep Baseball Association; see the Resources section).

Since goalball and beep baseball were developed to make use of hearing instead of vision to track balls and maintain orientation within a given playing area, they are generally not pursued by people with deafblindness. However, modifications have been made at the authors' sports camps that enable students with deafblindness to play both games, as described later in this chapter.

It is difficult to describe the intricacies of a new sport to a person who has never seen it, let alone to convey the excitement and action of a fast-moving game or the skill of talented athletes. Readers are therefore urged to consult videos of goalball and beep baseball (many are available on the Internet) to supplement the information provided in this chapter.

GOALBALL

History

Goalball is a fast-paced, physically challenging sport played exclusively by blind or blindfolded athletes. It was developed by Austrian Hanz Lorenzen and German Sepp Reindl to meet the rehabilitative and competitive needs of veterans who were blinded during World War II (IBSA, n.d., "Goalball"). Its popularity began to grow in earnest, however, after its debut in the Toronto Paralympic Games in 1976, where the U.S. team competed for the first time. The game has become extremely popular among athletes with visual impairments and has the second highest participation of any sport among the members of the USABA (Ponchillia, Strause, & Ponchillia, 2002). The USABA holds a national goalball championship in which 12 men's and 8 women's teams qualify through a set of tournaments held in representative regions around the country.

Description

Goalball is played by two teams of three players on an indoor court similar in size to that of volleyball. The object of the game is to throw the ball across the floor and over the other team's goal line, while the opposing team tries to prevent this from happening by either blocking the throw or by deflecting the ball out of bounds (known as "blocking out." The ball is about the size of a basketball and contains bells; players track the location of the ball by its sound. Because the degree of vision among people with visual impairments varies so greatly, all players are required to wear eyeshades during play so that no players have an advantage. Complete up-to-date goalball rules are available from the IBSA website (http://www.ibsa.es/eng/deportes/goalball/reglamento.htm).

The Court

The goalball playing court is a rectangle approximately the same size as a volleyball court (18 meters by 9 meters). The court is divided into six distinct areas: team, landing, and neutral areas for each team. Players of opposing teams do not run up and down the court. Rather, they remain in the *team areas* that encompass the outer 3 meters of both ends of the court.

The next 3-meter area toward midcourt is designated the *landing area.* A ball thrown by a player must first strike the floor in this area to avoid a throwing penalty. The two remaining 3-meter areas on either side of the midline are the *neutral areas.*

The boundaries of the goalball court and between the different areas are marked by cord held in place with vinyl gymnasium tape, so that players can feel the lines with their feet or hands. Each team area contains three pairs of orientation lines, also marked with cords, used by the players to indicate their position on the court and to maintain their orientation.

Teams face one another, with the player designated as the *center* placed slightly ahead of and between two players called *wings.* All three players defend a goal net at their backs that is approximately chest high and that spans the entire width of the court along the goal line.

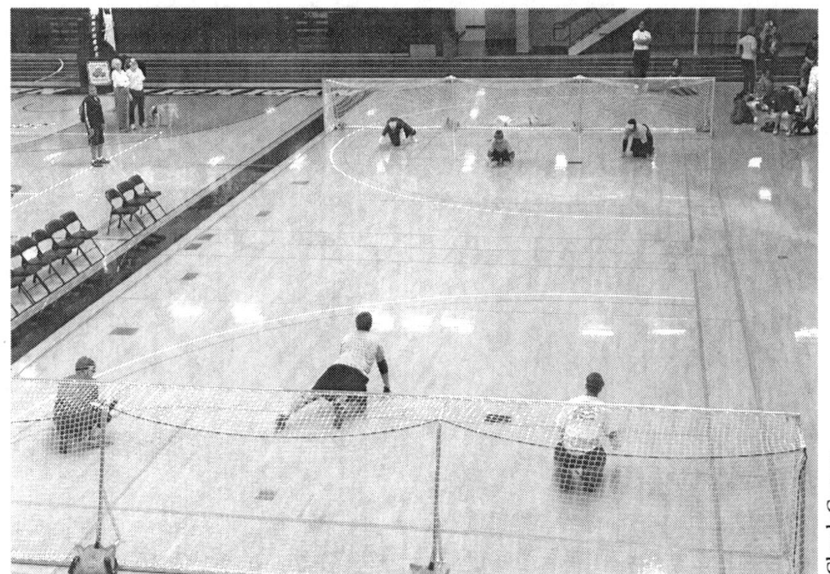

Chuck Comer

The goalball court with both teams in position. Taped lines indicate boundaries and mark the positions for the players.

The center normally straddles the 0.5-meter center orientation line. Its counterpart, the rear center line, extends a half meter from the goal line into the team area midway between the sidelines). The wing lines extend into the team area from the sidelines midway between the goal line and the front line of the team area; they serve as place markers for the wings. The third, unnamed, pair of orientation lines is placed on the front line of the team area 1.5 meters from the sideline. They are significantly shorter (0.15 meters) than the others and play a relatively minor role, mainly helping the center identify where the wing lines end.

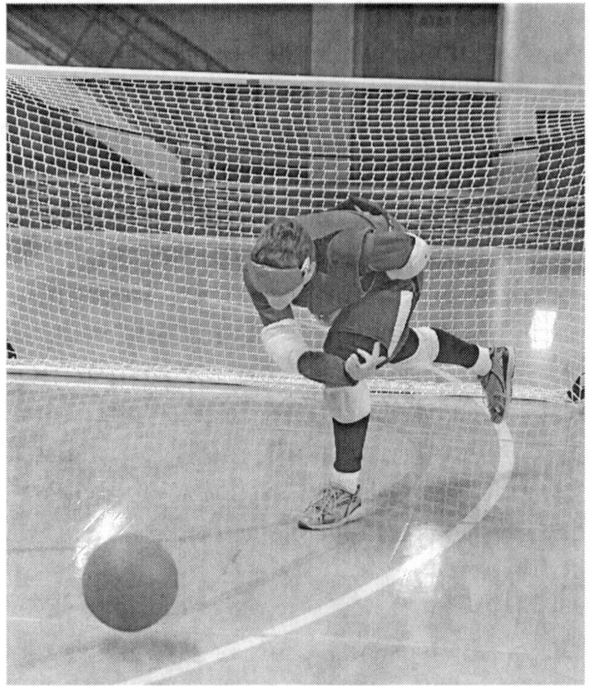

Chuck Comer

Practicing throwing. The goalball is most commonly delivered in the same manner as a bowling ball.

Scoring

A score is accomplished when a player on one team throws the ball between or over the opposing defensive players and it crosses their goal line into the net. The ball is rolled back and forth continuously between teams until a goal is scored, an infraction occurs, a penalty is called, the ball is sent out of bounds, or a team calls time out or brings in a substitute player.

Throwing

A goalball is most commonly delivered in the same manner as a bowling ball. A thrower generally uses a few running steps before releasing the ball underhand near the surface of the playing floor. Beginning players often start by throwing the ball without the approach and then work toward adding the run up, since the more powerful throw resulting from the running approach is more likely to score. Experienced players often modify the throw to gain more ball speed. The most common of these modifications is a discus-like spin and throw. After blocking the other team's throw, each team has 10 seconds to throw the ball; the ball must touch the floor of the court in that team's "landing area" to be a legal throw. No team member may make more than two consecutive throws.

Blocking

Proper defensive blocking form consists of a player dropping down or sliding into a position on his or her side on the playing floor that places the body at a 90-degree angle to the approaching ball. Players extend arms and legs, with wrists, elbows, shoulders, hips, knees, and ankles totally extended in order to block a rolling ball. A bent knee or elbow often results in an offensive score, because a speeding ball can be deflected off bent body parts and up and over the defender.

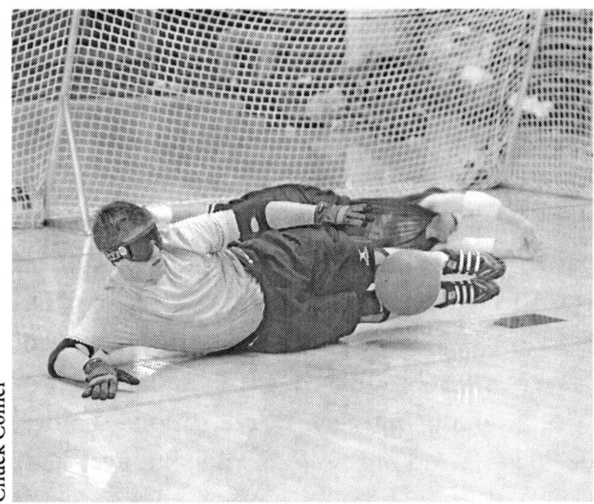

Chuck Comer

Practicing blocking in goalball. This player needs to practice fully extending his arms.

Substitutions and Time Out

Each team is allowed three substitutions during the playing time of a game, when a player on the bench replaces one of the players on the court. Substitutions made at the halftime break in play are unlimited, however, and do not count as one of the three allotted per game. Three time outs are also permitted per game.

Rule Violations

Goalball infractions are minor rule violations that result in losing possession of the ball, while penalties are major violations that result in a single member of the offending team being required to defend the entire goal line alone against a penalty throw (see Sidebar 9.1). Penalties result in the offending player becoming the sole defender during a penalty throw, much as is done in a free kick in soccer. Major penalties include a team taking more than 10 seconds to return a throw after blocking (10-second violation), throwing the ball in the air beyond the team's landing area (high ball violation), and having the same player throw the ball more

SIDEBAR 9.1

Goalball Infractions and Penalties

Infractions

Infractions are minor rule violations that cause the team to lose its turn to throw and include the following:

- Premature throw: Throwing the ball before the referee indicates the ball is in play
- Dead ball: not pursuing a blocked ball and having it stop dead
- Pass out: passing the ball out of bounds
- Ball over: blocking the ball back across the midcourt line

Goalball Penalties

Penalties result in the offending player defending the entire goal against a free throw from the opponents. In the case of a team penalty, the last player to throw the ball defends the goal. Actions resulting in penalties include the following:

- Short ball: a ball that does not reach the defending players
- High ball: a thrown ball that lands outside the landing area and in the neutral area
- Long ball: a thrown ball that lands in the opponent's landing area on its second bounce. This does not give the opposing team enough time to respond.
- Eyeshade: touching the eyeshade during play without the referee's permission
- Third-time throw: a player throwing the ball three consecutive times. Only two throws in a row are permitted.
- Illegal defense: a defender moved into the landing area to block a ball
- Unsportsmanlike conduct: unsportsmanlike behavior by a player or team
- 10 seconds: a player or team taking more than 10 seconds to return the ball after first blocking it

than two times consecutively (third-time throw violation). (See the complete list of penalties in Sidebar 9.1.) The outer perimeter of the 18-by-9-meter playing area is surrounded by a 1.5-meter-wide strip known as the *line out area.* If a ball is blocked out of the playing area and remains in the line out area, the clock continues to run, but if it is blocked out beyond the line out area, the referee calls, "Line out" and the clock is stopped.

Matches last a total of 24 minutes and are divided into two equal halves with a 3-minute break in between. In case of a tie, two additional overtime periods of 3 minutes each are played. If the match is still tied at the end of overtime, the winner is determined by a "shoot out" in which the players of each team face one another one-on-one, each getting a chance to throw once.

Goalball Equipment

Aside from the audible goalball itself, the main equipment necessary for the game is eyeshades and appropriate knee and elbow pads. Cord and tape are needed to mark the boundaries. While nets are used for the goals in regulation games, many beginning teams mark the goals with bright traffic cones during training. Sidebar 9.2 describes in more detail the equipment necessary for individual players and for initiating a goalball program.

The eyeshade or occluder is an important part of the game. In competition, eyeshading is done under formal conditions. Before a game begins, the referee inspects each player's eyeshade for integrity, such as looking for pinholes, loose fit, or other windows of sight. Referees then hand them back to players, who must face their own goal and place the eyeshade over their eyes, and then the referee inspects them again. Players may not touch the eyeshade after this inspection unless they request it of the referee. Adjustments to the eyeshade are permitted only with players' backs turned to their opponents. If eye patching under the eyeshade is also done, it occurs before a game, before the occluder is put in place, and is inspected by an official. This degree of detail is followed in large part because of a history of players with residual vision being accused of "peeking" during play. In recreational games, occlusion need not be so formal, but eye shading needs to be total. The best means by which to ensure this is by using ski goggles that have had their lenses taped over with black tape, because it is easy to see under or around a cloth or homemade eyeshade. Students' concerns about blindfolding are discussed later in this chapter.

Competitive Options

The USABA is the national and the IBSA is the international governing body for goalball competition. The USABA and its state affiliates generally offer three or four regional qualifying tournaments each year, and the national championship event follows their completion. Regional tournaments are open to all teams with proper uniforms, but in recent years, the national tournament can be reached only by an outstanding performance at one of the regional events. Players on elite teams, such as the USA Paralympic Goalball Team or the USA Junior Elite Goalball Team, are also selected according to their performance at USABA tournaments. Both senior and junior teams earned medals in recent Paralympics and IBSA World Games.

SIDEBAR 9.2

Equipment Required for Goalball

- *Eyeshades:* Goalball is a game that requires no vision. Therefore, the rules require each player's eyes to be occluded by an eyeshade. In the United States, most players use ski goggles with the lenses covered with tape, but elite competition also requires that players wear eye patches under the goggles.
- *Elbow pads:* Beginning and advanced players alike require protection for elbows. The quality of the padding naturally increases with the size of players and the intensity with which the game is played. Therefore, middle school, high school, and adult players generally use high-quality volleyball pads.
- *Knee pad:* The same considerations apply to the quality of knee pads. Consequently, middle school, high school, and adult players generally use good-quality volleyball knee pads.
- *Hip pad:* Hip pads, such as those worn by hockey players, hockey referees, or football players, are normally used by larger or more advanced players, because it is common to slide on one's side several feet along the playing floor to stop an opponent's throw. Beginning players, who do not yet use such sliding maneuvers, often do not wear these pads. However, their use is recommended.
- *Shoes and clothing:* Any good basketball or other gym shoes are fine for goalball. Most players wear shorts or pants and shirts made of synthetic materials that tend to facilitate the defensive slide maneuver. Players wear shirts with sleeves of varying lengths, chosen more or less through personal preference.
- *Goalball:* Goalballs are sold by several vendors in the United States and Canada. The official ball is available from the USABA (see the Resources section).
- *Cord:* Cord of approximately ⅛ inch (0.003 meter) is used to mark the boundaries and orientation lines of the goalball court, placed under the center of a 2-inch-wide strip of vinyl floor tape. Various materials including Venetian blind cord, lengths of small-diameter vinyl irrigation pipe, or cotton rope have been used for this purpose.
- *Vinyl gymnasium floor tape:* Two-inch vinyl floor tape is used to tape the cords along the boundary and orientation line on the goalball court. It is designed to be removed easily from gymnasium floors without pulling up the finish or leaving gum residue on the floor.
- *Goal nets:* Goal nets are used in nearly all competitive events nowadays, but they are generally too expensive for developing teams to purchase for use in practices. Small traffic cones can be used to mark the left and right corners of the goal line to substitute for goal nets. In such cases, the cones should be placed on the outside edge of the boundary; if the ball touches the cone, it is called "out."
- *Whistle:* A referee's whistle is necessary for any team that is working toward competition, because the referees use whistles to communicate with players: one whistle blast means stop or start of play during a game, two whistle blasts mean a goal has been scored, and three whistle blasts are used to start and end periods.

ROLE MODELS

GOALBALL

Tyler Merren

Tyler Merren was recently referred to as "the Michael Jordan of U.S. goalball" by fellow players, an apt comparison. He plays every position, is a superb defensive player, and throws a rocket-like serve on offense. Also, like Jordan, he is not showy or egocentric. Rather, he is the gentle husband and father of three children who spends much of his time helping others learn the game of goalball or track and field or other sports.

Tyler is from an athletic family. His natural athletic prowess began to be affected by his Leber's congenital amaurosis by the time he was 14 years old. The degenerative eye condition was slowly taking his vision and decreasing his ability to play the ball sports he loved. His parents learned about one of the sports education camps for athletes with visual impairments, and immediately signed him up. After he learned ways to continue to compete in familiar sports and was introduced to goalball, Tyler embraced the opportunity to excel in sports again. A natural goalball player, he immediately began to play regularly on a local goalball team.

With a new confidence and attitude, Tyler organized an assembly for his entire school, where he and his teammates gave a presentation on goalball with the help and support of his teachers. At the beginning of the assembly, Tyler explained his vision loss to the entire student body, described the effects on his ability to see his way around, and told the students about his involvement in goalball. Using goalball as a tool to demonstrate that he was still capable of playing sports, he recruited members of the football team to play blindfolded against him and his goalball teammates (also blindfolded). The students roared their support when Tyler and his teammates handily beat the sighted team, and Tyler has soared since that time.

As a student at Western Michigan University, Tyler played on the goalball team, which won two national championships. Tyler was selected for the U.S. team in 2001, just two years after learning the game, and has been on the team since, becoming part of the team that turned the U.S. international goalball fortunes around in the mid-2000s.

Robin Theryoung

Low vision from albinism seemed to get in the way of sports for Robin Theryoung until she learned about goalball at a sports education camp. With a new ability to engage in active sports that did not depend on fine visual acuity, Theryoung fell in love with goalball. As a blindfolded goalball player, Robin used her long arms and legs to her advantage on women's goalball teams, and her enthusiasm for the game is infectious. After earning her bachelor's degree from Albion College and dual master's degrees in blindness and low vision studies at Western Michigan University, Robin moved to Colorado Springs, Colorado, and played with the Colorado Bandits. Working as an orientation and mobility instructor, Theryoung worked out daily to improve her fitness and her goalball skills. Her hard work paid off as she and her USA Women's Goalball teammates were the first to be accepted in the Resident Athlete Program at the U.S. Olympic Training Center in Colorado Springs. She and her teammates have earned numerous medals in elite international competitions, including a gold medal from the Goalball World Championships in 2006 and the Paralympic gold medal in 2008.

Teaching Tips

Developing Skills and Sports Concepts

Goalball is not only an exciting competitive sport but also an excellent activity for developing physical conditioning and skills, as well as sports concepts in children. It is excellent for teaching basic sports skills, including all aspects of throwing, reaching and extending, rotating and diving, tracking sound, and controlling body speed. Perhaps more important, it is the ideal game for teaching the often neglected sports space concepts of directions, levels, pathways, location, and extension and the force concepts of time, rate, and flow, described by Graham, Parker, and Holt/Hale (2009) and discussed in Chapter 1. As discussed in that chapter, children with early-onset visual impairments who attend the authors' sports camps often have difficulty with such concepts. Such developmental lags quite frequently can be assessed and remediated through goalball. The cases of Dorian and James presented in the opening vignette illustrate this point and demonstrate how goalball can be used to develop sports concepts of space and effort.

■ *Dorian's coach began to teach Dorian the spatial and movement concepts he lacked, starting with reacting more quickly to sounds. The coach began by placing Dorian in proper starting position at the center line, throwing the goalball down on the floor in random directions approximately 2 feet away, and asking Dorian to slap the ball with the palms of both hands as quickly as he could. At first, Dorian reacted slowly and reached out to the ball with just one hand, but after three weeks of 20-minute daily drills, he began to reach with both hands and could consistently touch the ball almost immediately with the fingertips of both hands. As his skill improved, the ball was moved farther and farther away from him until he was able not only slap to it quickly with the palms of both hands but also to slide his body along the floor to reach it.*

The coach continued the reaction drills as a warm-up before regular goalball practices. After three months of the reaction drills and playing in practices, Dorian moved to the ball nearly as quickly as James. However, Dorian had developed the habit of jumping at the ball head-first instead of placing the front of his entire body perpendicular to the ball's line of travel. He was still confused about the relationship between the ball's pathway and the pathway he needed to take to intersect its trajectory. The coach initiated a second drill to help Dorian learn these concepts and to become proficient at predicting the pathway of a moving object. Again, the coach placed Dorian on defense at the center line, went to the other end of the court, and started throwing moderately fast balls from the center line, the left wing line, and then the right wing line. At first the coach told Dorian to only listen to where the ball was traveling, rather than trying to block it. Then the coach asked him to predict where the next set of throws would pass him by yelling, "Left," "Right," or "At me" as soon as he knew. Next, Dorian had to predict whether the ball would pass him on his far left, on his left, right at him, on his right, or on his far right. Once Dorian was able to consistently predict where the ball would pass him, the final drill required him to actually block the ball, starting close to either his left or his right side and gradually increasing the distance as his prediction skills grew.

As with the earlier reaction drill, this trajectory drill became an everyday part of goalball practice for Dorian. The six months of training significantly decreased the difference in skill level between Dorian and James until it became hard to tell them apart on the defensive end of the court. Dorian not only had learned to be a competent goalball player but also had learned concepts about movement, effort, and timing that could serve him in other sports as well as in his everyday travel. ■

Tips for Teaching Beginners

Goalball can easily be simplified for a physical education class or for recreational, beginning, or young players with a few simple modifications, such as eliminating the need for expensive equipment, simplifying the rules, or mixing veteran players with beginners. The following are some modifications that have been helpful in simplifying the game:

- *Play on tumbling mats to avoid need for equipment:* To eliminate the need for expensive hip, elbow, and knee pads, use tumbling mats instead of the bare gym floor as the team areas. The mats can be marked with the four raised orientation lines under tape, just as the team area of the court would normally be marked.
- *Decrease court size:* For small children under the age of 8 to 10 years, decrease the court to two-thirds the normal length to promote scoring. The width of the court should remain the standard 9 meters.
- *Use minimal rules and instruction:* Play initial games with the bare minimum of instruction. Children tend to learn the game's concepts best and become accustomed to navigating the court by throwing and blocking the ball back and forth with supervision. Introduce the rules and work on individual skills after the students have become comfortable with these elements. Do not enforce infraction or penalty rules during beginning play until players have a good understanding of the basic concept of the game, but be sure that players all get the opportunity to throw.
- *Have players observe games before playing:* If there are more players in the group or class than slots in the game, have the athletes who are waiting to play next sit behind the boundary line of the court at the three player positions, so they can learn "listening skills."
- *Use an experienced player or coach at center:* If there are experienced players in the group, place one at the center position of each team to help manage the game and assist the new players. Alternatively, placing an instructor who is not wearing an occluder at the center position works well for teaching the game to beginners.
- *Mix genders with young players:* Use mixed teams of boys and girls in games played by young players (up to 12 years of age).

Instructors should be aware that some children who are resistant to playing goalball, particularly those with residual vision, may have an aversion to wearing the eyeshade. (See the section "The Eyeshade and Low Vision" in this chapter.) Instructors who suspect this as the source of a child's reluctance can allow the child to play a few games without the eyeshade. However, the child should not be permitted to play the center position, since he or she would likely dominate the game by easily blocking every ball.

Starting a Goalball Activity or Program

Students with visual impairments, who may not have the same opportunities as their classmates to take part in sports or other physical activities in school or in after-school programs, can benefit tremendously from the chance to participate in a program for playing a sport designed around their abilities such as goalball. Initiating and managing a local goalball program for beginners or inexperienced players on an informal basis is well within the capabilities of teachers, parents and other family members or caretakers, and other advocates. One of the most successful youth goalball programs in the country was started by a group of four or five teachers of students with visual impairments and the students' parents. It began as an after-school program for a few children, and due to its popularity, it grew to a statewide program that offered three or four one-day tournaments annually, each of which commonly attracted more than 50 children. The competition was divided into age and skill groups of beginners (approximately 6 to 8 years old), intermediate (approximately 9 to 12), and advanced (older than 13 years). Suggestions to help get a local program started are listed in Sidebar 9.3.

SIDEBAR 9.3

Suggestions for Starting a Local Goalball Program

Setting up a goalball program does not have to be difficult. The following are some suggestions from teachers who have been successful in starting local programs. In addition, the tips for teaching goalball to beginners outlined in the text will be helpful when starting a program with learners who are new to the sport.

- Include the siblings and friends of the students with visual impairments in order to increase the number of players and teams; likewise, use mixed teams of boys and girls in games played by young players up to 12 years of age.
- Look for a gymnasium or large room in a local school, church, park, or other private agency that is large enough for a goalball court plus at least four additional feet on the sidelines, to prevent players from running into walls. Attempt to find a gym that does not have extremely loud heating or cooling fans or a gym that has fans that can be turned off during play.
- If insurance coverage is needed, require players to join USABA and obtain coverage from the organization.
- Look for local sporting goods stores or other retailers as potential donors of knee and elbow pads. All players require at least a set of good elbow and knee pads (volleyball quality if possible). Also, older or more experienced players need to wear hip protection, because they slide across the floor on their sides to block throws. Generally, football running back, hockey player, or hockey referee pads are used, although there are also specialized goalball pants (see the Resources

(Continued on next page)

SIDEBAR 9.3 *(continued)*

section). If pad donors cannot be found, economical pads can be found at many used sports equipment stores (see playitagainsports.com).

- If there are no donors or funds available for obtaining pads, eliminate the need for them by using tumbling mats as the team areas instead of the bare gym floor. The tumbling mats can be marked with the center and wing orientation lines under tape, just as the team area of the court would normally be marked.
- Use a regulation ball if at all possible, as there is no good substitute (see the Resources section).

BEEP BASEBALL

History

Although beep baseball was invented as early as 1964, like goalball, it did not gain popularity until the mid-1970s. According to the National Beep Baseball Association Hall of Fame website (History of Beep Baseball and the NBBA, n.d.), a Montana Bell engineer modified a fast-pitch softball in 1964 to emit a series of beeps that made it possible for players to track the ball using only hearing. This was followed by the development of beep baseball rules by the local Telephone Pioneers. The growth in popularity resulted from the introduction of a newly developed 16-inch beep baseball in the mid-1970s, which made it easier to hit with a swung bat. In addition, the rules were modified in 1975 by members of the Twin Cities–based Braille Sports Foundation, which made the game more interesting and more playable. Popularity grew, resulting in the players and supporters organizing the first Beep Baseball World Series in St. Paul, Minnesota, in 1975. The series has been continued since that time. The National Beep Baseball Association (NBBA), which was formed by these early pioneers, has also developed its own Hall of Fame, in which it describes its history and most outstanding players (www.halloffame.nbba.org).

Description

Beep baseball, like goalball, is played under blindfold in order to remove vision as a factor in ability to play the game. Unlike goalball, which was specifically designed for players who are blind or blindfolded, however, beep baseball is a modification of an existing game. Like baseball, it is played on a traditional ballfield diamond, and the ball is pitched to a batter, who tries to hit it with a bat. When the ball is struck by the batter, the player runs to a base, and the fielders attempt to get the runner out, but if the fielders are not successful, runs are scored. Several adaptations have been made to the game, however, to make it possible for players with visual impairments to track the ball using hearing and to maintain safety among the players running in the field. Following the AccesSports model described in Chapter 5, the adaptations include making the targets—balls and bases—emit sounds and changing rules to make scoring easier and the game safer to play.

Overall, aside from the eyeshades and the beeping ball, the biggest differences are that there are only three bases, including home base,

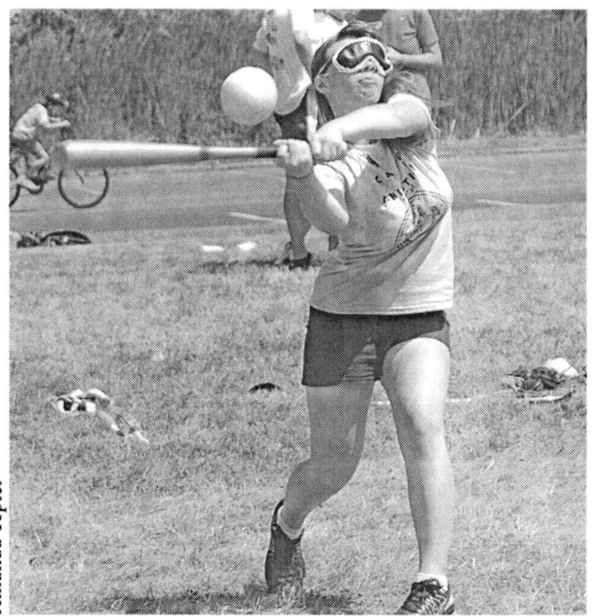

Amanda Tepfer

A blindfolded player batting a beep baseball.

which also emit sounds; there are only six players on a team; and the pitcher is on the same team as the batter. Games have six innings and four strikes, instead of three. When the ball is struck toward the six fielders, the umpire randomly selects and activates the sound beacon of either first or third base. The batter reacts to the sound and runs as fast as possible toward the tone coming from the base, attempting to touch it before a fielder grabs the ball. A run is scored if the batter touches the base before the fielder has caught the ball, but if the fielder catches the ball first, the runner is out. Runners do not circle the bases, and fielders are not required to throw the ball to tag the runner at the base to make an out. Finally, each team has one or two sighted spotters, members of the team who do not play themselves but assist the team when in the field to provide helpful information about the batter before the ball is in play, designate which fielder will field the ball, and prevent collisions. The pitcher and catcher are also sighted and do not bat or play the field; they are on the same team as the batter. The rules and terminology of beep baseball are outlined in Sidebar 9.4.

The following are the specific adaptations to the targets and rules.

Target Adaptations

- The ball emits rhythmic and continuous beeps when the pin is pulled from the on-off switch mechanism.
- Rather than the flat pads used for bases in standard baseball, the bases in beep baseball are vinyl-covered foam towers that emit continuous tones when activated by the umpire. They range from 48 to 54 inches high and have a cylindrical, square, or cone shape of 8 to 10 inches in diameter.

Rule Adaptations

The rules of beep baseball are modified significantly to make the game safer and scoring simpler. Those rules modifications that are required to play an informal game can be summarized as follows:

- There are only two bases in addition to home base, first and third base.
- The pitcher is on the batter's team.
- The pitcher announces in a cadence, "Ready, pitch!" releasing the ball on "pitch" to let the batter know when to swing. The pitcher aims for the spot where the bat will connect with the ball if the batter swings on command.
- Each team is required to have at least one spotter, a sighted member of the defense who helps the fielders orient to a batted ball.
- A catch is defined as holding the ball in hand above the ground and away from the body.

SIDEBAR 9.4

Basic Beep Baseball Rules and Terminology

In beep baseball, a game in which the main players are blindfolded, a batter from one team attempts to hit a beeping ball into fair territory and then tries to reach a buzzing base before the other team is able to field the ball. The following is an outline of some of the rules and terminology that govern the game:

Bases: There are three bases: home base (plate), first base, and third base. First and third bases emit a steady buzz when activated; home plate does not emit a sound.

Batting/batter's box: the 4′ x 8′ area near and on either side of home plate where the batter stands with both entire feet when batting. The lines are considered part of the box. When the head umpire calls "Play," the batter has 30 seconds to occupy the batter's box.

Catch: the act of a fielder in getting secure possession of the ball, in hands or glove, above the ground, and away from the body. In the rare event that a defensive player catches a live, batted fly ball in flight prior to the ball touching the ground, this will automatically retire the side.

Fair hit: a batted ball that settles on fair territory on or between base lines and on or beyond the 40-foot line or that contacts fair ground on or beyond the 40-foot line.

Fielder: any one of the six players of a team when it is not at bat (defensive team). The fielders are referred to by number, with F1 being the infielder at first base; F3 the infielder at shortstop; F5 the infielder at third base; F2 the outfielder in right field; F4 the outfielder in center; and F6 the outfielder in left field. There is no specific distinction between outfield and infield positions in beep baseball. The terms *infield* and *outfield* are used in these rules to distinguish between positions 1, 3, and 5 and 2, 4, and 6, respectively, although a team may place the players occupying these positions anywhere on the playing field. P is pitcher (nonfielding position), C is catcher (nonfielding position), and Sp is spotter (also a nonfielding position).

Home run: a batted ball that travels at least 180 feet in the air over fair territory; the runner must also run to and touch the activated base.

Inning: that portion of the game which includes a turn at bat for each team. A regulation beep baseball game is six innings. A team's half inning at bat ends when there is a third out or when a fly ball is caught or, in the last half-inning of a game, the winning run is scored.

Mask rule: The batter-on-deck must have a blindfold in place prior to entering the on-deck circle. The penalty for the on-deck batter not having a blindfold in place prior to entering the circle is a strike on the current batter. Once the batter-on-deck has the blindfold in place, it should not be lowered or removed without permission from the umpire until that person has completed his or her turn at bat by scoring, striking out, or being put out. If a batter or batter-on-deck removes the mask illegally, he or she is declared out, although the umpire may issue up to two team warnings before charging the penalty strike or declaring the batter or batter-on-deck out.

No pitch: a batted ball that touches the pitcher or his clothing. The count to the batter remains the same as it was before that pitch.

On-deck circle: a circle for each team, 5 feet in diameter, located a safe distance to the side of and behind home plate where the next batter will stand while awaiting his or her turn at bat. When the head umpire calls "Play," the on-deck batter will have 30 seconds to occupy the on-deck circle. The penalty for a batter not being at the plate or an on-deck batter not being ready in the circle within 30 seconds is a strike on the current batter.

Passed ball: a pitch that is not swung at by the batter. A batter is allowed one passed ball without penalty. Additional passed balls are considered strikes.

SIDEBAR 9.4 *(continued)*

Put out: the act of a fielder in retiring a runner by legally fielding the ball before the runner has legally touched the activated base.

Run: the score made by a runner who legally advances to and touches the activated base before being put out by the defense.

Spotter: a nonplaying member of the defensive team who assists the defensive team in the field. Each team must have one but not more than two spotters. The spotters take a position on the field in fair territory prior to the umpire calling "Play." The spotters may assist the defense by positioning themselves on the field prior to each pitch. Spotters may advise if a batter is right- or left-handed, male or female, or may provide any additional information that the spotter feels is necessary for the players to know, before the umpire calls "Play" or before the first pitch to that batter. The spotter may use only the numbers 1 through 6 when designating which player is in the best position to field a batted ball. If the spotter attempts to convey any other information or give any other verbal or physical assistance to aid a player or players in locating the ball, the umpire awards the offensive team a run.

Exceptions to spotter interference include:

1. In the event a ball in flight presents a chance of injury to a defensive player, the spotter should call out a warning.
2. In the event that two fielders are going to collide, the spotter should call out a warning.
3. If a runner and a fielder are going to collide, the spotter should call out a warning.
4. A spotter may knock down an unusually hard hit ball traveling toward a defensive player.

Strike out: the result of the batter having four strikes charged against him or her.

Source: Adapted from NBBA Rules of the Game, the National Beep Baseball Association, 2011, retrieved from www.nbba.org/rules/index.htm.

- A run is scored if the activated base is touched by the batter/runner before a catch is made.
- Catching a fly ball (which is extremely rare) retires the side.
- There are only six fielders.
- The game consists of six innings.
- A fair hit occurs when the ball settles, that is, when a fly ball hits or a ground ball stops rolling on or between the base lines and on or beyond the 40-foot line (measured from home plate).
- A batter is allowed four strikes and one pass (balls not swung at) per at bat.
- A home run occurs when a batter hits the ball in the air a distance of 180 feet and then safely touches a base.

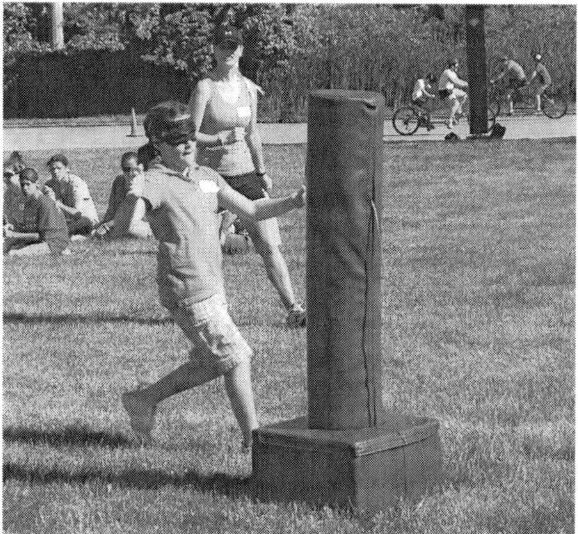

Amanda Tepfer

Running to a base after a hit. The bases in beep baseball emit a continuous tone so that blindfolded players can locate them.

The complete rules of beep baseball are available at the NBBA website (www.nbba.org).

Sighted spotters in the field have the responsibility of alerting the fielders as to where the ball is heading after a batter hits it, so the defensive players can converge there. Generally the short infielders are stationed near the left, right, and middle of the infield, while the three outfielders are similarly placed in the traditional left field, center field, and right field positions. Each of the fielders' areas are designated by a number; the infield, from right to left, consists of areas 1, 3, and 5; the outfield consists of areas 2, 4, and 6. Spotters are limited to calling out the number of the area in which the ball will land. The traditional placement of the six fielders is often modified by a team. A common configuration involves moving a particularly outstanding defensive player out of the infield into short center field.

ROLE MODEL

BEEP BASEBALL

Ray Marshall

Ray Marshall is perhaps the best beep baseball player to ever take the field. Ray was such a legend that he was sought after by teams from across the United States. As a result, he played for the Albuquerque True Sight, the Phoenix Outlaws, and the Chicago Cobras during his 15-year career. He led the True Sight to eight NBBA titles and won numerous awards.

Ray Marshall's awards do not really tell the whole story, however. Ray was a defensive genius, according to other players. He was everywhere on the field, making put out after put out, snatching away balls that appeared to be hits at the last second. It was his fielding that led the Albuquerque team to a record six straight titles. Kalamazoo player Dave Gordon once said, "It's just demoralizing having Marshall out there in the field. You just know if you don't get the ball up in the air and over his head, you're out. It's like magic!"

Ray's "sixth sense" for knowing where the ball is also made him an outstanding goalball player. He was an important founding board member of both the NBBA and the USABA.

Teaching Tips

Beep baseball, like goalball, can be used to teach basic physical skills building and basic sports concepts, as well as to help children with visual impairments develop ear-hand coordination. Beep baseball's basic skill set differs somewhat from that of goalball, however, including overhand throwing, catching, and striking. Overhand throwing can be taught using the techniques presented in Chapter 4. (A step-by-step lesson plan for teaching throwing is in Chapter 7.) Catching a ball in a glove or with both hands is a rare experience for players with limited or no vision, so it is also essential to teach catching skills starting with an introduction to the glove and moving through fielding beeping ground balls. Striking a pitched ball is difficult and depends on having a skilled pitcher. Batting skills might more easily be introduced using a batting tee. If the learner is not familiar with the motion of swinging a bat, it must be taught first, perhaps starting with a step-by-step breakdown of the motions, as described in Chapter 4, and using a large workout bag or other cushioned surface as a backstop for the bat.

Because a beep baseball game can accommodate so many players, with two teams of six each, plus sighted pitchers, catchers, and spotters, it is suitable for a middle or high school physical education class. It is also an ideal way to include the sighted classmates of a student with a visual impairment in one of his or her games. Because the game involves bats and players with occluded vision who cannot see the bats being swung, however, special rules need to be established for when and where it is acceptable to swing the bat and when and where it is not. It is also recommended that specific verbal commands be established to alert fielders to cover their faces for protection from an airborne batted ball when necessary. For many beep baseball players, however, the thrill of playing baseball far outweighs the risks posed by the game, particularly when the hazards are significantly reduced by implementation of these simple safety precautions.

THE EYESHADE AND LOW VISION

Since both goalball and beep baseball are games designed specifically for players with visual impairments, wearing an eyeshade to occlude vision so that all players are on a level playing field, so to speak, is a crucial part of the game. Occasionally, however, the idea of wearing an eyeshade can discourage a child with low vision from participating in a game that requires it. A small number of students with low vision at the sports camps have refused to participate in goalball or beep baseball activities because they will not wear a blindfold. Some say that the eyeshade frightens them, some say that they do not want to be blind, and others seem not to understand the source of their aversion.

Teachers or coaches can usually help students overcome such fears by addressing them with the student or the group before introducing a game that requires occlusion. It is rare for a student to continue to refuse to wear an eyeshade after such a discussion. If a student continues to refuse to wear one, he or she can be allowed to play without it for a time, and the teacher or coach can then attempt to reinstate it as the student becomes more comfortable. It is important, especially for young students or students just starting to play, that the students learn to like the game first, before worrying about enforcing the rules. Most students in that situation eventually become involved with the game and agree to use the eyeshade. A student who is permitted to play with vision should not be placed at the center position in goalball or center field in beep baseball, however, because it would be unfair to the players on the opposing team. Occasionally, students are excused from games requiring occlusion at the sports camps because they simply cannot overcome their fear. In such cases, they are offered alternative activities, and reports of the student's fears are given to the local vision education teachers with recommendations for counseling services.

ADAPTATIONS FOR STUDENTS WITH DEAFBLINDNESS

The benefits derived by students with visual impairments from playing games such as goalball and beep baseball, such as development of physical and cognitive skills, as well as enhanced social skills, independence, self-determination, and self-confidence, are equally important for students with deafblindness. As noted earlier, although these sports depend on the use of hearing, adaptations can be made to make them accessible to students with hearing impairments. The following adaptations have been used successfully at the authors' sports camps.

Goalball

- Permit the use of residual vision. Students with hearing impairments and low vision are allowed to play without occlusion; however, they are limited to the wing positions.
- Use a spotter to indicate the position of the ball and timing of the throw. A spotter indicates information about the ball by touching the player with deafblindness on the back. That is, a touch on the left side of the back indicates that the ball is being thrown from the wing to the left; in the middle of the back for the center; and the right side of the back for the wing to the right. The moment that the ball is released is indicated by double tapping the player on the back.
- Hand the ball to players with deafblindness, after the ball has been blocked by a teammate, rather than passing it to them.
- Increase the 10-second rule for the length of time a player is allowed to hold the ball before throwing it to 15 seconds.

Beep Baseball

- Use spotters. Use a long tap stick to tap a batter with deafblindness when the bat should be swung.
- Use a batting tee. Allow the player to bat the ball off a tee.
- Use a guide runner. Use a guide runner to accompany a runner with deafblindness to either first or third base after a hit.
- Permit the use of residual vision. Allow players with deafblindness to use their residual vision to field balls.
- Use a spotter in the field. Use a spotter to guide the fielder who is deafblind to the ball.
- Adapt the rules for declaring a runner out. Count it as an "out" if the ball is simply touched, rather than fielded, before the batter reaches a base safely.

Such adaptations of the rules can ensure that individuals with deafblindness have the opportunity to play these games along with their friends and enjoy the same benefits.

CONCLUSION

Goalball and beep baseball have probably done more to educate the public about the athleticism of people with visual impairments than any other competitive game. USABA-sponsored goalball tournaments and NBBA beep baseball events, with their large numbers of athletes with visual impairments, seem to have attracted more mainstream news coverage than individual participants who are visually impaired in mainstream athletic events.

As information about sports designed for people with visual impairments becomes more widely available, it is hoped that more children and adults will be introduced to the advantages of goalball and beep baseball through the kinds of programs described in this chapter. In addition to the benefits of increased physical and conceptual skills that playing these games helps develop in their players, the national organizations for each sport provide networks for learning, developing, and playing in elite competitions. Equally important, people with visual impairments or deafblindness can identify with these sports and experience the pride that comes with saying, “I'm a beep baseball player” or “I'm a goalball player.” For teachers who work with children with visual impairments or deafblindness, these games are also important tools for teaching sports concepts and physical skills and particularly to help remediate the sports concept and physical skill difficulties of students with severe early-onset visual impairments in the education system.

For those who may sometimes prefer less competitive activities, there are many other active pursuits that can be enjoyed during leisure time with similar benefits. As demonstrated in the following chapter, virtually any recreation activity can be enjoyed by people with visual impairments or deafblindness.

10 Recreational Activities and Their Adaptations:

TOWARD A POSITIVE QUALITY OF LIFE

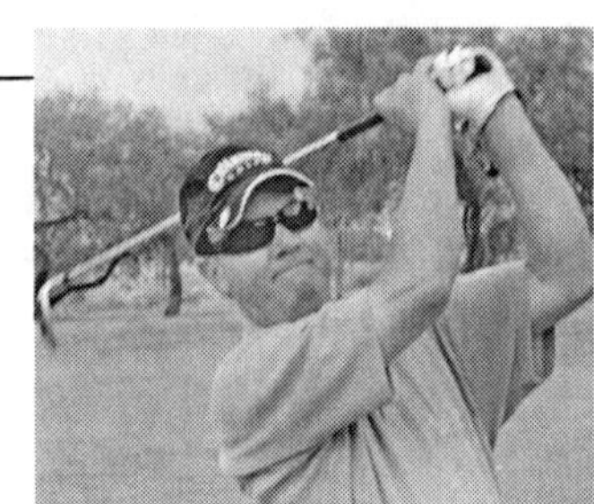
Earl Dotter/American Foundation for the Blind

IN THIS CHAPTER

- **Defining Recreation**
- **The Importance of Recreation**
- **Recreational Goals in Education and Vocational Rehabilitation**
- **Adaptations for Recreational Activities**

Soo Lee is a college student pursuing a career in rehabilitation counseling. She has extremely low vision as the result of a childhood disease. One of her classmates invited her to a weekend cross-country ski event called Ski for Light. Curious and excited about an opportunity for recreation in the middle of winter, Soo Lee registered for the program and carpooled north with several other people to stay at the ski lodge where the event was held.

The snow was deep and the thermometer reading was low, but Soo Lee learned the basics of cross-country skiing from Ski for Light volunteers and not only was able to compete in the beginner's division of the competition that was held at the end of the weekend, but also managed to stay on her skis the length of a long slope through the woods. Her experience was short, but the effects were lasting. She often mentions her ski experience during her graduate work and says it makes her smile every time she thinks about it.

■

Rebekkah, a young adult who was born with total blindness, was adopted at age 14 by a family from a packed orphanage overseas. However, Rebekkah was usually kept still in her crib or in a closed room because the adults did not know how to "manage" a child with blindness, and her adoptive family was found to be unfit. Rebekkah was later placed in a foster family.

When Rebekkah was 18, she was accepted into a center-based vocational rehabilitation and independent living training program. As a result of her early isolation, she had an unusual lack of knowledge about daily life, but she seemed eager to learn. She particularly enjoyed her newfound freedom to become involved in recreational activities offered in the evenings. Everything was new and enjoyable to her, particularly shopping, snowshoeing, bowling, and attending the new multiplex theater with audio-descriptive capabilities that allowed her to hear descriptions of what was happening in the action scenes. On a recent outing to a bowling alley, Jorge, the recreation instructor, showed Rebekkah how to use a bowling rail as a guide to maintaining a straight line on the approach to the lane.

■

Robert began losing his peripheral vision and night vision shortly after he began driver training in his teens. He was devastated to learn that the retinitis pigmentosa associated with his Usher syndrome had begun, as the eye care specialist had predicted. He had been born with a severe hearing impairment and had learned to communicate with American Sign Language, but now he was becoming blind as well as deaf.

As he neared the end of high school, Robert was referred to a vocational training center for people with blindness or low vision, where he received training in the center's business enterprise program. Shortly after high school graduation, he began operating his own vending stand in a federal office building. The work was fulfilling and demanding, but at the end of the workday and on weekends, Robert found himself isolated and bored and sought recreation and fitness activities. From a local disability resource center, he learned about an accessible bowling league, as well as a consumer organization for people with visual impairments that had regular meetings and a variety of recreational activities, including bus trips to tourist locations, a tactile art gallery in a nearby city, and a local parks program. Once Robert made contact with recreational and fitness opportunities, he felt he had a much more enjoyable and active lifestyle outside of his job. ■

Recreational activities are an important part of life for everyone, as illustrated by the experiences of the three individuals profiled in the vignettes, and recreational activities that involve active movement have particular benefits for health and well-being. In general, recreation offers participants pleasure and relaxation, reduces stress, provides opportunities for socializing, and increases feelings of satisfaction and well-being. Recreation that incorporates physical activity provides these benefits plus the advantages of improved health and fitness.

Recreation is also a primary component of the expanded core curriculum, as noted in Chapter 3, the components additional to the general education curriculum for students with visual impairments or deafblindness that enable them to access that curriculum and to learn the skills necessary to be independent, productive, educated members of society. The activities involved in recreation can also supplement other components of the expanded core curriculum, such as socialization, orientation and mobility (O&M), independent living, and self-determination. A focus on recreation can have far-reaching effects on the lives of individuals with visual impairments, involving them in pursuits that enhance their self-esteem, independence, sense of purpose, and enjoyment of life. As the examples presented in this chapter show, once the everyday hurdles of transportation and orientation to the locale are mastered, nearly any activity can suit individuals with visual impairments or deafblindness.

DEFINING RECREATION

Recreation, leisure, and *therapeutic recreation* are terms often used interchangeably. All relate to the use of free time that is not otherwise dedicated to work, school, or other obligatory tasks such as daily living activities. The literature provides in-depth definitions for each term (Kaplan, 1975; Leitner & Leitner, 1996), but for the purposes of this text, the term *leisure time* is used to describe any free, unobligated time that can be used in discretionary activities, and *recreation* is used to describe preferred pleasurable and enjoyable activity conducted during leisure time.

Recreational activities can be sedentary in nature, such as knitting, chess, playing a musical instrument, or social networking on the computer. Although these activities are worthwhile and important, this chapter focuses on more active recreational activities that enhance physical fitness and well-being, such as skiing, bowling, hiking, rock climbing, boating, or bicycling.

Therapeutic recreation is often used to describe organized activities for targeted groups, such as people with disabilities or residents of assisted living communities. Therapeutic recreation uses treatment, education, and recreation services to help people with illnesses, disabilities, and other conditions to develop and use their leisure in ways that enhance their health, independence, and well-being. Although much of active recreation has therapeutic outcomes, the discussion in this chapter does not address therapeutic recreation per se; rather, this chapter is primarily aimed at addressing the following questions:

- What can people with visual impairments or deafblindness do for active recreation?
- How can these activities be adapted, and how can the activities be taught?
- What resources are needed to perform and teach these activities?

THE IMPORTANCE OF RECREATION

Soo Lee, Rebekkah, and Robert, described in the opening vignettes, found their recreational pursuits helpful in relieving stress, improving their quality of life, and helping them to feel better about themselves and their skills. Research bears out that their experiences are like those of most people who can benefit from involvement in recreational activities.

People's lives today are much busier and more tightly scheduled than in years past. Work, commuting, and family activities all seem to require a high level of multitasking and juggling of priorities. The negative effects of these activities can therefore lend more impetus to relaxing or enjoyable recreational activities that have health benefits and help buffer the adverse effects of stressful, busy lives (Iso-Ahola & Park, 1996; Tsai, 2005). Recreation can increase individuals' quality of life or life satisfaction, thought of as the general well-being of individuals and societies and people's personal satisfaction (or dissatisfaction) with the conditions under which they live. Since recreation is a highly social phenomenon frequently organized around friendship or family groups, social psychologists have found that recreation buffers the effects of stress on both physical and mental health (Biddle, Fox, & Boutcher, 2000; Schuster, Hammitt, & Moore, 2006; Iso-Ahola & Park, 1996).

Research has shown that recreation is an important factor in quality of life for everyone, including elders and people with disabilities (Barnett & Webber, 2008; Johnson, 2009; Leitner & Leitner, 1996; Lieberman & MacVicar, 2003; Tsai, 2005). Today's Americans are healthier overall and are likely to live many years longer in retirement, and will therefore have more time and more need for recreational activities; in fact, according to Wellner (1998), the huge baby boom generation will probably stay active longer than today's older Americans. Zabriskie, Lundberg, and Groff (2005) studied individuals with disabilities who participated in community-based therapeutic recreation and adapted sports programs, and found that participation positively influenced quality of life, overall health, and the quality of family and social life. The study also showed that participants with disabilities were willing to learn new activities and skills, and furthermore, seemed to enjoy ongoing community-based programs.

The interrelationship of active recreation and fitness (discussed in Chapter 11) is well known (Johnson, 2009; Morris, Sallybanks, Willis, & Makkai, 2003). Quality of life is positively affected by even moderate physical activity, and individuals who engage in recreational activities will likely benefit by having improved cardiovascular function, better ability to sleep, improved self-esteem, increased stamina, and decreased stress levels (U.S. Department of Health and Human Services, 1999), all of which not only improve quality of life (Lieberman & Taule, 1998) but also have positive benefits in other daily activities. When an individual has better flexibility, strength, and stamina, activities of daily living will be easier and less stressful on the body, as one's body is more used to these types of movements. Thus, research supports the value of encouraging active recreation for people of every age and ability.

RECREATIONAL GOALS IN EDUCATION AND VOCATIONAL REHABILITATION

Given the documented value of recreational activity that increases physical activity and improves fitness, it is important for professionals who work with individuals who are visually impaired or deafblind to make sure that such activities are included in the services provided to them, whether they are children, adults, or older adults. As discussed at the beginning of this chapter, recreation is a key component of the expanded core curriculum and must be part of students' educational plan along with O&M, socialization, independent living, and self-determination. Including goals for recreation and leisure offers the opportunity to help students integrate recreational activity into their lives, both now and in the future. Adolescents with visual impairments should be given the opportunity to determine which recreational activities they want to do in their free time, how often, where, and with whom. Recreational goal setting should also be included in any planning for a student's transition to life after high school (Lieberman, Modell, Ponchillia, & Jackson, 2006; see Chapter 3).

Similarly, goals related to recreation can be incorporated in programs for adults who have visual impairments and who receive professional services. Individuals who become disabled as adults generally receive vocational rehabilitation services focused on enabling the person to become employed, and a formal plan of services known as an Individualized Plan for Employment (IPE) is prepared as part of this process. While the goals of the IPE are mainly job related, it is also necessary to include recreation in the course of lessons or other activities. For example, during O&M lessons—those focused on learning travel skills—the instructor might help the individual who has a visual impairment apply O&M skills on a route from home to work but also include the route from work to a bowling alley or community recreation and fitness center. Lessons from a vision rehabilitation therapist who teaches independent living skills might include Internet searches for adapted recreation equipment or could reinforce use of low vision devices and techniques during a lesson on a recreational activity.

Adults who lose their vision and do not plan to return to work, such as those who are already retired, receive what are known as independent living rehabilitation services to help them carry out everyday activities as independently as possible. It is common to include leisure-time goals in the Independent Living Plan that is formulated with them. Attempts to meet recreational goals would likely incorporate and reinforce the use of skills such as O&M techniques, organizational methods, spatial awareness, and use of low vision or tactile techniques, as well as overall adjustment to vision loss.

In addition to the health and fitness benefits of recreation activities discussed earlier, the benefits of including recreational goals in educational or rehabilitation plans for individuals with visual impairments or deafblindness include self-empowerment, growth of self-esteem, use and reinforcement of learned adaptive skills, and improved quality of life. In addition, in educational or rehabilitation settings the individuals are able to benefit from the expertise and resources of professionals trained in working with individuals with blindness or low vision, such as teachers of students with visual impairments, vision rehabilitation therapists, or O&M specialists, who can assist other professionals, such as recreation instructors, fitness coordinators, or nursing home activity directors, as they provide their services.

When individuals receive services in a rehabilitation center rather than at home, the programs typically offer opportunities to learn recreational skills. Recreation is usually included as part of the vocational rehabilitation process because the activities give individuals the opportunity to apply their newly learned coping and adaptive skills. Center-based programs may also have adaptive recreation instructors who are available for consultation for community sports and recreation professionals who wish to include participants with visual impairments or deafblindness. When such activities are learned as part of the rehabilitation experience, individuals are more likely to engage in the activities when they return to their home communities. Activities that are likely to be included at a rehabilitation center include tandem cycling, hiking, walking, wall climbing, swimming, horseback riding, kayaking or canoeing, fitness activities, goalball, and downhill, cross-country, or waterskiing. One training center even makes use of a local go-cart track where their clients can drive two-driver go-carts!

ADAPTATIONS FOR RECREATIONAL ACTIVITIES

The examples of recreational activities provided in this chapter were chosen to illustrate the variety of active and social pursuits that individuals with visual impairments and deafblindness may engage in. Most of these activities can be done with family, friends, or neighbors. They can be taught by physical educators, parents, teachers, vision rehabilitation therapists, or even O&M instructors. However, activities that require considerable skill and involve a degree of risk, such as skiing, horseback riding, swimming, or dogsledding, should be taught by someone who is skilled at that activity and familiar with the adaptations for people with visual impairments. Only a handful of the potential activities and sports played by people with visual impairments are discussed here, since virtually any activity one might name can, and probably will, be adapted for the enjoyment of someone who is visually impaired. For example, tennis played with a beeping ball, played for many years in Asia, Russia, and Great Britain, has recently been gaining popularity in the United States (Lin, 2012).

To find information and instructors for any of these activities, potential participants can start with the list of organizations that sponsor and provide information about specific sports in the Resources section at the end of this book. A search for local recreation services using the AFB Directory of Services on the website of the American Foundation for the Blind (AFB; www.afb.org) can also be helpful. Local agencies that provide services for people with visual impairments or national organizations that provide information and referrals are additional sources for such information (again, see the Resources section or the AFB Directory of Services for contact information). Friends and acquaintances who are involved in a particular activity can also help an individual get started in learning the skills involved or can accompany them to the activity and act as a guide.

For each of the activities discussed in this chapter, suggestions are provided about how to introduce and teach the activity to individuals with visual impairments, any adaptive equipment needed, and modifications and adaptations that will help to ensure enjoyment, success, and safety. However, readers will also find it helpful to refer back to Chapters 4 and 5 to review methods of instruction and ways to determine what adaptations or modifications may be useful.

Snow Sports

Snowshoeing, Nordic (cross-country) skiing, Alpine (downhill) skiing, sledding, snowboarding, and ice skating are all activities that get people out in the fresh air in wintertime. All can be done as either recreational activities or competitive sports. These activities also have many side benefits, such as socializing and enjoying traditions such as sipping hot cocoa on the trail or chatting fireside at a ski lodge. Table 10.1 provides a summary of suggested adaptations for teaching snow sports to people with visual or hearing impairments.

TABLE 10.1. Adaptations for Teaching Snow Sports

Snow Sport	Prerequisite or Basic Skills Needed	Instructional Modifications	Equipment Adaptations
Nordic/ Cross-Country Skiing	Directional concepts (left, right, clock-face directions) Ability to tie shoelaces or use Velcro and other fasteners	Initial instruction about equipment and basic commands given indoors Guide skis in parallel tracks beside the skier, in front to serve as sound or visual beacon, or behind to give directional guidance Guide gives verbal descriptions of track or trail ("slow left curve to 2 o'clock, down slope straight," "deep dip," "low hump") Guide tells skier "Track left" or "Track right" if skier loses track and ski is outside the groove and, describes where skis need to be pointed by using the clock method, for example "ski tips to 11 o'clock"	Sun filters and visor High-contrast bib, hat, or other clothing Bells or other sound source for guides to use as a beacon
Downhill (Alpine) Skiing	Directional concepts Ability to use buckles, Velcro, and other fasteners	Orientation to equipment and adjustments given indoors Teach "Sit" command to stop instantly in case of emergency Orientation to chair lift or tow rope One or two guides ski behind, next to, or in front of skier	Sun filters and visor Safety vests in high-contrast color with labels saying "Visually Impaired Skier" and "Ski Guide" Novices may benefit from ski poles, longer poles, or tethers with guide and skier holding onto either end For skiers who are deafblind, a vibrating buzzer on each wrist can be used to indicate the direction of turns

TABLE 10.1. (Continued)

Snow Sport	Prerequisite or Basic Skills Needed	Instructional Modifications	Equipment Adaptations
Snowboarding	Directional concepts Ability to buckle	Basic instruction and explanation of terms given indoors Orientation to tow rope or chair lift Verbal feedback about conditions of hill and obstacles	Sun filters and visor Bright or contrasting vest or pinnie Bells or other sound source
Snowshoeing	Ability to buckle or adjust harness	Guide walks in front of, next to, or behind Guide may give verbal feedback	Sun filters and visor Trekking or cross-country ski poles for balance Contrasting jacket or pinnie Bells or other sound source
Ice skating	Directional concepts Ability to tie shoelaces	Examination of skates indoors Human guide using a guide rope Guide provides verbal cues about upcoming turns or obstacles	Sun filters and visor Commercial ice skating "trainer" device, a rubber- tipped walker, or folding chair to push in front for stability Short guide rope knotted on both ends

Teaching Snow Sports Indoors First

In general, initial instruction for snow sports is best provided indoors for individuals with visual impairments. As suggested in Chapter 4, the individual with a visual impairment or deafblindness should be given the opportunity for overall tactile or visual and haptic inspection of the equipment rather than having someone simply strap on the snowshoes or clip feet into ski bindings for them. It is easier and more comfortable to examine bindings, adjustors, and other parts with ungloved hands indoors before going outdoors in the cold; participants are less likely to get chilled or to risk frostbite than if they must stand outside with bare fingers to examine a ski or snowshoe binding or to learn the correct way to slip their hands through the strap of trekking or ski poles. It is particularly important for individuals who are deafblind to be in a relatively warm place if they and an interpreter need to be able to use their hands to communicate in sign language. It will also be helpful to explain basic commands and techniques in a relatively quick introduction indoors. Otherwise, a first experience with snow sports can turn into a negative one that may affect future participation.

Prerequisite Skills

For most of the snow sports discussed here, it is important for participants to have good directional skills, such as left, right, and in front, so that they can follow instructions from a guide. The clock-face method of indicating directions, in which 12 o'clock is used as the direction being faced, is frequently useful for many outdoor sports; the face of a clock is mentally superimposed over the landscape, and the positions of the numbers are used to describe the direction of an object or a turn in the path (e.g., "There is a tree at two o'clock"). The clock-face method is generally considered more accurate than simply using the terms, "ahead and right" for 2 o'clock, since it indicates how far right one should focus.

Another important skill for most snow activities, as well as other activities that require special footwear, is good shoe-lacing or boot-buckling skills so that individuals can get ready independently. Making sure that equipment is properly fastened is an important safety concern. If a participant is not yet able to manage the lacing or buckling task, someone can assist him or her, because taking time to teach that prerequisite skill would interfere with the primary goal of learning to skate, snowshoe, or ski. It is nevertheless important that the individual gets the opportunity to examine the boot or skate before it is laced on so that he or she will understand the parts of the footwear (blade, ski binding, ice skate toe picks or rake, and so forth) as they relate to learning the new skill. In the rare event that a person with a visual impairment and, perhaps, limited life experience does not know how to tie shoes, a referral can be made for lessons from a vision rehabilitation therapist or teacher of students with visual impairments; or perhaps alternative solutions can be used, such as Velcro closures.

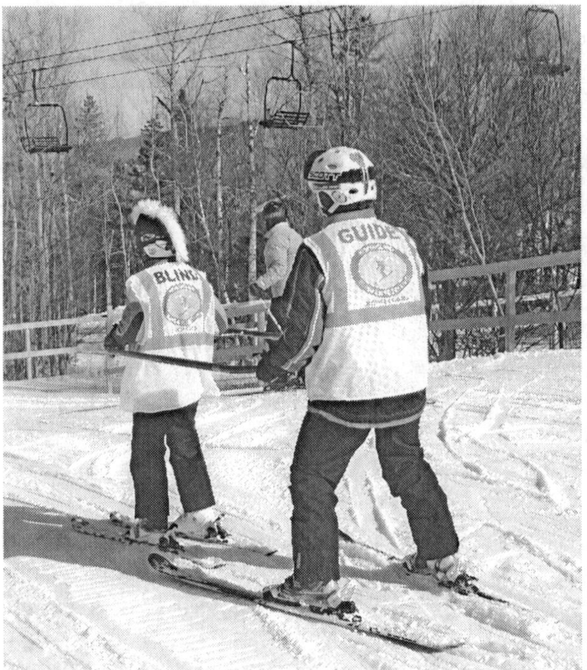

New England Blind and Visually Impaired Alpine Ski Festival

This guide skis behind the beginning skier and uses two poles and his voice to guide her, while their bright yellow vests alert others to the presence of a skier with visual impairments.

Adapted Equipment

Each winter sport and activity typically requires its own equipment, such as skis, poles, skates, snowshoes, and so forth. Such equipment does not generally require special adaptation for participants who have visual impairments. However, individuals who are light sensitive may require special sun filters and visors to protect them from the glare. Guides typically wear bright, contrasting colors or a black and white striped referee's vest as well as a vest or pinnie that might say "Ski Guide" in bold, black letters. Skiers or other participants who have visual impairments might also have a vest with the words "Visually Impaired Skier" on it so they are visible to others on the slopes or trails who can avoid skiing in their paths. Guides may also carry a sound source, such as bells, to make it easier to follow them. It is also recommended that people wear helmets for downhill skiing, snowboarding, and ice skating.

For people who are deafblind, it is important not only to show them the parts of the equipment and the function of each but also to make sure they know what each part is called in sign language and how it is spelled. It may take time and patience to fully understand the equipment.

Cross-Country Skiing

When Soo Lee was shown how to cross-country ski, her guide first asked her to examine the ski boots and the ski bindings to see how the toes clip in. Soo Lee could see and feel how the bindings matched up with her boots. Then, the guide had Soo Lee use touch to examine how he slid his wrists into the straps of ski poles and gripped them. Once Soo Lee understood, she practiced it a few times until she felt comfortable. The guide asked Soo Lee to release her bindings and then relatch her boots into the skis enough times to feel comfortable with the procedure. Then they reviewed her understanding of descriptive directional terms such as "track left (move skis left to place them in the track grooves)," "track right," "snowplow," and "ski tips toward two o'clock."

Once Soo Lee and her guide were sure she could manage the equipment and understood some of the basic terms, they went outside. Though Soo Lee had some vision, she was unable to see variations in the trail such as dips or bumps. Her guide skied beside and a bit ahead of her, and described the trail ahead so Soo Lee could anticipate drops, bumps, and hills.

When Robert went to the annual state Ski for Light event, he arranged for Lorna, an American Sign Language interpreter, to go along. Lorna worked together with the guide to explain the basics to Robert while they were indoors. They found a well-lit area of the lodge where Robert could see Lorna's hand movements, the guide, and the equipment. Robert was able to use his remaining vision to view the instruction. After a bit of explanation about the upcoming outdoor lesson, they were ready to enjoy cross-country skiing.

Robert wore sun filters and a cap with a bill so he could avoid glare; his guide wore a bright orange vest that had "Ski Guide" in bold black letters. Robert preferred having his guide ski in front of him so Robert could use his guide as a visual beacon.

Cross-country or Nordic skiing involves skiing across the countryside in varied terrain, rather than in designated downhill runs. The boots and skis are somewhat different from those used in downhill skiing. Some cross-country ski facilities provide groomed trails with tracks, which are premade grooves into which the skis fit, for the skiers to follow. The experiences of Soo Lee and Robert illustrate different ways guides may work with beginning skiers, depending on their needs and preferences.

As mentioned earlier, it is good practice to introduce students to the equipment and terminology while they are still inside. Some cross-country ski boots have extensions at the toes that clip into the bindings on the skis, and it can require quite a bit of practice to get the boots properly seated and the bindings latched, as well as to release the bindings when necessary. If the beginning skier has sufficient vision, the guide can explain the equipment verbally; otherwise, the guide can use physical guidance to manipulate the student's hands on the equipment or tactile modeling to have the student feel the guide's hands as he or she manipulates it.

Students also need to learn how ski poles are held and be introduced to the descriptive terminology that the guide will use on the trail, such as *track left, track right, snowplow,* and *ski tips toward two o'clock.* Some descriptive terms and phrases often used, such as *S curve* and *Put your ski tips into a V shape,* are based on the print alphabet and may not be meaningful for a few individuals who understand only braille rather than print. In this case the skill needs to be demonstrated through tactile modeling to the participant and he or she taught the appropriate cue for that skill so he or she knows how to do it, when to use it, and why. For example, the V shape position for the skis (ski tips together) is used to slow down or stop. Skiing an S curve is used to ski down a hill in a controlled fashion. The terms, "ski tips to 2 o'clock" or "11 o'clock" are used to help the skier with a visual impairment reorient his or her skis parallel to the grooves of ski tracks common on groomed trails, so the suggestion "track left" or "track right" can then be given to get the skis back into the tracks.

In cross-country skiing, guides may ski next to the skier, if there are parallel tracks, or in front, wearing high-contrast clothing or carrying a sound source such as bells. Guides can also follow the skier, offering verbal directional guidance. Verbal description of the trail should include curves, dips, bumps, and hills and the location of the track if the skier has slipped out of it.

Alpine (Downhill) Skiing and Snowboarding

> *Alpine (downhill) skiing is one of the rare opportunities available which allows the blind individual to move freely at speed through time and space. An opportunity to embrace and commune with the primal force of gravity, thus experiencing the sheer exhilaration of controlled mass in motion, in a physically independent setting.*
>
> —Brian Santos, Paralympic downhill skier (www.ibsa.es/eng/deportes/alpineskiing/presentacion.htm)

Downhill (Alpine) skiing and snowboarding are discussed together here, as they are both done on snow on mountains and require some of the same preparations and adaptations. While skiers glide downhill on two narrow skis facing down the hill, snowboarding involves gliding down a slope while standing sideways on a single board, with one shoulder facing down the hill. In both sports, the feet are in boots that are attached with bindings to the board or ski. Most people who learn to ski start out slowly on smaller hills, and they increase the height of their hills, their speed, and their skills as they practice and improve. They may start out on a small hill and progress to hills that entail using lifts to get to the top. Individuals who are visually impaired can improve just as sighted people do and can reach skill levels that put them in major competitions if they choose to go that route.

Skiers or snowboarders with low vision may need a guide to ski in front of them. As with other winter sports, both the skiers or snowboarders and their guides generally wear identifying bright vests to make it easier for others on the slopes to see and avoid them. Skiers with little usable vision as well as beginners are typically guided with one or more long poles. One technique is to have both skier and guide ski side by side, both holding onto a long bamboo-like pole as though they were standing side by side at a railing. Other skiers and guides use two ski poles or longer poles, one in each hand. In that case, the guide typically skis behind while holding onto the uphill ends of poles, and the skier with a visual impairment holds onto the opposite end of the poles. This allows the guide skier to direct the learner verbally.

The use of clearly defined terminology is important for clear communication and safety while skiing. The agreed-upon terms should include one that directs the learner to "sit" or "drop and stop" immediately in the event of danger. When this is understood, the participant and guide can feel comfortable knowing that they can stop quickly in the face of any obstacles or danger on the slopes.

In addition to an orientation to the equipment, as required for other snow sports, the use of a chair-lift or rope tow to ascend hills in downhill skiing and snowboarding also requires orientation and instruction if a student is successful enough at skiing or snowboarding to graduate to higher hills. Ski resort operators will often arrange to stop or slow the equipment so new learners can become familiar with it. There are several types of ski lifts to which skiers may need orientation.

Individuals with deafblindness who want to ski or snowboard will use the same techniques of dressing inside, positioning with the poles, and learning to start and stop correctly. The details of how to communicate on the slope will have to be developed by the instructor, the participant, and an intervener or interpreter (see the discussion of communication in Chapter 4). Because these sports take place in the cold and most people need to wear gloves, communication has to be well planned and purposeful to be both safe and meaningful. For example, if a participant is going to be skiing down a hill holding the end of a pole or tether, the instructor might explain that when the participant gets to the flat area, the instructor will tap the participant on the right shoulder and give the participant feedback about his or her performance. This type of planned instruction and communication will allow the participant

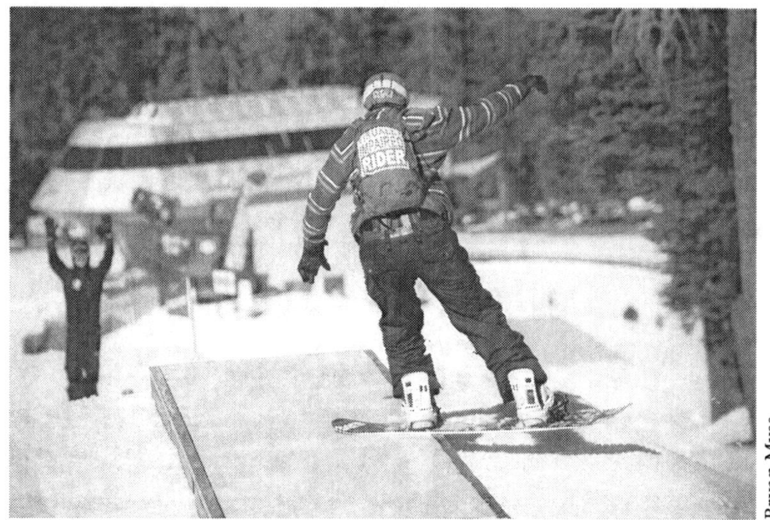

Bryan Myss

Champion snowboard rider Thomas Patrick Wolfe performing a trick called Backside Nosepress to Switch Out, while a coach signals that it is safe for him to proceed.

ROLE MODEL

SNOWBOARDING

Thomas Patrick Wolf: Snowboard Champion Extraordinaire

Diagnosed with retinitis pigmentosa at age 10 and legally blind by age 25, Thomas Wolf features on his resume his status as an accomplished artist, skater, and national snowboard champion. His love of the extreme sport of snowboarding led him to take home a silver medal from the 2008 USA Snowboard Association Nationals in superpipe. He also competes in slopestyle, halfpipe, and boardercross. His resume also includes twin master's degrees from Western Michigan University in orientation and mobility and vision rehabilitation therapy. He is employed by U.S. Department of Veterans Affairs, teaching blinded veterans.

As an artist, he enjoys photography, acrylics, three-dimensional images, and abstract prints. His acrylic painting expertise on snowboards led to having one of his snowboard designs accepted as one of 30 in the Whistler, British Columbia, Canada, International Snowboard Design Competition.

to experience the sport but still know when he or she can gain relevant feedback. The same guidelines apply to snowboarding.

Typically, two guides are needed with skiers who are deafblind. The guides usually ski 6 to 10 feet behind the skier with deafblindness and use tethers to communicate when turns are coming up, when to slow down, and so forth and to help the skier stay in control. For example, tugging on the left or right sides of the tether signals which direction to turn to the skier who is deafblind. If the skier is totally deaf and totally blind, the process of learning how to ski will likely take a long time, and more direct contact with the skier is necessary. For an advanced skier with deafblindness, subtle "vibrating" buzzers can be placed on each wrist and activated by remote control to indicate the direction of the turn and stops and a tether is not necessary. Usually, only one guide, who skis behind the skier, is needed if the individual is an experienced skier.

There are a number of national and state organizations that promote ski opportunities for people with visual impairments or other disabilities, including the USABA, which coordinates national and international competitive opportunities (see the Resources section). Thanks to the efforts of the Professional Ski Instructors of America and the American Association of Snowboard Instructors (PSIA-AASI), which has produced *Adaptive Snowsports Instruction* (2003), a manual for Alpine, snowboard, and Nordic adaptive instruction, most ski resorts can provide instruction to skiers with visual impairments and their guides.

Snowshoeing

Snowshoeing is another sport that allows people to get outside in the winter and obtain some exercise and fresh air. Because snowshoeing does not necessarily involve a lot of speed or steep descents, some people are more comfortable with snowshoeing than with activities such as downhill skiing. Snowshoes are essentially wide, flat aluminum frames, covered with fabric, that attach to a person's boots. The width of the snowshoes are especially useful in very deep, soft snow, because they enable the user to stay on the surface, eliminating the drudgery of moving through snow in hiking boots or even cross-country skis. Snowshoes also have sharp metal edges under the toe area to help grip the ground in icy or rough terrain. Poles are often used to help with balance, and they also increase the amount of exercise for the arms.

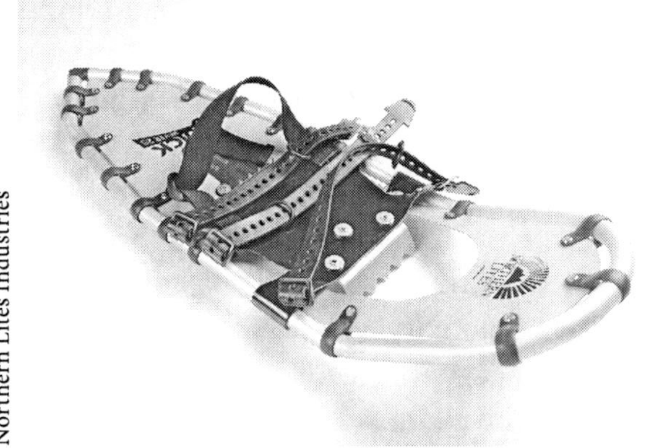

Northern Lites Industries

Snowshoe bindings such as these that are easy to get on and off and stay firmly fastened can make a big difference in a snowshoer's comfort.

As with other snow sports, it is easier if the snowshoes are put on while the participant is inside, if possible, as adjusting snow-covered straps and aluminum bindings by touch without gloves in below-freezing temperatures can be awkward and painful. Ideally, snowshoes should be easy to put on and should stay on reliably without readjustment even after miles on the trail. Snowshoes with straps made of strong, pliable rubber that exert constant elastic pressure on the top of the boots are less likely to loosen under conditions of rigorous use than the more common rigid nylon straps that most snowshoes use (see the Resources section).

A snowshoer with a visual impairment commonly uses two ski poles to maintain balance and to monitor the trees and other objects in his or her travel path. Some follow a guide, while some individuals may prefer the guide to be behind or beside them, where it is easier for the guide to give verbal directions. An individual with deafblindness may benefit from the use of such ski poles, with one end of the poles held by a guide in front or on the side to give tactile feedback when necessary for communicating the presence of hills, ice, turns, or dangerous areas.

Ice Skating

Ice skating is also a winter sport that is popular among people with visual impairments or deafblindness. It is usually done on the ice in an artificial indoor or outdoor rink or in a rink set up on the frozen surface of an outdoor body of water. As a result, the major difficulty faced by skaters with limited vision is staying within the boundaries of the ice rink and avoiding collisions with other skaters.

Learning to skate is not significantly affected by lack of vision, so adaptive techniques other than guiding the skater are usually not required. Beginners, regardless of visual condition, often skate while pushing a chair or other

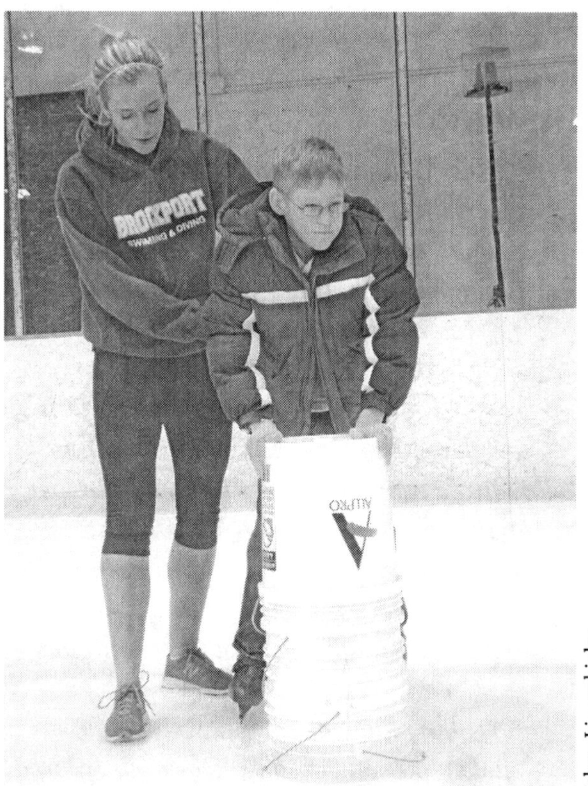

Kelsey Linsenbigler

Beginning ice skaters often practice while pushing an object such as this stack of overturned buckets or a chair to help with balance and to monitor the ice immediately in front of them.

similar object along in front of them, which gives added balance and helps monitor the ice immediately in front of them, much as a long cane helps a walker monitor the sidewalk. The guiding techniques used in running, such as using a guide wire or a human guide (see Chapters 8 and 10), are also effective in an ice rink.

Ice skating on the clear frozen surface of a large lake that is free of people and obstacles can afford individuals with limited vision a unique opportunity to go as fast as they desire on their skates without being guided by anyone. Winter sports instructors may well want to take advantage of such a situation for their students, because the opportunity to move at speed freely and independently is otherwise rarely available to them.

Bowling

Rebekkah, whose early childhood experiences were described earlier in this chapter, enjoyed learning to bowl, but during her orientation to the equipment she was initially reluctant to examine one of the pins, fearing that she would be stuck by something sharp. Jorge, the recreation instructor from the rehabilitation center, realized that Rebekkah's limited life experience had led her to mistakenly believe that the bowling pins were similar to sewing pins, and that he needed to be careful not to make assumptions about her concepts.

Once he had reassured Rebekkah by describing them as smooth wooden pins shaped like soda bottles, Rebekkah enjoyed using her hands to examine the pins, the bowling ball with its three holes, the ball return, the gutters, the foul line, and the smooth, oiled boards of the lane, as well as the special guide rail that helped her line up with the center of the lane. Jorge used verbal description, tactile modeling, and physical guidance to teach her the basic skills of bowling.

Ten-pin bowling is an excellent community recreational activity, one which people of all ages can engage in together, and bowling alleys are found in most communities. Once an individual with a visual impairment has had an initial orientation to the facility and some instruction in the activity, he or she can generally bowl without much assistance from others, except for feedback about scores. Leagues for bowlers who have blindness can be found in many communities. The American Blind Bowling Association is the official North American sanctioning organization for ten-pin bowlers who have visual impairments or blindness (see the Resources section).

Probably the only prerequisite skill for bowling is being able to lace up the bowling shoes, as with ice skating and some of the other activities mentioned in the section on snow sports. Bowling also requires little adaptation except for lining up with the center of the lane and managing the scorekeeping control panel, if it is accessible.

As always, each bowler needs to be assessed to determine how much basic knowledge of the sport he or she has and how much instruction will be necessary. If the individual has no knowledge or skills and lacks sufficient vision to see the entire lane length, orientation to the parts and layout of a bowling alley and the bowling lane is important for safety and to obtain an overall understanding of the activity. The configuration of the lane, including the set pins, lane, gutters, and foul line should be presented. This can be done using a tactile scale model or, after getting permission, with a hands-on orientation, taking the individual down the lane in his or her socks to haptically investigate all the parts.

Other aspects related to safety should also be among the first details covered, including how to hold and work with the ball and the ball return. For example, it would be important to teach how to search for a ball resting in the ball return area without having one's fingers in position to get banged by another bowler's ball as it shoots out of the ball return. Next is familiarization with the throwing end of the lane, including how to approach the lane with its step up to the alley, orientation to the ball return, position of a guide rail, if one is used, and how to return safely to one's seat after stepping off the lane. It is also important to point out that bowling lanes are oiled past the foul line, so if a bowler moves over the foul line, bowling shoes should be wiped off in order to avoid slips. New bowlers need information about how to select a ball that fits the hand and is the correct weight, how to hold the ball, and how to score. Terminology such as *strike, spare, frame, line, hook, reset,* and *gutter* should be introduced to new bowlers. The experience of Rebekkah on her first bowling trip, described at the beginning of this section, points out the importance of carefully explaining new concepts to individuals with visual impairments and not making assumptions about their previous experience or familiarity with them.

If possible, orientation to the scorekeeping station should be included, although it is unlikely bowling alleys will routinely have accessible scoring consoles. Scorekeepers can give feedback by calling out the numbers of the pins knocked down or still standing. A tactile graphic depicting the arrangement of the ten pins with their accompanying numbers will be helpful for new learners, so that they can grasp where the remaining pins are located in order to determine in which direction their ball needs to go to hit them.

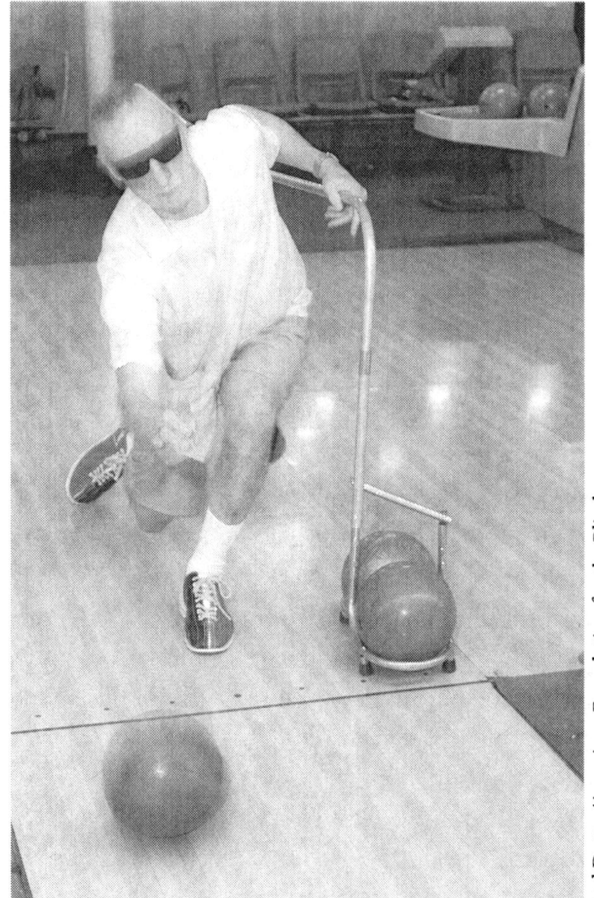
Earl Dotter/American Foundation for the Blind

A bowler slides his hand along the top of a bowling guide rail to maintain a straight line toward the alley during his approach, while delivering the ball with the other hand.

Instruction about bowling techniques can include modeling and physical guidance. Verbal description can be helpful, too, for example, "When you release the ball, your thumb should point the way down the alley toward the pins. After you release the ball, the thumb should point toward twelve o'clock." Beginning bowlers often simply stand at the foul line to deliver the ball without using any approach. After they get used to delivering the ball, they can begin working on the approach.

A common tool for bowlers who are blind is a lightweight portable bowling guide rail to help with lining up during their approach to the lane, although bowlers who have functional vision may not need this assistance. The guide rail provides a tactile indicator at waist height of a straight line down the alley. A bowler who needs the assistance of a guide rail usually slides one hand along its smooth surface while delivering the ball with the other hand. A beginner who is not using an approach may hold onto the guide rail at the foul line while delivering the ball with the other hand. Guide rails are typically placed along the first board outside the width of the lane, are lined up with the gutter, and extend back from the foul line toward the entry to the approach, so that the dominant hand is in the center of the lane. A right-handed bowler uses the rail for a guide with his or her left hand and vice versa for a left-handed bowler. Bowling teams with both right-handed and left-handed bowlers need two rails. Guide rails are sold by the American Blind Bowling Association (see the Resources section).

Other ways to help bowlers who have a visual impairment line up with their dominant arm in the center of the lane include placing a tactile marker on the floor, such as a strip of carpeting, or setting up a guide rope strung from a chair or the table to the center of the lane for the bowler to trail. Instructors or people bowling with the participant with a visual impairment need to be sure the string or rope does not get in the way of any sighted bowlers in the same lane.

Bicycling and Tandem Cycling

Cycling is probably one of the best choices of an activity for lifelong fitness and recreation; it can be enjoyed by everyone, young and old. Few adaptations are required when teaching someone who has a visual impairment. Although tandem cycling is probably the easiest way to enjoy the activity for individuals with visual impairments or deafblindness, children and adults who have low vision may see well enough to cycle independently or by following someone else wearing high-contrast attire, especially in a quiet park, cul de sac, or large, empty parking lot, or around a track. Riding solo can give an individual a wonderful feeling of independence; however, it is always advisable for someone with sight to be present to ensure safety, particularly if the rider has severe limitations in visual acuity or peripheral vision. In this case a guide can ride either in front for the person who is visually impaired to follow or behind to give the individual verbal cues. If the person with a visual impairment is deafblind, the use of a tandem bike is the safest option.

For tandem cycling, a sighted "captain," who rides in the front, and helmets for both riders are the only necessities besides the tandem bicycle. The person who is visually impaired sits on the back, shares pedaling work, and is referred to as the "stoker."

As explained in the discussion of competitive tandem cycling in Chapter 8, a new rider needs to be oriented to all the parts of the bicycle, including the seats, handlebars, front and back pedals, gearshift, brake mechanisms, and toe clips. A good way to begin instruction is to have the beginner use a stationary exercise bike to learn how to pedal and to get a feel for stroke rhythm, frequency, and proper pedaling force. If it is feasible, the individual can take a spinning class at a local gym or health club to become comfortable with pedaling and to build stamina. (See Chapter 11 for more information about spinning, stationary exercise bikes, and bicycle riding as a fitness exercise.)

The other aspects of learning tandem cycling involve maintaining balance on a bike and communication between the stoker and the captain. Before riding together, it is crucial for the participants to develop specific signals (verbal or tactile) for turning, slowing down, speeding up, stopping, or emergencies to avoid confusion and injuries, particularly for individuals who are deafblind.

When an individual is first beginning to ride, the captain can straddle the bike with feet on the ground to hold it steady while the stoker mounts and gets his or her foot in the pedals. It is important for the captain to be an experienced rider to help provide stability for the beginner. Once the stoker is comfortable on the bicycle, both parties can start together, mounting from the left side, with the left foot on the ground and the right foot on the pedal. When the captain gives the command to start, both push down on the right pedal together to get going; then they sit down and get their balance, and then resume pedaling. See Chapter 8 for additional details about teaching tandem cycling.

Tandem bikes come in a wide range of prices, but the Rush-Miller Foundation (see the Resources section) assists children ages 5 to 17 with visual impairments to obtain their first bike. Tandems are available in recumbent versions, too, which have seats similar to chairs in which the rider reclines instead of sitting up straight or crouching over; the pedals are forward of the riders instead of beneath them.

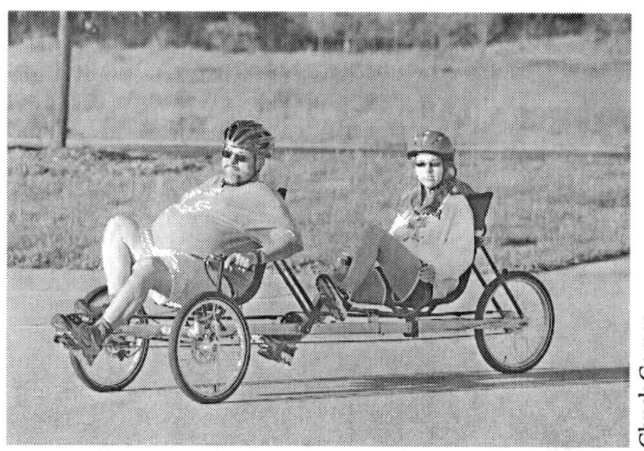

Chuck Comer

A recumbent tandem is one way to enjoy recreational cycling.

Another alternative is a two-person bicycle on which the participants ride side by side (sometimes known as a sociable). Surrey bikes have a bench seat, three or four wheels, and an awning, while duo bikes have two separate seats side by side and three or four wheels. In side-by-side bicycles the sighted participant is responsible for steering and stopping. This style is more conducive to communication during the ride, which is particularly helpful if the participant is deafblind and using signing. The stability of a three- or four-wheeled bike helps with the comfort level of the participant and offers support to riders who may have poor balance or other disabilities. Local bicycle shops do not usually sell these bikes, but they can direct a customer to specialty stores or catalogues that do.

Another alternative is a "child in front" tandem, known as a Buddy Bike (see the Resources section), that places the stoker in the front seat, while the rear rider controls the steering. It is shorter in length than a standard tandem and has a lower front seat so both riders can safely enjoy the view. It is sturdy enough to support two adults of average weight.

When seeking information about local tandem cycling opportunities, good places to begin are bicycle shops and clubs. Quite commonly, there are club riders who own tandems and who would appreciate the opportunity to share rides or information. The USABA and other organizations provide recreational as well as competitive cycling opportunities for athletes with visual impairments (see the Resources section for more information).

Golf

Golf is an increasingly popular sport with many benefits for health and socializing. Generally, those who have golfed previously will need little orientation, while someone new to the activity is likely to need both an overview of the game and specific explanations, the extent of which will be determined by an assessment of the swing and knowledge of the game.

The only prerequisites for playing golf are a desire to play and patience—the same prerequisites for sighted people. The United States Blind Golf Association (USBGA; see the Resources section) provides information on its website and gives specific rules about the degree to which golfers can receive assistance in competitive situations. In general, golfers who have visual impairments must follow the rules of the United States Golf Association, with one exception: the club may be grounded in a hazard; in other words, the club may touch the sand in a sand trap prior to swinging, which is not allowed for sighted golfers.

Visual impairment generally affects the ability to see the location of the game's targets—that is, the ball and the next hole—so routine

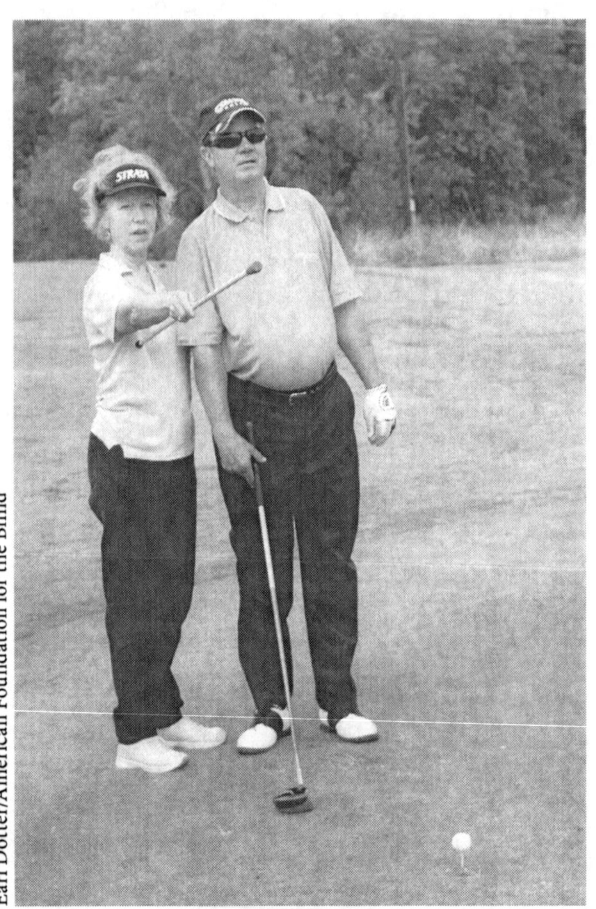
Earl Dotter/American Foundation for the Blind

A golfer's partner and guide helps him line up a shot.

ROLE MODEL

GOLFER

Patrick Malloy

Patrick Malloy, a golfer who is blind, was honored in 2011 as the male winner of the Royal Bank of Scotland's Achiever of the Year and awarded a $10,000 scholarship. He was selected for his accomplishments as a mentor and coach at First Tee of Philadelphia, an organization that uses the game of golf to promote life skills and educational values for youths. As an intern at the organization, Malloy also converted multiple copies of the First Tee curriculum into braille. Malloy is attending Muhlenberg College and hopes to go to law school to specialize in disability law.

adaptations include reaching down to touch the ball and using a coach or spotter. As a coach and new golfer work together, they develop a method for providing sighted feedback and matching performance to it. One way for a coach to assist the golfer in "addressing" the ball—that is, positioning the golfer and the club behind the ball and getting aligned prior to taking the stroke—is to take hold of the club from behind the golfer, in order to position the club properly behind the ball and assist the golfer in adjusting his or her direction and stance in relationship to the ball (Andrews, n.d.). As always when working with an individual who has a visual impairment, however, the least intrusive method of instruction that will convey the necessary information is recommended (see Chapter 4); if a learner seems to require physical guidance, the coach should ask the golfer's permission. The USABA has additional suggestions for adaptations in addressing the ball, lining up to aim the shot, striking the ball during the swing, knowing the distance to the green, and knowing where the hole is while putting; these are presented in Sidebar 10.1. Coaches should also provide as much feedback as possible about the direction, distance, and characteristics of the hole, as well as the distance the ball travels after a shot, to enable the golfer to learn over time how his or her form and the particular clubs used affect the direction of the ball and the distance it travels.

SIDEBAR 10.1

Adaptations for Playing Golf

Golfers who cannot see the ball require adaptations to addressing the ball, lining up to aim the shot, striking the ball during the swing, knowing the distance to the green, and knowing where the hole is while putting. (For simplicity's sake, a right-handed golfer is used as the example here.)

- *Addressing the ball* requires ensuring that the club face is set so that it strikes the ball at a perfect right angle. If the club face is left open (rotated clockwise), the ball will slice away to the right, and if the club face is too closed (rotated too far counterclockwise), the ball will hook to the left. Right handers without vision address the ball properly by taking the proper left-hand grip on the club, leaning down, and placing the club head squarely behind the ball with the right hand, then standing up and keeping the left-hand grip steady. The club is then set to be swung properly. A modification of this technique is to simply place the club head behind the ball and then stand up and take the proper grip with both hands.
- *Lining up* to hit the ball in the proper direction can be done by having a caddie lay a club on the ground that is aimed at the direction of the desired placement, then having the golfer line up his or her toes along the club shaft.
- *Predicting distance* is done as it is with a beginning golfer who can afford a caddie, which is have a caddie who is familiar with the course predict the distance. The choice of club for proper distance is something that must be established with much practice.
- *Putting* can be assisted by using the end of the flagstick to "bang" around in the cup, to give the golfer a sound target. If the ball is extremely close to the hole, the golfer can place the left hand in the hole and tap the ball in with the putter held in the right hand.

Source: Adapted with permission from "Golf: Modifications and Suggestions for Training and Competition," United States Association of Blind Athletes (USABA), http://usaba.org/index.php/sports/sports-adaptations/.

Instruction for new golfers should include terminology, golf etiquette, and methods of keeping score. Adaptations for golf may include use of low vision devices to spot the target or sound devices placed at the hole to provide direction. The use of a clock-face analogy may be useful in describing the terrain, for example, "Tree at 1 o'clock," or "Flagstick and cup at 12 o'clock." Personal Global Positioning System (GPS) devices with accessibility features can be useful for orientation on the course. Competitions sponsored by the USBGA and the International Blind Golf Association (IBGA) use the same visual classifications (B1, B2, and B3) as the USABA and IBSA organizations (see Chapter 8).

Sailing

Sailing is the art of maneuvering a vessel that is propelled by the wind through the water. This is done by changing the trim (that is, the position) of the sail or sails, the rudder, or the rigging to change the speed and direction of a boat. A number of organizations and individuals are involved in teaching and promoting sailing by those with visual impairments or deafblindness (see the Resources section), including Blind Sailing International (www.blindsailing.org), the national and international governing body for competitive international sailing by persons who are visually impaired or deafblind.

The amount of instruction or modification needed to engage in the sport of sailing will depend on the craft, whether the individual will be sailing alone or with others, and the body of water (whether, for example, sailing on a quiet lake or a lake with many docks and other watercraft; whether in the open ocean or in a busy seaport with shipping lanes). Orientation to the craft while docked is beneficial to those who are unfamiliar with the vessel. Even if an individual is familiar with sailing in general, he or she will still need to be oriented to an unfamiliar boat. As with any boating activity, wearing flotation devices, using safety harnesses when sailing offshore, and learning to sit on the windward side of the boat or how to hike on a sailing dinghy are important concepts to share with the participant. (In sailing, *hiking* refers to shifting one's weight to the side of the boat to counteract the boat's heeling, or tilting, as a result of the wind.) The instructor should be someone with extensive sailing experience and should be a person who can explain what happens and where and why the participant should be positioned during the sailing of the boat.

ROLE MODEL

SAILOR

Kris Scheppe

Kris Scheppe was born with a love of the water and is open to trying anything new and adventurous. Diagnosed at a young age with retinitis pigmentosa, which results in a gradual loss of peripheral vision, Scheppe started sailing at age 11 with his family on a lake in North Carolina. After moving to Wisconsin, he gained sailing experience on Lake Michigan cruising the Wisconsin coast. Kris has logged many sea miles sailing various boats through the Caribbean. He currently lives on a 36-foot sailboat, "Blind Victoria," which he is equipping to sail nonstop around the world. (See his website www.blindcircumnavigation.org for more information about his quest.) In his spare time, Scheppe runs his own technology business.

Sailing is an easily adaptable sport and does not require much modification. It is important to have an awareness of where the wind is coming from; this can be accomplished by feeling the wind on one's face or wetting a finger and noticing which side is coldest. Boats that are steered with a tiller usually are easier to handle for someone with a visual impairment than boats with a steering wheel, as it is easier to feel feedback from the rudder with a tiller.

Sighted guides are used to direct sailors with visual impairments and make them aware of surrounding obstacles. Using the clock-face analogy to indicate direction is the best way to give instructions about where to steer or to describe where objects are positioned. It has also been shown to be possible to navigate sailboats on large bodies of water by using an accessible GPS device. Basic sailing terms can also be taught and used to guide in trimming the sail (adjusting the angle of the sail to the wind) and steering. Clear communication among all crewmembers is essential for the safe and efficient operation of a sailboat. For sailors sailing alone, familiarity of the body of water is essential.

Waterskiing

For people who love waterskiing, it is important to know how to successfully introduce it to a skier with a visual impairment. As an activity that does not require using vision to spot a target, few adaptations are necessary for waterskiing. Skiers with low vision may need a sun visor to remain comfortable if bright light causes discomfort. Knowing how to swim is a prerequisite to waterskiing (swimming as a sport or as a fitness activity is discussed in detail in Chapters 8 and 10).

Water-ski clubs that have hosted clinics for new skiers with blindness or low vision suggest giving the skier the opportunity to examine ski equipment visually and by touch on dry land first. Skiers who are visually impaired need the same basic information as any new skier about putting on the skis and adjusting the bindings, holding the tow rope, body positions, boat signals, and safety. The instructor can begin with the skier standing in the skis in shallow water near the shore to demonstrate how to hold the tow rope and to give feedback on body position. The guide can pull slowly on the rope so the skier can get an idea of how to hold on when the rope is under tension. Verbal signals and boat and water-ski safety information should be reviewed before the first attempt on water. As with any water sport, a life jacket should be worn.

The crew consists of one or two instructors, the learner, a driver, and a spotter. The spotter rides in the boat, watches and communicates

ROLE MODEL

WATER-SKIER

April Shinholster Martin

April Shinholster Martin, who is totally blind from a congenital eye condition, won the Royce Andes Award presented to a promising new national skier by the Water Skiers with Disabilities Association Western Region in addition to earning the National Women's Slalom Ski Championship in the same year. The Royce Andes Award is given to athletes who not only exhibit great skill but also inspire others to try, to learn, and to compete.

with the skier, and notifies the driver if adjustments need to be made to the boat's speed or if the skier has fallen. A learner usually starts by skiing with a boom, a bar that extends from the left side of the boat. The boom is long enough for the instructor to ski beside the learner with a visual impairment. Once a skier masters skiing with a boom, the skier may ski independently with a regulation length tow rope behind the boat. The instructor sits at the back of the boat and gives the skier verbal instruction.

For those who choose not to ski, riding behind the ski boat while sitting on a large inner tube attached to the boat is a lot of fun. More information about water-ski instruction and competitive events is available from the Water Skiers with Disabilities Association and the International Waterski and Wakeboard Federation Disabled Council (see the Resources section).

Kayaking and Canoeing

Kayaking and canoeing are similar water sports with positive social and health benefits. In many cases, family and friends can all participate, and as it is common to have two or more paddlers in the same boat, paddling with a guide is common.

A kayak is a long boat that has an opening for one or two seats. The paddle has a blade at both ends, frequently set at an angle to each other, and is held in the center. Both sides of the paddle are used to propel the boat through the water as well as to steer.

A canoe is a long open boat with seats inside. In canoeing it is common for two, three, or even four people to paddle together in one boat. Paddling in a canoe is done on both sides; the single paddle has a handle at one end and a blade at the other, which is used to paddle and steer.

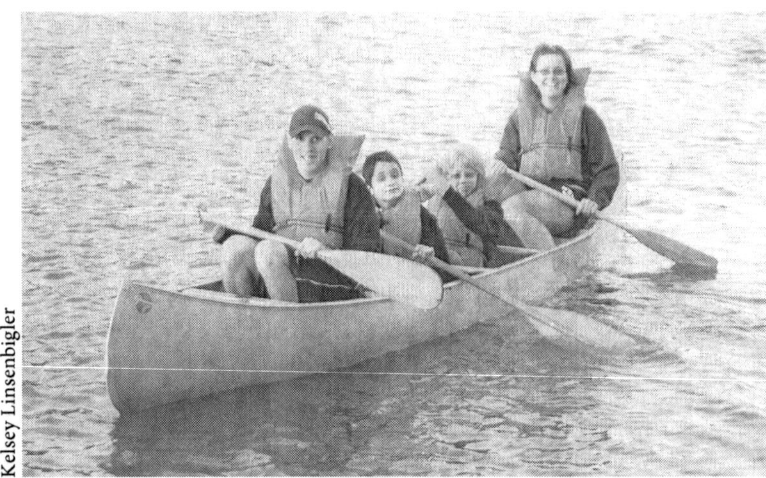

Kelsey Linsenbigler

Canoeing, pictured here, or kayaking, can be chosen for a relaxing day of recreation with friends or family or for a thrilling ride through fast-moving water and rapids.

Very few modifications or adaptations are needed for paddlers with visual impairments. Some flatwater paddlers canoe or kayak alone on lakes, depending on their vision, on GPS devices, or on sound sources such as a radio or beeper device that can be remotely activated to help them return to shore. Paddling alone should be done only by experienced paddlers who are familiar with the waterway and during safe weather conditions.

Whitewater canoeists and kayakers who choose to paddle down flowing rivers are more likely to paddle with others who can spot hazards such as downed trees, submerged rocks, or rapids. It is recommended that those who attempt whitewater kayaking or canoeing seek instruction from experts in the additional skills necessary, such as "wet exits"—exiting a kayak while upside down in the water after it has tipped over—or lining—pulling the craft along the river from shore.

Someone who has not previously paddled should be oriented while on dry land so he or she can be shown the parts of the craft and the basic paddling motions. Instructions about transferring from land to the watercraft, tipovers, and water safety should be included in the initial instruction. Before going out onto the water, it might be helpful to demonstrate, either by modeling or by physical guidance, how the new paddler can steady the boat from the dock or shore for the other paddlers to enter and how to steady the boat while seated inside. If kayaking with a spray skirt—a waterproof cover that is worn around the waist and covers the cockpit of the kayak to keep water out of the boat and the paddler from getting soaked—instruction is necessary in how to don the spray skirt and seal it around the cockpit when seated in the kayak. Flotation devices such as life preservers are important for all paddlers. Persons who wear electronic devices such as hearing aids should be advised to remove them if tip-overs are likely; alternative methods for communicating may then be necessary.

ROLE MODELS

ARCTIC KAYAKERS

Paul and Susan Ponchillia

Author Paul Ponchillia grew up boating and canoeing and continued these activities after he lost his vision in adulthood. Paul and co-author Susan Vlahas Ponchillia, who shared his love of the outdoors, camping, and canoeing, began a series of trips that took them, Paul's dog guide, and their canoe to northern locations such as the Boundary Canoe Waters in northern Minnesota and various bodies of water in Canada. As they gained more skill, they began kayaking in more challenging and remote locations in their new tandem sea kayak, which provided a drier paddle because it had spray skirts and drier storage for their gear. On sunny days, Paul's dog would nap in the sun in one of the storage compartments; on cold and rainy days, she would sleep under a spray skirt between his feet while he paddled.

The Ponchillias' enjoyment of northern landscapes and remote water has since taken them to Greenland, Iceland, Baffin Island, Great Slave Lake in Canada's Northwest Territories, glacier-covered Ellesmere Island near the North Pole in Nunavut, Canada, and to a remote fly-in island near Kodiak, Alaska. Whether the Ponchillias took a short paddle across the lake near their home or paddled through chunks of icebergs in an icy environment, Paul's blindness never hindered their enjoyment of moving through the water propelled by their own physical skills.

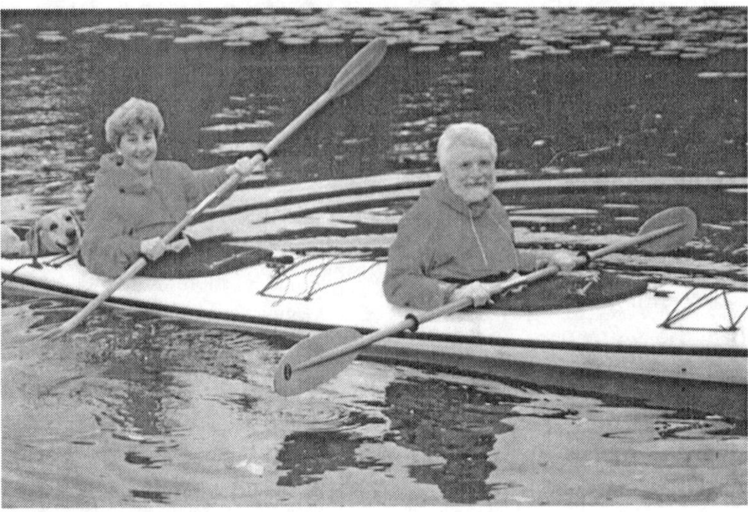

Paul and Susan Ponchillia and Paul's dog guide Ginger kayaking in the wilderness.

Individuals who are deafblind may need an interpreter in another boat next to their boat for clear communication.

Someone who has never seen paddling done before may not understand how the craft is propelled with a paddle. In that case, it may be useful to have the individual paddle with his or her hands first, as if trying to "pull the water toward you." Once that concept is understood, substituting a paddle for one's hands will make more sense. Orientation to the paddle should include how to hold it so that the blade is vertical when it is pulled back through the water and it exerts the greatest possible force.

Several organizations sponsor outdoor programs for people with visual impairments or deafblindness that include canoeing and kayaking (see the Resources section). Many local canoeing and kayaking outfitters are able to make arrangements to provide programs for paddlers with visual impairments. The American Canoe Association sponsors adaptive paddling workshops for instructors, outfitters, recreation program providers, and rehabilitation professionals. A book published with the American Canoe Association, *Canoeing and Kayaking for People with Disabilities* (Zeller, 2009), includes information about adaptations for people with visual impairments.

CONCLUSION

As the sampling of recreational activities presented in this chapter illustrates, individuals with visual impairments or deafblindness are able to take part in virtually any active recreational activity, and opportunities to do so are becoming increasingly available. It is important for professionals in the areas of physical education, recreation, and visual impairment to be cognizant of the importance of recreational activities for health and well-being and to encourage individuals who have visual impairments or deafblindness to find recreation options that suit them.

Although the recreational activities described in this chapter all contribute to improved health and fitness, sometimes it is important to focus on activities specifically geared to that goal. The next chapter discusses adapting a variety of fitness activities for individuals with visual impairments or deafblindness.

11 Fitness

A LIFELONG PURSUIT

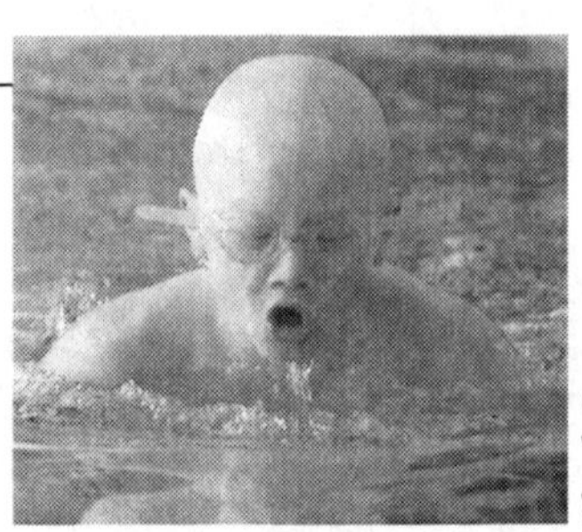
Chuck Comer

IN THIS CHAPTER

- **Importance of Fitness**
- **Assessment**
- **Accessing Fitness Activities**
- **Programming for Fitness**
- **Goal Setting and Evaluation**
- **Running and Walking**
- **Rollerblading**
- **Bicycling**
- **Swimming**
- **Aerobics and Jazzercise**
- **Electronic Exercise Games**
- **Weightlifting**
- **Exercise Machines**
- **Trampoline or Rebounder**
- **Jumping Rope**
- **Yoga**

■ Fitness or Exercise Balls

■ Fitness at Home

■ *Jacobe, 11 years old and totally blind, was very excited about his first day of middle school. He and his mobility instructor, Ms. Patterson, had familiarized themselves with the layout of the school over the summer. As a result, Jacobe knew how to get from the bus to his classes, to the cafeteria, to the gym, and to the rest rooms. Jacobe and his classmates had 5 minutes to get from one class to the next, which seemed to Jacobe like a very short time. By the end of the first day, Jacobe was exhausted. Although he had gone to a Lions Club camp in the summer, where he took part in activities like boating, hiking, and bowling, nothing had prepared him for the amount of walking required during his school day. The next day he felt even more tired, and on Wednesday he told his mother that he did not want to go to school.*

When his mother learned that Jacobe wanted to stay home from school because he did not want to face the frustration of navigating the halls while he was so tired, she called Ms. Patterson, who then met with Mr. Gustoff, the physical educator. Mr. Gustoff had not yet met Jacobe, but he knew about him and was preparing to include him in the general physical education class.

As a result of the teachers' discussion, Mr. Gustoff developed a conditioning program for Jacobe to do at home and embedded fitness into his classes. He talked with Jacobe about the value of increasing his stamina, the conditioning program, the goals, and the time it takes to reach them. For the first few weeks, Jacobe was still exhausted by the walking in addition to his conditioning exercises, but by Halloween, he was keeping up with his friends in the halls and was not out of breath by the last few periods of the day. In fact, Jacobe was considering going out for the track team in seventh grade and planned on attending a summer sports camp for students with visual impairments.

■

Beth was thrilled to complete her independent living training with a vision rehabilitation therapist. They had worked together to meet the goals necessary to manage her budget, buy groceries and prepare meals, and do home management tasks. She was done with school, done with her vocational training, and settling into her new job as a medical office receptionist and getting her nearby apartment organized. One of the concerns that she and the vision rehabilitation therapist discussed during training is that Beth did not have much strength in her arms and got winded easily when they walked together on lessons about going to the grocery and taking her clothes to the laundry room. Beth was not able to easily carry a saucepan of boiling water from stove to sink when she drained pasta, and it was difficult for her to lift a half-gallon milk container. At work, unlike the other people she worked with, she lacked the strength to lift a replacement bottle of water onto the water cooler. She had to leave early for her morning bus in order to walk there in time because she would get winded and have to stop if she had to walk quickly. She knew from her discussions with the vision rehabilitation therapist that she could take charge of improving her fitness and it would make life easier for her. In addition to making life easier, Beth wanted to be fitter, because she knew she'd feel better.

Devin had been extremely overweight throughout his childhood as a result of a condition known as Bardet-Biedl or Laurence-Moon-Bardet-Biedl syndrome. Various physical issues contributed to the overweight, and his vision problem further hampered his desire to be fit and have energy. As a young adult, he found himself more limited by his weight than by his vision problem.

To Devin's relief, bariatric surgery helped him lose enough weight to move about more easily. He applied for a scholarship at the local YMCA and sought the assistance of the staff there to begin working on fitness activities. The staff did not know much about blindness and low vision, but were willing to assist him in meeting his fitness goals. He advocated for himself by explaining what he could and could not see, and he described the techniques that they could use to guide him and make explanations. He started a spinning class. Initially, he was only able to keep up with the class during the warm-up, but each time he attended he stayed on the bike even if he pedaled slowly. Gradually, he increased his endurance.

Experiences like those of Jacobe, Beth, and Devin are not uncommon among children and adults with visual impairments. Research has shown that children with visual impairments often lag behind their sighted peers in health-related fitness (Houwen, Hartman, & Visscher, 2009; Kozub & Oh, 2004; Lieberman & McHugh, 2001; Lieberman, Byrne, Mattern, Watt, & Fernández-Vivó, 2010). And, as discussed throughout this book, a variety of difficulties, from lack of physical skills and training to inaccessible exercise facilities, stand in the way of both children and adults with visual impairments getting the regular physical activity that might improve that situation (Stuart, Lieberman, & Hand, 2006).

As adults, individuals who have been excluded from fitness opportunities as children may have difficulties like Beth's. She had no physical impairments besides her blindness, yet her lack of arm strength interfered with simple daily activities, and her lack of stamina and overall low level of fitness hindered her life at home and at work. This chapter presents some of the many ways in which individuals with visual impairments or deafblindness can participate more in health-related fitness activities, so that children like Jacobe and young adults like Beth can make smooth transitions to new stages of life and possess the endurance they need for any endeavor.

IMPORTANCE OF FITNESS

Fitness can be defined as the state or condition of being fit, or physically sound and healthy. Being fit can help a person function all day without undue fatigue. A basic level of fitness is important to fulfill the physical needs of activities of daily living (McGregor & Farrenkopf, 2000). Being fit can also contribute to looking good and feeling good about oneself (Corn, Bina, and Sacks, 2009).

Research has shown that individuals with visual impairments utilize more energy to do the same activities of daily living as their sighted peers (Kobberling, Jankowski, & Leger, 1989).

Given this greater effort on the part of individuals with visual impairments, it would seem that they need even higher levels of health-related fitness than their sighted peers. In addition, the lack of fitness among individuals who have visual impairments may contribute to their lack of employment. Over 60 percent of working-age adults with visual impairments are unemployed or not even in the labor force, according to at least one measure (AFB, 2012). Although there are many variables that contribute to this low rate of employment, one reason may be that employers do not see individuals with visual impairments as having the stamina to fulfill the physical demands of a particular job (Lieberman, Byrne, Mattern, Watt, & Fernández-Vivó, 2010) or activities of daily living (McGregor & Farrenkopf, 2000). An improvement in health-related fitness will increase stamina and help people be more energetic and capable on the job. Improved health-related fitness can also promote many areas of the expanded core curriculum for students with visual impairments, such as independence, orientation and mobility, self-determination, recreation, socialization, and career development.

Working on one's fitness can be done in free time or can be embedded into daily living skills. For example, Beth incorporated walking into her daily routine so she could improve her stamina and basic level of fitness. Incorporating biking or walking into one's commute is an excellent way to maintain fitness daily. Another option is to incorporate fitness into recreational activity time. An individual might go for a walk, swim, ride a bike, kayak, or work out at the gym before work, during lunch, or after work. Planning fitness activities with friends helps ensure that consistent habits are formed and goals are met.

ASSESSMENT

On the first day Jacobe attended physical education class with Mr. Gustoff, he was assessed on push-ups and the mile run. He was able to do four push-ups, and ran and walked the mile in 18 minutes. Comparing his scores to the minimum standard deemed healthy for children who are blind and 11 years old on the Brockport Physical Fitness Test, he was just below the standard of 8 to 20 for his push-ups, and he was also considerably below the standard of 12 minutes for his mile run time.

Mr. Gustoff decided to embed endurance activities into the warm-ups and closure activities in his class and to start off each class with upper-body strength games and activities such as crab walk, push-up games, or gymnastics-type drills. He also copied instructions for upper-body strength activities for Jacobe to do at home. In addition, Mr. Gustoff obtained two talking pedometers, one for home and one for school, so Jacobe could keep track of the distance he traveled at school and in physical education class as well as at home and on weekends. Jacobe's parents encouraged him to keep a daily log so he could chart his improvement.

To determine the strengths and weaknesses of a student's health-related fitness, instructors need to have some way to assess their abilities. The Brockport Physical Fitness Test (Winnick & Short, 1999) is a valid and reliable assessment to determine whether children and adolescents with visual impairments can meet the minimum standards deemed healthy for individuals of the same age and with the same disability. The areas of the Brockport Physical Fitness Test and the measurements used (described in more detail in Chapter 3) are the following:

- abdominal strength and endurance: curl-ups
- cardiovascular endurance, measured by a 1-mile walk/run
- body composition, measured by height, weight, and a skinfold measure
- upper-body strength and endurance: push-ups and pull-ups
- flexibility: sit and reach, back extension test, and back saver test

The results of the Brockport Physical Fitness Test can be used to set goals and objectives for individuals with visual impairments at any age. If a student does not achieve the minimum deemed healthy according to the standards for individuals with visual impairments for their gender and age, they need to focus on that area to improve their health-related fitness. For example, Beth would very likely not pass the push-ups test of upper-body strength. Her program would then focus on activities that develop upper-body strength such as weight training, push-ups, pull-ups, yoga, or Pilates.

ACCESSING FITNESS ACTIVITIES

Robert, a vending stand operator with both hearing and visual impairments, whose interest in recreational activities was described in Chapter 10, began a membership at the YMCA so he could use the weight training equipment and the pool for lap swimming. Communicating with the staff and other participants was difficult at first, but the staff learned ways to work around the communication issues using a variety of solutions such as finger spelling, notes written in large, bold print, gestures, and a device that had a print display to show what Robert typed in braille. Robert also engaged the services of an interpreter for certain occasions, such as when he first received his orientation at the YMCA. He worked with the staff there so they knew exactly how to assist him in improving fitness while keeping him safe. The fitness activities at the Y were a good complement to the recreational activities he attended through the consumer organization for people with visual impairments.

When Robert joined the Y, he decided what he wanted to do, found a way to participate in that activity, and set goals for himself. There are many ways to incorporate fitness into the lives of individuals who are visually impaired. However, as already noted, there are also barriers that can discourage many people from attempting such activities, and they may need assistance to overcome them. Professionals who work with individuals with visual impairments or deafblindness—whether they are children in school, adults in rehabilitation programs or the community, or older adults—can help them on the path to becoming involved in physical activities, starting by encouraging them to think about the kinds of activities they might enjoy. To begin, the following questions can be considered:

- Do you prefer to be active in individual or group activities?
- Do you prefer indoor or outdoor activities?

- Do the activities you enjoy seem to be more moderate or vigorous in nature?
- Do you prefer activities that are more competitive or more recreational?

Once an individual has decided which activity best suits his or her individual needs, he or she needs to determine specifically how to pursue this activity, that is, where and when he will do it, and with whom. The additional questions listed in Sidebar 11.1 can help people with visual impairments or deafblindness think about how to make the choices and take the concrete steps necessary to the gain access to the activities they would like to do in their own community. (For more information on accessing fitness and other recreational activities, see Lieberman, Modell, Ponchillia, & Jackson, 2006).

Like Robert, Jacobe was successful in targeting an activity that he enjoyed and overcoming the obstacles to participating in it:

> *Jacobe had ridden a tandem bike at the Lions summer camp and really liked it. He was able to borrow a bike from the camp for a few weeks and rode with his sister and friends several days a week. Jacobe loved the freedom he felt on the bike and was very disappointed when he had to give it back. The camp director suggested he go to the local Lions Club to ask for money to buy a bike, although tandems cost quite a bit more than regular bikes, and he was not sure they would be able to afford it.*
>
> *Jacobe spoke to the Lions Club members about his love of biking and how he had learned how to bike at the Lions Camp. Moved by Jacobe's excitement, they teamed up with two other clubs to buy Jacobe the tandem bike. Now he could ride whenever he wanted, as long as he found someone to go with him!*

SIDEBAR 11.1

Accessing Fitness Activities in the Community

The following are some questions to consider when discussing potential fitness activities with an individual with a visual impairment or deafblindness:

- What activities are available in the community that the participant would enjoy?
- Which activities are accessible or could be made accessible to the participant?
- How will progress in the activity be measured?
- How will the individual travel to and from the chosen activity?
- How much will the activity cost?
- How can staff members be educated about the needs of an individual with a visual impairment or deafblindness?
- Who will participate in the activity with the individual? How will they support the participant in engaging in that activity?

For children:

- How can parents get their child involved in community activities with nondisabled peers?
- Are any helpers available for the child with a visual impairment or deafblindness if he or she is involved in an integrated group activity?

PROGRAMMING FOR FITNESS

There is a tremendous variety of activities that promote fitness, include walking, running, hiking, swimming, biking, yoga, kayaking, bicycling, lifting weights, aerobics, and Jazzercize, as well as using exercise machines such as the elliptical trainer, step machine or stair climber, or stationary bike. Swimming, biking, and track and field are some of the most preferred activities for children with visual impairments (Lieberman, Robinson, & Rollheiser, 2006), but children often do not have the opportunity to make their own choices when it comes to home or physical education (Robinson & Lieberman, 2004). It is important to allow a person who is visually impaired to try different types of activities to determine which ones they like best (McGregor & Farrenkopf, 2000), both because it reinforces their self-determination and because they are more likely to stick with activities they have selected.

Some individuals seem to not prefer to move and sweat. In this case, getting a talking pedometer and incorporating additional walking into their day may be the best way to get them moving and to show them that they can indeed walk 1 to 2 miles in a day and perhaps lose enough weight to feel more comfortable moving. Other ideas for encouraging reluctant exercisers include describing activities in a positive manner, stressing the enjoyment of the experience, involving a student's friends or family members, and teaching the prerequisite skills (McGregor & Farrenkopf, 2000).

To ensure that individuals with visual impairments possess the stamina they need for activities of daily living, as well as promoting fitness for a lifetime, there are many modifications or workarounds that can be made to promote success. The AccesSports Model, outlined in Chapter 5, aids in determining important parts of a given activity that may need to be adapted. Some of the following information has been covered in detail with regard to teaching sports and physical activities in schools. Therefore, the following sections provide a summary of a variety of activities in which individuals with visual impairments can take part to promote fitness as well as modifications that can help them participate. (See Chapters 8 and 9 for additional discussion of adaptations.)

GOAL SETTING AND EVALUATION

Some people participate in fitness activities for fun and socialization. The involvement is done for the purpose of enjoyment and participation. Other people participate for the purpose of reaching goals and improving on existing performance.

Participants can set goals related to decreasing the time a given activity takes, increasing distance traveled, increasing number of repetitions performed, or increasing speed. One's goals depend on what one wants to achieve. If a person wants to walk the Cystic Fibrosis 10 Kilometers (6.2 miles) walk-a-thon to raise money with his or her friends, that person would increase the distance that he or she walked each week. For example, Devin can now walk 3 miles with his family and feel pretty good. The walk-a-thon is in 6 weeks. He would try to increase about a half mile each week in order to be able to walk the whole walk-a-thon by the time it is held.

In another situation,

■ *Martha is on her ninth-grade swim team and she wants to swim in the local tournament. She would time herself on the chosen events and try to swim faster and faster in each practice. Martha may also set a goal to swim a time that would allow her to compete with juniors of her age who have her level of visual impairment so she can qualify for the Junior National Swim Tournament through the United States Association of Blind Athletes (USABA). She would make that time her goal and work toward cutting her time down to qualify for that tournament.*

RUNNING AND WALKING

Running and walking both offer numerous health benefits. Walking is an effective way to improve fitness, transport oneself from place to place, and improve socialization opportunities. The following are some guiding adaptations for walking and running. Participants should have the opportunity to try each method to determine which methods they prefer. An individual may prefer one technique for walking or jogging and another for sprinting. Chapter 8 provides additional information about running adaptations as they are used in competition.

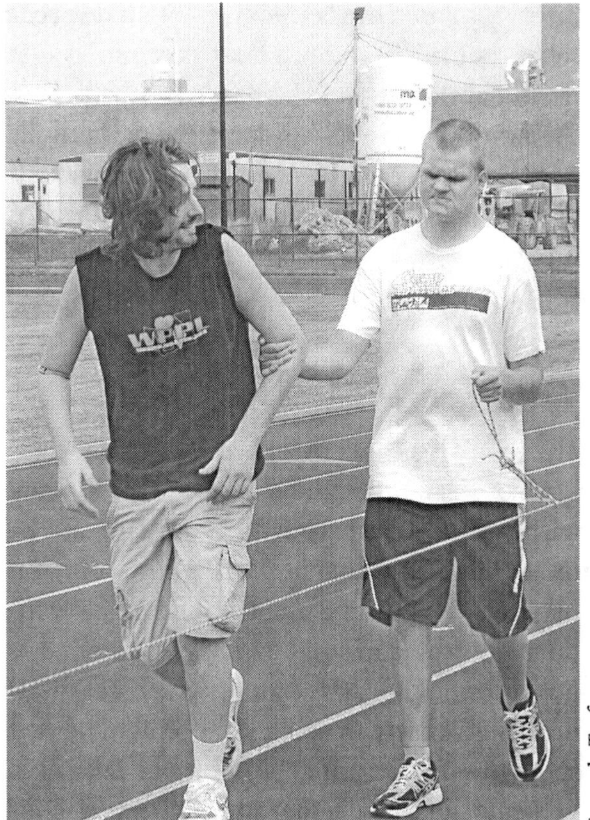

Amanda Tepfer

A runner using both a guide wire and a sighted guide.

Guide Wires

A guide wire is a rope or wire that is suspended along a running course that a runner who is visually impaired can use as a guide. A guide wire system can be set up attached to any stationary, permanent structure, for example, on a track or in a backyard or driveway attached to short poles or in a gym attached to eyehooks in the wall. The rope must be pulled taut at waist height or low to the ground. So that the walker or runner does not have to hold directly onto the rope, a loop of rope or a tether that slides along the guide wire can be attached with a carabiner (a metal ring of the sort used in rope climbing) or key ring, or a 4-inch-long piece of PVC tube can be threaded on the rope for the participant to hold. A warning knot placed at least 2 feet from the end of the rope will alert the individual to the end of the runway; a change in the texture of the floor or ground surface can serve the same purpose.

Human Guide

When using the human guide technique for running, the individual with a visual impairment usually holds the guide runner's elbow with thumb and fingers on either side of the arm (as described in Chapter 4), or he or she may choose to hold onto the guide's shoulder. The pair also can hold hands, or a person with low vision can follow the runner if the guide wears a brightly colored shirt or pinnie. The guide needs to be trained in guiding and communication techniques, and should be able to run faster than the runner who is visually impaired so the guide does not hold back the runner. For individuals with visual impairments who are running for fitness, it is safest if the terrain is smooth, with few obstacles, roots, rocks, or holes.

Tether

The tether is a short rope, a towel, or a shoelace held between the guide and the individual with a visual impairment. Each end of the tether has a knot that helps the runners hold it between their second and third fingers. Wrapping the tether around each person's hand is not recommended, as injuries (such as shoulder dislocation) can occur if the tether is jerked suddenly if one runner stumbles or falls. It is better to hold the tether loosely so that runners can let go if necessary. The guide runner gives voice commands to indicate turns or obstacles. With this technique also, the guide should be able to run faster than the runner with a visual impairment. (See Chapter 8 for use of a tether in racing.) In addition to having all the advantages of running with a human guide, which is faster than other adaptations, runners using a tether have more space around them and feel more independent than with other guiding techniques (Lieberman, Butcher, & Moak, 2001; Lieberman, 2011).

Calling

The calling method can be used for beginning instruction in running as well as in sprint practices. The runner who has a visual impairment runs independently, unrestricted by holding onto anything, toward a person who is calling out to him or her, acting essentially as a sound beacon. The caller can stand at the other end of a gymnasium or track for a short run or for distances can run behind, beside, or in front of the runner holding a bell or keys, or using verbal instruction. The calling method for runners on a track is described in detail in Sidebar 11.2. This technique does not restrict the runner. He or she has the feeling of being independent and able to move as fast as desired without worrying about running into anything. Arm motion can be full and natural.

Running with a caller can slow a runner down somewhat because of the need to focus on where the caller is. However, it works well for practice running and can assist runners who do

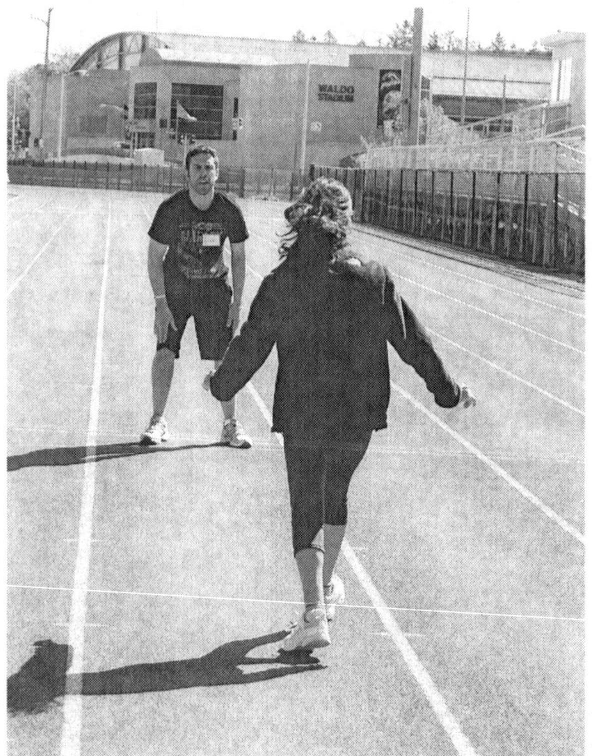
Chuck Comer

A runner follows the voice of a caller in the same lane.

SIDEBAR 11.2

The Calling Method for Guiding Runners

Calling is a method of guiding a runner, usually used on a track under conditions similar to those of sprint racing. Although it is not permitted in formal competitions, it can provide someone with a severe visual impairment or blindness a rare opportunity to run without being tethered to a guide and has been described as "wonderful" by many who have experienced it.

Before the sprint, a runner is generally placed in lane 4 or near the middle of the track. The caller stands in the same lane at a distance of about 30 yards for beginners and faces the runner. The caller helps the runner line up correctly by using cupped hands to yell, "Point at me, here, here, here!" When the runner is properly aligned, the command to begin is given: "Runner to your mark, set, go!" As the runner starts, the caller repeatedly yells the runner's lane number through cupped hands: "Four! Four! Four!" If the runner veers out of the proper lane, the caller yells the new lane number with more urgency ("*Five! Five! Five!*") until the runner returns to the original lane. If the runner veers by more than one lane—for example, from lane 4 as far as either lanes 2 or 6—the caller stops the run immediately. If calling is being used in a formal race, as the runner approaches the finish line, the caller stops calling and moves out of the lane, yelling, "Finish!" as the runner crosses the line.

In the case of a 100-meter sprint, two callers are required. The first is placed near the 50-meter mark and moves out of the lane when the runner approaches, at which time the second caller picks up the calling just short of the finish line.

Note that only one sprinter can run at a time using calling. If runners are competing, the best running time among them determines the winner.

not have guide runners who are fast enough to keep up. As noted in Chapter 8, callers are used in training only; this technique is not allowed in continental, world, or Paralympic competition.

Running without Assistance on a Track

Someone with low vision can often run independently on a track that has enough contrast between the lines and surface. This technique works best when the track is not crowded, and adults should monitor young student runners who are running unassisted to ensure that they do so safely. Runners who are visually impaired should have at least two lanes. The individual can run independently or side by side with a friend, using full arm swing and potentially an efficient biomechanical gait.

Running on a Treadmill

Treadmills are found in gyms, hotels, schools, and fitness centers around the country, and they are generally available and accessible to people with visual impairments. They provide the benefit of running independently without guides. Runners can run with full arm swing and can keep a record of speed and distance as they are recorded by the treadmill. The controls on a treadmill may need to be marked with some kind of tactile marking such as raised dots or brailled plastic tape. Unless the treadmill has audio output, the runner may need assistance to know the distance and time of the exercise session, although talking pedometers (discussed later in this chapter) or apps on cell phones can be used to give distances and times for runs or walks.

For safety or comfort, people may want to use treadmills with handrails. The runner need not hold onto the handrails, but the rails let the participant know when he or she has moved too far to one side or the other. Participants should start out slowly to get a feel for the motion of the treadmill and increase speed gradually.

Accessible Pedometers and Heart Rate Monitors

When people are involved in a running or walking program, it is useful for them to have feedback about their performance. There are several ways to measure walking or running activity. A pedometer measures steps and distance. There are a number of talking pedometers that measure walking steps, total distance traveled, and calories burned in a day. Some provide music that speeds up or slows down depending on the walker's cadence. Talking pedometers can be found at local sporting goods stores and on the Internet. The American Printing House for the Blind offers a Walk-Run for Fitness Kit that includes a talking pedometer along with a guidebook, an adjustable tether, and a guide wire system (see the Resources section).

In addition to a talking pedometer, the participant may also want to wear a heart-rate monitor. Heart-rate monitors give the participant immediate feedback about heart rate, that is, the number of heartbeats per minute, which offers information about how hard the person is working. Increasing one's heart rate while exercising increases the capacity of the heart to work and its efficiency and improves stamina for everyday activities. Depending on an individual's fitness goal, he or she may want to set his or her target heart rate at about 70 percent of maximum heart rate. Maximum heart rate is typically calculated by the formula 220 – age. Multiplying that by 0.70 gives the target number of heartbeats per minute at 70 percent of the maximum rate.

Jacobe wants to wear his heart-rate monitor to be sure he is walking or running within 70 percent of his maximum heart rate. Since he is 11 years old, his maximum heart rate is calculated as 220 – 11 or 209 beats per minute. His target rate is 70 percent of that number, or 209 × 0.70 = 146.3 beats per minute. Therefore, Jacobe can exercise wearing his heart-rate monitor and try to keep his heart-rate in the area of 140 to 150 beats per minute.

Using heart-rate monitors and talking pedometers helps ensure that participants work to their potential no matter what the activity (Beets, Foley, Tindall, & Lieberman, 2007; Lieberman, Stuart, Hand, & Robinson, 2006). Both devices are most effective when participants develop goals and work toward them. Holbrook et al. (2011) found that talking pedometers are most accurate when worn on the hip opposite any mobility aid an individual might be using, such as a cane, human guide, or dog guide.

As mentioned previously, there are now applications for cell phones or other mobile devices that can give distances, speeds, and calories burned during exercise. Most phones have audio output that would make the information accessible for individuals with visual impairments. There are also wrist bands that record steps, distances, and energy expenditure; the wrist bands themselves do not have audio output, but they have a free application that syncs the information with a phone that can then provide the audio output.

ROLLERBLADING

Rollerblading is an active, fun, enjoyable sport that can be executed on any flat, smooth surface. Rollerblading can improve cardiovascular endurance, leg strength, and balance. Since even the most experienced rollerblading athletes have accidents, it is important to always wear a helmet when rollerblading as well as wrist guards and elbow and knee pads. Rollerblades and pads can be purchased at any sporting goods or variety store or online.

The same adaptations used in running can be used for rollerblading, including a sighted guide, tether, or guide wire. The participant can also skate while trailing the wall of a building. See Table 11.1 for steps to teaching rollerblading. Rollerblading performance can be measured by time, distance, speed, or all three factors.

BICYCLING

Bicycling is a great low-impact fitness sport that is good for people of all ages and all abilities. There are many ways to bike to meet individual needs.

TABLE 11.1. Steps for Teaching Rollerblading

Steps	Instructor's Role	How to Measure
1. Put skates on and stand up	Help learner put skates on and hold learner's hand	How long learner can stand without falling
2. Skate on a rug or a padded surface that does not allow the wheels to spin too fast. Do this against a wall.	Hold learner's hand or allow learner to hold instructor's shoulder	How far or how long learner can skate on the padded surface
3. Do the previous step without the wall	Hold learner's hand or allow learner to hold instructor's shoulder	How far or how long learner can skate on the padded surface without holding the wall
4. Skate on a smooth floor while holding the wall	Allow learner to hold on to instructor or peer as much as necessary. A walker on wheels* can also be used for stability.	How far or how long learner can skate on the smooth surface while holding the wall or a walker
5. Skate without holding the wall for brief periods with physical assistance	Allow learner to hold on to instructor or peer as much as necessary. A walker on wheels can also be used for stability.	How long or how far learner can skate without holding the wall but with physical assistance
6. Skate independently without physical assistance	Promote independence as much as possible, although a walker can also be used if necessary	How long or how far learner can skate independently

*A shopping cart or a wheelchair can be substituted if a walker on wheels is not available.

Riding Independently

Individuals who have low vision may be able to ride a bicycle independently in a quiet park, in a cul de sac, or around a track, offering a significant feeling of independence. Even when an individual with low vision can ride independently, it is always safer if someone with sight is present and watching for obstacles or hazards.

Tandem Bicycles

Tandem cycling is covered in detail in Chapters 8 and 10. Someone who is interested in riding for fitness may find that contacting a local bicycling club, university, or community club is a good way to find a partner with similar interests. Before riding together, as noted previously, the participants need to develop specific signals, either verbal or tactile, for turning, stopping, or emergencies. It is important that individuals who are deafblind create a method of communicating to the guide rider a wish to turn and to stop. As noted in Chapter 10, surrey or duo bicycles, bicycles on which the participants ride side-by-side, are more conducive to communication if the participant is deafblind.

Stationary Bicycles

Anyone who has some functional use of his or her legs can use stationary bikes independently. Stationary bikes are found in health clubs and at schools and can be purchased for the home, and the participant does not have to worry about weather or having a sighted guide. Many stationary bikes display the distances pedaled and amount of time ridden. As with treadmills, the controls may need to be marked using some kind of tactile marker or braille. In addition, unless the machine has audio output, the cyclist may need assistance to know the distance and time of the exercise session.

Many health clubs offer "spinning" classes where all the participants ride a stationary bike and the instructor calls directions for increasing speed, doing hill work, or maintaining a certain pace. Spinning classes are generally easily accessible for a person with a visual impairment.

A bicycle stand, also known as a turbo trainer, can turn an ordinary bicycle into a stationary bike. The stand is a sturdy frame that sits on the floor. With the front tire of a bicycle removed, the bike snaps onto the frame. The pedals now can spin with or without resistance, while the bike does not move. These stands can be purchased at many sporting goods stores.

SWIMMING

Swimming is an effective fitness activity for individuals who are visually impaired or deafblind. Even beginning swimmers can receive an aerobic workout in the water by swimming laps or participating in water aerobics (aerobic exercise classes in the water) or similar activities. Exercising in the water improves range of motion, muscle strength, balance, stability, locomotion, and cardiovascular endurance; a school or community pool is a good place for socializing as well. Swimming can be enjoyed for recreation and fitness alone, or an individual can choose to take part in high school or community competitions or, through the USABA, in regional, national, or international competition, as described in Chapter 8.

There are few barriers to participating in swimming activities for people with visual impairments or deafblindness. Swimmers can move freely in the water without worrying about obstacles, especially when lanes are clearly marked with lane lines. Lane lines are ropes with small rings of plastic along the entire length of the lane that float on top of the water to divide the lanes for safety. Chapter 8 provides additional details about adaptations for competitive swimming.

Beginning Swimmers

Beginning swimmers need to learn basic swim skills to enhance their confidence in the water, including buoyancy (floating), kicking, arm motions, and breath control. Goals for beginning swimmers may include treading water, floating on front or back, kicking while holding onto the wall or a kickboard, holding breath for increasing lengths of time, or blowing bubbles in the water.

Adaptations for Swimming

The following are some ways to adapt swimming activities to ensure that every person can participate in swimming as a fitness activity.

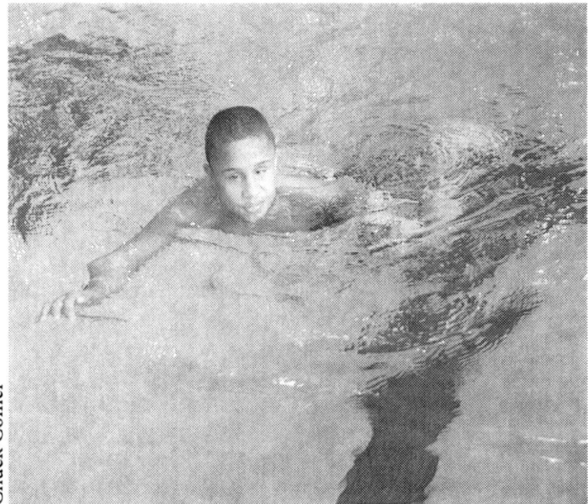

Chuck Comer

Treading water is a basic skill for beginners to learn and is also an effective exercise.

Flotation Devices

There are a variety of flotation devices, from kickboards to water wings to swimming "noodles" (long cylindrical pieces of foam), that swimmers can use to help them stay afloat while exercising in the water, if this makes the swimmer more comfortable. Swimmers can still receive an aerobic workout and even swim laps while using a flotation device. Kickboards are particularly helpful for lap swimming, because the board hits the side of the pool before the swimmer's head (Lepore, Gayle, and Stevens, 2007; see the section on Lap Swimming).

Treading Water

Treading water is an effective aerobic workout for individuals who do not feel comfortable swimming laps. The participant can tread for a specified period of time or use a treading motion to travel a given distance. Although treading water is typically used to stay in one place, the same motion can also be used to produce movement if that is the goal. Putting a waterproof radio on the deck to signal the shallow end of the pool or the corner of the pool may be helpful. When treading water, swimmers do not have to worry about bumping their heads on the wall of the pool. It is easier to communicate with individuals who are deafblind when they are treading water than when they are swimming laps.

Lap Swimming

Swimming can be a particularly efficient fitness activity because when done continuously it maintains one's heart rate at a high level for a sustained period of time. Many people do this by swimming laps—that is, swimming the length of the pool, turning at the end wall, and

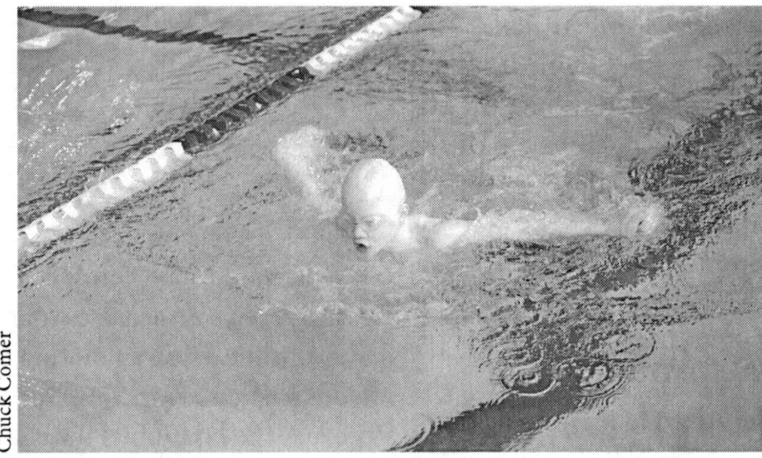
Chuck Comer

Swimmer doing the butterfly stroke. The main issues in lap swimming for fitness are staying in lane and knowing when the end of the pool is near.

swimming back. Any stroke can be used for lap swimming. Turns can be accomplished either by stopping and pivoting at the wall or by doing a front flip in the water (called a flip turn). Either turn is fine, although the flip turn is faster and is often used in competition.

Turning

Individuals with visual impairments or deafblindness may need an adaptation to lap swimming so that they know when they are about to reach the wall at the end of the pool and need to turn to avoid hitting their heads. Some swimmers with low vision may be able to make use of the visual clues provided in most pools to alert swimmers to the impending wall, such as an overhead flag or line painted on the pool bottom at designated distances from the end wall. For individuals who cannot use visual cues, the following are three ways to signal a swimmer when to turn:

1. An instructor or friend can tap the swimmer's shoulder with a kickboard when the swimmer is 3 to 4 feet from the wall.
2. An instructor or friend can tap the swimmer on the head with a *tap stick* (a long pole with a tennis ball or a section of a swimming noodle attached to the end) when the swimmer is 3 to 4 feet from the end of the pool (Lepore, Gayle, & Stevens, 2007). Tap sticks are used in international competition for athletes who are blind (see Chapter 8).
3. A sprinkler can be placed at either end of the pool to disturb the water 3 to 4 feet from the wall to warn the swimmer when to turn (Scheib & Ponchillia, 1999; see Chapter 8 for a more detailed description). The location of the sprinkler can be adjusted to the preference of the swimmer, who would then count strokes to know when to make the turn.

Trailing

Trailing involves using the wall and lane lines as guides for swimming laps the length of the pool to ensure that the swimmer will stay in her or his lane and swim the straightest line to the end of the pool (Lepore, Gayle, & Stevens,

2007). Trailing may slow the speed of new lap swimmers, but with practice, swimming in a straight line usually becomes natural.

Keeping Track of Distance and Laps

Devices such as counters, rings, or braille or large-print flip cards can be used to help swimmers keep track of the number of laps or distance they have covered. Lap-counting devices are sold, with or without stopwatches, that record each lap with the click of a button, but these are unlikely to have a speech feature. Another counting method is to place a basket with a specific number of plastic pool rings at the shallow end of the pool where swimmers start. The swimmer picks up one ring, swims to the other end of the pool, drops the ring into another basket, and swims back, completing a two-lap cycle. If a swimmer starts with 10 rings, he or she will know that 20 laps have been completed when all the rings have been dropped off at the far end of the pool. Because holding a ring while swimming can be difficult, some swimmers choose to use flip cards instead. The flip cards, mounted on a ring and placed at the shallow end of the pool where the swimmer starts, are marked with large-print or braille numbers. When the swimmer returns to the shallow end, having completed two laps, he or she flips over two cards. Whether swimmers use counting devices, count their own laps, or swim for time periods, their goal remains to keep track of performance and to maintain or improve fitness levels.

AEROBICS AND JAZZERCISE

Aerobics involves performing certain movements, with or without music, that increase one's heart rate. Any amount of movement can elevate the heart rate, and if it is continued for more than 5 minutes, it is considered aerobic. Therefore, aerobics can be done at a variety of levels. Aerobics movements frequently involve jumping and moving the arms and legs simultaneously to increase the heart rate. Jazzercise is a type of fitness training that combines aerobic exercise and dancing to jazz music. People who prefer less of an impact on their joints utilize low-impact or step aerobics, which still has fitness benefits without the impact of jumping. Regardless of the type of aerobics engaged in, the aim is to elevate the heart rate and have fun (McGregor & Farrenkopf, 2000; Lieberman & Taule, 1998).

Aerobics or Jazzercise is often done in a group setting or class, but it can also be done at home with a video or with music and with family and friends of all ages. The initial routine may have to be taught or described to an individual with a visual impairment or deafblindness by a peer tutor, paraeducator, or instructor, but the participant can then exercise independently, performing eight-count or four-count routines and combining different moves.

Some people who are blind have a tendency to rotate while doing aerobic movements, particularly during high-impact aerobics. Therefore it can be helpful to create tactile boundaries for these participants so they can remain oriented and know where they are in relation to the rest of the class. This can be done using rope held in place with gymnasium tape or having them do the workout on a carpet square.

One reason why many people like aerobics and Jazzercise is the upbeat music that accompanies most classes. In many of these classes, individuals with visual impairments or deafblindness will also enjoy the music. However, the music can sometimes interfere with learning the skills. It is often much easier to practice the movements initially without music. Individuals who are deafblind may appreciate the music more if the vibrations are enhanced by placing the speakers face down on a wooden floor, if possible, or having them hold a balloon, which will pick up the vibrations, while they are performing the skills.

High-Impact Aerobics and Jazzercise

In high-impact aerobics and Jazzercise, both feet leave the floor at some point during the movement. An individual can do jumping jacks, kicks to the front, or jog in place; bring the knees up and clap under the leg while jumping with the other leg; and do pendulum leg swings out to the sides, side jumps and front jumps in alternating directions, and other such movements. An individual must be in good condition to sustain this activity for a period of time.

Low-Impact Aerobics

In low-impact aerobic exercise, the participants keep one foot on the ground at all times to lessen the impact on the joints. An individual can march with high knees, kick to the front, bring a knee up and clap under the leg, march in place while bringing arms up and down, do toe touches to the front, right and left, or just walk briskly around the room. The goal is for the individual to move and keep his or her heart rate elevated. Anyone who is ambulatory can successfully participate in this activity.

Step Aerobics

The participants in step aerobics engage in a series of moves in which they step on and off a platform that is 4, 6, or 8 inches high at varying tempos and in different directions. The participant imitates the movements made by the instructor. Step aerobics is adaptable to any level of ability. An individual who cannot step up onto a platform can do the same movements without a step.

Wheelchair Aerobics

People who are in a wheelchair can participate in aerobics by moving their arms up in the air or out to the sides, punching down, or twisting at the hips for eight counts or more to elevate their heart rate. If they are able, they can move their legs at the same time as their arms.

Teaching Aerobics

An aerobic move can require a lot of words to describe, for example, "Bring the right elbow to the left knee," "Lunge forward and punch to the right and then to the left," "Kick to the front and touch your toes," or "Move to the right and left two steps and clap." These moves are often referred to with short verbal cues that can be timed to the music, such as "Elbow to knee," or simply "Punch." Most moves are consistently done for 8 to 10 counts to the music that is playing. When people are learning the moves in aerobics, it is helpful if the instructor does the moves in the same order and repeats them often, starting without music and progressing to full counts with the music as the participants learn them.

The authors recommend teaching the moves needed for many aerobics or Jazzercise classes using the teaching styles of tactile modeling or physical assistance (O'Connell, Lieberman, & Petersen, 2006). (See Chapter 4 for more information on these teaching styles.) Once the moves are clearly understood by the participant, then they can be taught using only a verbal cue for the movement (Ponchillia, Powell, Felski, & Nicklawski, 1992).

An instructor would use physical guidance with individuals who do not have sufficient vision or hearing to understand verbal instructions about the movement. The instructor explains the move and moves the participant's limbs through the desired movement pattern, either with a light tap or with fully assisted support. The instructor can then simplify the description of the pattern of moves with one touch cue or a sign cue that the participant will understand. For example, if the instructor wants the participant to march in place for eight counts as part of a low-impact aerobics routine, once the participant understands the concept, the instructor can say, "Marching," make the sign for soldier, or tap the individual's knee to signal marching. The participant then knows to march for eight counts, and then the instructor will give a new cue for the next move. Depending on the ability and condition of the participant, the instructor can also set up routines in which a given eight-count move is always followed by another specific eight-count move, and so on. Once the participant understands the moves, the instructor should promote independence by trying to fade out the touch cues. Sidebar 11.3 provides a simple teaching method for the steps that might be used to teach a front kick as part of an aerobic exercise routine.

SIDEBAR 11.3

Techniques for Teaching a Front Kick

The following steps provide an example of how an aerobic movement can be taught to a participant with a visual impairment:

1. Explain the move and demonstrate it, if the participant can benefit from a visual demonstration.
2. If necessary, have the participant use touch to observe the instructor or another class member kicking to the front with right and left legs.
3. Ask the participant to kick to the front with the right and then the left leg.
4. Offer correction of the placement of the participant's foot in the kick, first verbally and, if necessary, by having him or her touch the instructor's or another participant's foot and leg.
5. If necessary, physically guide the participant's leg into a high kick position so he or she can understand kinesthetically where the foot belongs when doing the kick.
6. Have the participant practice kicking to the front for eight counts with each leg.
7. Embed the front kick into a routine.
8. When the participant is comfortable with the routine, add music.

ELECTRONIC EXERCISE GAMES

Thanks to advances in technology, a number of computer and video games have been developed that may engage people in fitness activities. In some of these games (sometimes known as exergames), a form of physical activity is the input for progressing in the game. For example, in a game called Dance Dance Revolution, played on a television or computer screen, arrows on the screen move up and down, right and left in different sequences to music. The participant must step on the arrows of a matching pad in the order and sequence in which the arrows appear on the screen. Adaptations for people with visual impairments include eliminating background objects on the screen and focusing on just the arrows, slowing down the arrows, and having another person give verbal directions about which arrow appears (Gasperetti et al., 2010).

The Wii (Morelli, Folmer, Foley, & Lieberman, 2011) is another brand whose exercise games can be played by individuals with visual impairments either with or without adaptations, depending on the game, for play with other people with visual impairments or friends who are sighted. Games that can be played without adaptations are the Wii Hula Hoop, Wii boxing, and Wii jogging. A research project known as VI Fit (Morelli, Foley, Lieberman, & Folmer, 2011; Morelli, Foley, Columna, Lieberman, & Folmer, 2010) has adapted a number of other games to include more audio feedback and vibrotactile cues and makes them available on its website (www.vifit.org). The Wii tennis and Wii bowling games have been adapted for individuals with visual impairments and have proved to be very enjoyable (Boffoli, Foley, Gasparetti, Yang, and Lieberman, 2011). Another game called Pet-N-Punch, which is similar to the Whac-A-Mole arcade game, has also been modified with haptic and auditory cues.

WEIGHTLIFTING

Lifting weights is a simple and accessible way to improve muscular strength and endurance at home or in a fitness gym. At home the participant can have hand weights in amounts that are appropriate for the individual. Hand weights can be bought at any store that sells sporting goods. Other equipment that can be used in the home includes a weight bench and barbells. Resistance bands—large rubber bands that provide different amounts of tension when stretched—can be used to increase range of motion and strength as well and can be purchased from medical supplies dealers or physical therapist offices.

Jacobe's mother bought him 5-pound weights, 8-pound weights, and a yellow (low resistance) resistance band. With the help of Mr. Gustoff, he developed a routine of side bends, bicep curls, tricep curls, sit-ups, push-ups, front lunges, and lat pulls to do at home three times a week. He set goals and engaged in his routine listening to his favorite music or sometimes watching television.

Improvement in weightlifting can be measured by increase in the amount of weight lifted, in the number of repetitions (reps) of each exercise that is performed, or both. It is important to consult with a specialist to help with the participant's routine and work within the participant's physical abilities and individual goals.

EXERCISE MACHINES

A variety of exercise machines can be used for aerobic conditioning and fitness, either at a health club or at home. Treadmills were discussed earlier in this chapter as a way to do running or walking in the home, and stationary bicycles were discussed as an alternative to biking. A step machine or stair climber is another kind of machine, similar to a treadmill, but it simulates walking up steps in a consistent motion. Use of a step machine can improve an individual's cardiovascular endurance, leg strength, balance, and trunk stability. Like a treadmill, the display on a step machine can report the length of time exercised, number of steps taken, and calories burned. A step machine requires balance and stability, but it often has handles so the participant can hold on while exercising if necessary.

A similar machine, an elliptical trainer, simulates walking or running without the feet leaving the treads, so it provides a low-impact exercise. Most versions also work the upper body. Rowing machines are discussed later in this section.

These exercise machines can all be used in the home. Although they are not inexpensive, the types one would purchase for home use are less expensive than the industrial ones used in busy health clubs and, if used consistently, may be more affordable over the long term than a gym or health club membership.

Accessibility of Exercise Machines

As noted previously, the controls for some of these machines may need to be marked with tactile materials to make the machines accessible to people with visual impairments, and the displays that show information about length of time exercised and distance covered are not likely to be accessible. Programming particular workouts may be possible once a user has been oriented to the device, if the buttons that control resistance and other features are tactile and the machine beeps as the settings are changed. Burton and Huffman (2007) discuss these issues, as well as how to work with a health club to improve accessibility, and they provide additional resources on the topic.

Indoor Rowing

Indoor rowing is an especially good way to maintain fitness, because it provides an excellent cardiovascular workout and uses every muscle with every stroke: arms to pull, legs to push, and the torso to help provide power to both. Rowing machines can be used in a gym or health club or purchased for use at home. In many indoor rowers the seat slides on a shaft as the rower pulls back with the arms and pushes with the feet on a footplate, mimicking the action of rowing a racing shell (see Chapter 8).

The technique used in rowing is fairly simple, but if done incorrectly, it can cause injuries. For that reason it is important to learn the proper way to row. Sidebar 11.4 describes the steps involved in rowing and the movements used to accomplish each.

Although accessibility of the controls can be an issue with rowing machines as with other exercise machines, one manufacturer of rowing machines, Concept2 (see the Resources section), has adapted its machines to enable people with visual impairments or deafblindness to use its devices without assistance and to access virtually all of its functions. One option, Erg Chatter, runs on a laptop computer equipped with screen reading or screen enlargement software or with a refreshable braille output device. Once connected to the monitor via a USB cable (included in purchase), Erg Chatter enables the user to interact with the output device, for example, to hear one's stroke rate, split (the average time it would take to row 500 meters), or the elapsed time rowing. Erg Buddy provides the same feedback directly from the rower's monitor and allows the rower to run the program through an iPhone or iPad, eliminating the need for a laptop with access software.

SIDEBAR 11.4

Proper Indoor Rowing Technique

The rowing stroke can be divided into two major phases: the drive and the recovery. Within those phases, there are four steps: (a) the recovery, (b) the catch, (c) the drive, and (d) the finish. The drive is the work portion of the stroke; the recovery is the rest portion that prepares for the next drive. The body movements of the recovery are essentially the reverse of the drive. Blending these movements into a smooth continuum creates the rowing stroke.

The Recovery

- Extend arms until they straighten.
- Lean the upper body forward until shoulders are ahead of hips.
- Once the hands and the rowing handle have cleared the knees, allow the knees to bend and let the seat gradually slide forward.

The Catch

- Arms are straight; head is straight; shoulders are level and not hunched.
- Shoulders are in front of hips.
- Shins are vertical and not compressed beyond the perpendicular.
- Balls of the feet are in full contact with the footplate.

The Drive

- With straight arms and while maintaining the position of the upper body with shoulders in front of hips, exert pressure on the foot plate and begin pushing with the legs.
- As the legs approach straight, lean the upper body back until shoulders are behind hips and draw the hands back to the lower ribs in a straight line.

The Finish

- Legs are extended and handle is held lightly at the lower ribs.
- Upper body is slightly reclined with good support from the core muscles.
- Head is in a straight position.
- Neck and shoulders are relaxed, and arms are drawn past the body with flat wrists.

Source: Adapted with permission from T. Smythe, The Rowing Stroke: Concept2, retrieved 7/4/2012 from http://www.concept2.com/us/training/technique.asp.

One user of Erg Chatter (Blas, 2011) reported enhancing his workout by patching the iPod of his iPhone and the Erg Chatter output together, so he can listen to his workout statistics to the accompaniment of his favorite music.

TRAMPOLINE OR REBOUNDER

A trampoline is an exercise device consisting of a durable cloth stretched taut and connected to a steel frame using springs so that a person standing on the cloth bounces. A small version of a trampoline is known as a rebounder, which can be used in the home. An individual can run in place, jump, march, or do aerobic routines on a trampoline or rebounder to improve cardiovascular endurance, leg strength, balance, and trunk stability. Effort and improvement can be measured by time elapsed, number of jumps, or both. Music can be used as motivation and for enjoyment. Rebounders or trampolines can be bought at any sporting goods store or online.

Safety is a key concern when using trampolines or rebounders, because of the risk of falling. Safety measures include purchasing a rebounder with a handle bar, placing the rebounder against a wall, not jumping too high, and not having more than one person on the device at a time. If necessary the participant can use a spotter. Friends can take turns on the rebounder, and individuals can exercise on it while watching TV or listening to music.

JUMPING ROPE

Jumping rope aids in agility, balance, and aerobic and muscular endurance. It can be done slowly with little impact or quickly with high impact; it can be done to favorite music or to no music. It can be done with family and friends, and practice is rewarded with visible improvement in skill. Success can be measured by the number of jumps or the continuous amount of time spent jumping.

Individuals can jump rope in a driveway, in a yard, or in a clear garage. To remain in a safe area, the jumper can mark off the area with bright cones, a rope on the floor with tape over it, mats, or towels. A jump rope kit with a guidebook is available from the American Printing House for the Blind (see the Resources section). Methods of teaching jump rope are discussed in detail in Chapter 7.

YOGA

Life can be stressful for many individuals with a visual impairment or deafblindness. Probably the most important advantage of yoga is its teaching of relaxation, although yoga can also result in weight loss and improved strength and flexibility. It is probably safest to learn yoga in a class, where basic moves, proper positions, and appropriate body mechanics can be taught. Once these are learned, yoga can be practiced in the home and learned from a book or video.

Yoga instruction, like aerobics, can utilize the techniques of physical assistance and tactile modeling coupled with explanation. A special yoga mat with indentations has been developed for people with visual impairments. The indentations help yoga students feel where their hands, feet, and head should be placed in basic yoga postures (see the Resources section). The mat also has braille markings, a line down the middle horizontally, and a line across vertically for orientation. The mat comes with a DVD video that provides detailed explanations of the poses as well as beginner and intermediate classes.

Once having learned the basic yoga poses, the participant can train in the home or yard, alone or with friends and family. Yoga is an inexpensive way to improve fitness and to obtain relaxation.

FITNESS OR EXERCISE BALLS

A fitness or exercise ball can provide an overall body workout. Although fitness balls are not generally used for cardiovascular training, they are excellent for stretching and for strengthening core and upper- and lower-body muscles. The ball helps the user develop and maintain good body control and balance. Exercise balls are appropriate for people of all ages. They are excellent exercise tools for older people, because they encourage muscle strength and flexibility, free joint movement, core strength, and good balance, all of which are important in order to continue activities of daily living during later life.

Exercise balls are also easily used by people with visual impairments because the balls require little adaptation. An exercise ball that contains bells (one that can be found on the Internet is known as the Jinglin' Ball) makes it easier for people with visual impairments to find the ball if it rolls out of reach during the workout. Also, it can be difficult to know where the boundaries are for a workout area, and likewise where the furniture or other obstacles are, while engaged in an active ball exercise. The boundaries can be monitored by limiting the workout to the raised surface of an area rug or a tumbling mat or by strategically placing a music source at a known point in the room as an auditory base.

Attention should be paid to safety when using an exercise ball; because some routines require exercisers to sit or lie extended across the top of balls, the exercisers are at some risk of falling as the ball rolls. Trainers and teachers should assess a participant's balance before starting an exercise ball regimen, as research has shown that older people and those who are blind tend to have balance difficulties compared with younger, sighted individuals (Arnot & Gaines, 1984; Haibach, Lieberman, & Ritter, 2011), although this is not a reason to avoid the exercise ball as a fitness tool. As a rule, it is best not to begin a ball workout alone; rather, new fitness ball users should have an assistant to "spot" for them during their early attempts at learning to use the device.

Many exercise or fitness balls come with a list of exercises, and there are numerous sources for fitness ball workouts on the Internet. However, the movements and positions used during the exercise session are nearly always presented visually on the websites, as either photographs or videos, so an exerciser with a visual impairment or deafblindness will need an assistant or spotter to help the exerciser interpret the exercises, using verbal description and tactile modeling or physical guidance. Because it is difficult to find complete descriptions of these exercises, a beginning fitness routine of 10 fitness ball exercises is described in detail in Sidebar 11.5.

FITNESS AT HOME

Many individuals with visual impairments or deafblindness have difficulty traveling to places in the community for recreation and fitness activities such as an aerobics or yoga class (Lieberman & MacVicar, 2003). They may also be unable to find a sighted guide to help them in running, walking, or tandem bicycling. As an alternative, participating in fitness and recreation activities in the home can be an easy, safe, and rewarding endeavor for the participant and the family (Lieberman & Pecorella, 2006). Although there are many benefits to participating in exercise activities in the community related to socialization, friendships, goal setting, and the variety of activities available, doing these activities at home can also have many benefits. There are fewer barriers to exercising at home, where the individual has more control over time and scheduling, and lighting, noise, and transportation problems are nonexistent. A number of activities that have been described in this chapter can be engaged in at home, including the following:

SIDEBAR 11.5

Ten Fitness Ball Exercises for Beginners

The following exercise routine, performed using a fitness ball, includes some stretching as well as exercises that work different muscle groups for an overall workout, including the core, upper body, lower body, and lower back. The participant can start with one set of these exercises and work up to three sets. When he or she is comfortable with these 10 exercises on the fitness ball, new exercises can be added as desired.

Muscle-Stretching Exercises

1. Back and hamstring stretch

Starting position: Sit on ball with back straight. Place feet flat on floor slightly more than shoulder width apart. Place palms on knees.

Action: Straighten legs touching only heels on floor. Bend at the waist as ball rolls back, sliding palms down legs.

Finish: Hold 15 seconds. Return to starting position and repeat 10 times.

2. Side Stretch

Starting position: To stretch the right side, lie on the left side, placing the ball midway between the left shoulder and hip and keeping the trunk, hips, and right leg completely straight. Bend the left leg at the knee to about 90 degrees, pointing the bent knee straight forward like the hour hand at the 3 o'clock position, and touch the floor with the left side of the left foot. Keep the right arm lying straight along the top of the extended right leg.

Action: Keeping the left foot planted, bend the right leg and move the torso down toward the right foot. Then straighten right leg and simultaneously extend right arm over the head, stretching the entire right side of body. Continue to keep left foot planted.

Finish: Hold the stretch for 10 seconds and repeat 5 times. Then switch sides and repeat.

Core Muscle Strengthening

3. Core Rolls

Starting position: Sit on ball with back straight, feet flat on floor, palms on legs near knees.

Action: Keeping feet and hands planted, swivel hips so the movement of the buttocks rolls the top of the ball around in a circular motion, first clockwise to the right, then counterclockwise to the left. At the far side of each rotation, tighten the abdominal muscles.

Finish: Alternate 15 rolls clockwise with 15 counterclockwise, rest 10 seconds, and repeat two more sets.

4. Ball Crunches

Starting position: Sit on the ball, keeping feet flat on the floor at shoulder width.

Action: Place hands behind head, and roll hips forward until ball just touches the lower back. Squeeze abdominal muscles and roll backward, returning to original sitting position.

Finish: Complete 15 reps.

5. Core Crunches

Starting position: Start on knees behind ball, resting weight on the outside of the hands and arms on ball.

Action: Roll forward on forearms over the ball, squeezing the abdominal muscles, until weight is on the elbows, stomach touches the ball, and head comes up. The body is nearly straight.

Finish: Return to starting position. Repeat 15 reps.

Upper-Body Muscle Strengthening

6. Push-Ups

Starting position: Lie face down over ball, with hands on floor, arms straight. Place weight on ball on thighs just above knees and on hands. Body is straight, nearly parallel to floor, in a similar position to that used for traditional push-ups.

(Continued on next page)

SIDEBAR 11.5 *(continued)*

Action: Bend elbows, bringing face to near floor, and push up by straightening arms.
Finish: Do 15 reps.

Lower-Body Muscle Strengthening

7. Wall Squat

Starting position: Stand about 2 feet from wall with ball pinned between the wall and the lower back, feet shoulder-width apart and slightly ahead of hips.
Action: Keeping the ball pinned, roll down the wall by bending the knees and dropping the buttocks until thighs are parallel to the floor. Keep abdominal muscles tight and back straight.
Finish: Straighten legs and stand up, keeping back straight. Repeat 15 times.

Lower-Back Muscle Strengthening

8. Trunk Extension

Starting position: Start on knees hugging ball, with stomach pressed lightly against it.
Action: Raising chest and head, place pressure against ball with abdomen until back is straight or slightly arched.
Finish: Hold 10 seconds. Repeat 15 times.

9. Opposite Limb Extension

Starting position: Lie on ball on stomach with arms and legs extended, hands and feet touching floor for balance.
Action: While looking at the floor, raise right arm and left leg. Hold for 2 seconds. Switch sides, raising left arm and right leg.
Finish: Repeat 15 times for each arm-leg combination.

10. Ball Bridge

Starting position: Lie on back on floor, with backs of legs and ankles resting on the ball, knees bent.
Action: Using abdominal muscles and not arms, raise buttocks from floor until back and legs are straight. Hold for 10 seconds.
Finish: Repeat 15 times.

Sources: R. Arnot and C. Gaines, *Sports Talent* (Harmondsworth, United Kingdom: Penguin, 1984); Exercise Pictures (2006). Lifetime Fitness Routines. www.lifetime-fitness-routines.com/exerciseballroutine.html; Top 10: Fitness Ball Exercises. Ask Men. www.askmen.com/top_10/fitness_top_ten/36_fitness_list.html.

- weightlifting
- exercise machines, such as the treadmill, elliptical trainer, step machine, and indoor rower
- trampoline or rebounder
- jump rope
- exercise balls
- yoga
- electronic exercise games

Exercise videos to help individuals get started in almost any activity, from low- and high-impact aerobics and Jazzercise to weightlifting to yoga, can be found at local libraries, book stores, and sporting goods stores and on the Internet. While an individual with a visual impairment or deafblindness may need to sit very close to the screen to get the idea of what the on-screen instructor is doing or may need to ask a family member or a friend for an explanation and assistance, videos are still an excellent option to enhance a home fitness program.

CONCLUSION

There are many ways for people with visual impairments or deafblindness to access the benefits of physical activity, such as improved health and greater ease in performing everyday activities, including those at school or at work. The activities presented in this chapter are perhaps among those most easily accessed or adapted. As should be clear from the information presented throughout this book, however, with some ingenuity, enthusiasm, and knowledge of adaptations, individuals with visual impairments or deafblindness can participate in virtually any sport, recreation, or fitness activity. The results of doing so, not only for health and fitness but also for helping people achieve greater independence, confidence, and overall satisfaction with life, can be life altering.

12 Sports and Related Organizations of Special Interest

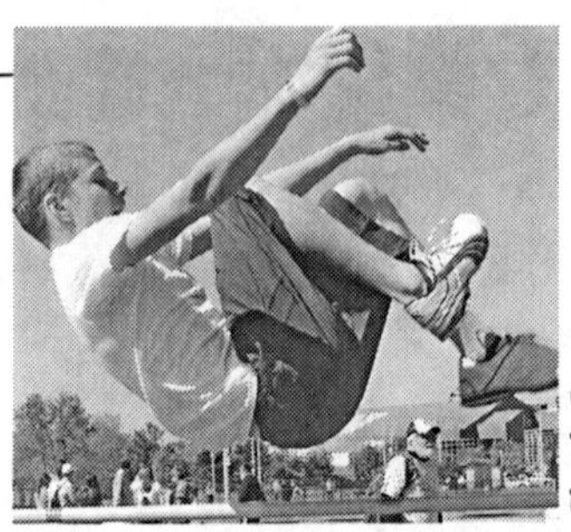
Chuck Comer

IN THIS CHAPTER

- **United States Association of Blind Athletes (USABA)**
- **Canadian Blind Sports Association (CBSA)**
- **Paralympic Games**
- **International Blind Sports Federation (IBSA)**

Individuals with visual impairments or deafblindness who want to participate in sports, recreation, or fitness activities can do so on a variety of levels: as individuals; in local programs or sports clubs, including those geared to people with visual impairments; or at the national or even higher levels of international competition.

Ideally, most communities would offer a wide variety of opportunities for participation in sports and recreation programs for individuals of all ages with visual impairments or deafblindness. In fact, this type of strong, comprehensive programming is available in many communities across the United States and Canada, such as in Atlanta, Colorado Springs, Kalamazoo, Ottawa, Philadelphia, Portland (Maine), Portland (Oregon), San Francisco, St. Augustine, Toronto, and Vancouver. Examples of activities offered in these programs include beep baseball, bowling, canoeing, dragon boating, goalball, kayaking, Nordic and alpine skiing, road racing, rowing, showdown, tandem cycling, and track and field events. Many of the organizations that sponsor the programming in these communities are affiliates of the United States Association of Blind Athletes (USABA) or the Canadian Blind Sports Association (CBSA). The affiliates act as early sports educators for area youths with visual impairments or deafblindness, hold local and state- or provincial-wide competitions, and also recommend and promote local athletes for national training and competitive activities held by the national organizations or the national Paralympic Committees. A few highly talented athletes progress from local to national and on to international competition, such as the Paralympic Games or the International Blind Sports Federation (IBSA) World Championship Games, through this network.

The programs in these communities are unusual, however; most local communities have little or no sports or recreational programming for their citizens with visual impairments, which puts a greater burden on the individual to find opportunities for physical activities. The organizations described in this chapter are working to fill this gap and to develop a strong network for sports and recreation for people with visual impairments or deafblindness. In the United States, many athletic programs for people who are blind or visually impaired are organized through one national organization: the USABA. Similar programs in much of Canada are organized through the CBSA. This chapter discusses these two organizations, along with the two international organizations that sponsor international sports competitions for people with disabilities: the International Paralympic Committee (IPC) and the International Blind Sports Federation (IBSA). In addition, there are many local organizations devoted to providing sports and recreation opportunities for people who are visually impaired or deafblind as well as organizations that focus on a wide variety of individual sports and activities. Information on these organizations appears in the Resources section at the end of this book.

UNITED STATES ASSOCIATION OF BLIND ATHLETES (USABA)

The United States Association of Blind Athletes (USABA) is a nonprofit membership organization that provides opportunities for participation and training and competition in the following sports for athletes who are blind or deafblind or have low vision: athletics (track and field), tandem cycling, showdown, goalball, judo, powerlifting, Nordic and Alpine skiing, swimming, wrestling, 5-a-side football, triathlon, archery, rowing, audio-darts, and ten-pin bowling. Its mission is to "enhance the lives of blind and visually impaired people by providing the opportunity for participation in sports and physical activity" (http://usaba.org/index.php/about-us/mission-and-vision/).The association also has a number of state affiliates across the United States, which are called sports clubs. USABA members range from children with visual impairments who are just beginning to develop their sports skills, to youths who are participating on their school or local club teams, to adults running in a local 5K race, to elite athletes who train for international competitions such as the Paralympic

Games. Since its founding in 1976, the USABA has reached thousands of individuals with visual impairments.

While not everyone who is visually impaired or blind has the ability or desire to be a Paralympian, the skills learned through sports are beneficial in all aspects of daily living, as has been emphasized throughout this book. Rather than focus on limitations, USABA "aims to provide people who are blind and visually impaired the tools to know their abilities by experiencing success through sports" and strives for a future in which all individuals who are visually impaired have the same opportunities to discover their potential and pursue their athletic dreams in the same way as anyone else.

The USABA arose as a result of the efforts of a few pioneers during and following the Paralympic Games of 1976 in Toronto (Dr. Eugenia Scott, personal communication, March 1, 2008). Early blind sports pioneers Charles and Josephine Buell and Arthur and Helen Copeland organized a group of track, swimming, and wrestling athletes who competed in the Toronto Paralympic Games. Scott reported that the first U.S. goalball team to compete internationally was formed "on the spot" in Toronto in 1976 from the track and swimming athletes, none of whom had ever seen a goalball, let alone an actual game, before that time. The first meeting to organize USABA occurred in August 1976 in the days immediately following the Toronto Paralympic Games.

USABA has emerged as more than just a world-class trainer of blind athletes; it has also become a champion of the abilities of American athletes who are legally blind. USABA believes that athletes who are blind or visually impaired can and should compete alongside their sighted peers and against other athletes who are blind and visually impaired. While many athletes who are blind or visually impaired have had great success, according to USABA, each year more than 50,000 youths with visual impairments are left on the sidelines in their schools' physical education classes, and fewer than half have the opportunity to participate on either school or club sports teams. Through programs such as the USABA National Sports Education Camps Project and Camp Abilities, USABA attempts to provide youths with the skills and confidence needed to participate not only in their physical education classes at school but also on sports teams alongside sighted youths. In addition to the Sports Education Camps, USABA provides clinics for youths and adults around the country in judo, tandem cycling, track and field, goalball, Nordic and Alpine skiing, and power lifting. USABA also hosts sports festivals where participants are exposed to a variety of sports during clinic sessions, and at the conclusion of the festival, participants can compete in a sports competition that includes peers with visual impairments and sighted peers.

The USABA website (www.usaba.org) provides information for people who are interested in becoming involved with the organization in development camps (where participants work on improving their performance), trainings, and competitions, as well as on the performance levels required to qualify for various competitions. As a reference resource, USABA, through its website, provides information about upcoming sports events and results of various competitions, including the USABA records for most sports, the results of past Paralympics, and the results of USABA-sanctioned goalball tournaments for the past several years. These records of the highest performance reached by athletes with visual impairments can serve as both goals and inspiration for young athletes. Of particular interest to coaches and teachers, from special educators to physical educators, are the descriptions of the adaptations necessary to make all the major sports activities accessible to athletes with visual impairments.

Most recently, the USABA has begun to serve military veterans who have come back from war with visual impairments. The USABA provides training and competitions for blinded veterans throughout the country.

CANADIAN BLIND SPORTS ASSOCIATION (CBSA)

Like the USABA, the Canadian Blind Sports Association (CBSA) was founded in 1976. It is the recognized national sports organization for goalball and primary advocate for Canadians who are blind or visually impaired. CBSA advocates within the Canadian sports system and has a number of provincial affiliates. Its mission and values are similar to those of the USABA. However, its promotion of accessibility differs somewhat from that of its U.S. counterpart, because barriers to access in Canada relate not only to visual impairment but also to the two official languages of Canada, English and French.

The CBSA leadership promotes a strategy advocating the participation of athletes with visual impairments, with the goal that "an increased number of persons who are blind or visually impaired [will be] involved in sport (as athletes, coaches, officials, volunteers) at all levels (community, provincial, national, and international)" (http://www.canadianblindsports.ca/eng/about/mission.htm). The organization also aims to have "employed and professionally trained coaches, trained officials and volunteers, and high-caliber sport science and sport medicine practitioners . . . reflecting a commitment to a technically and ethically sound and safe program" of sports.

CBSA, through its website, provides excellent information about the game of goalball and about the process of selecting coaches and players for the Canadian National Team. CBSA is in the process of expanding its information about other sports.

CBSA is connected within the Canadian sports system and internationally, and it is recognized by its members, other sports organizations, and the public as a valued representative of goalball and an expert on blindness for sports system participants who are blind or visually impaired. Organizations at the provincial level also provide events, training, and advocacy.

PARALYMPIC GAMES

The Paralympic Games are held in conjunction with the Olympic Games, differing only in that all the Paralympic competitors have a disability of one type or another. According to the website of the International Paralympic Movement (www.paralympic.org), "the Paralympics are elite sport events for athletes with a disability. They emphasize, however, the participants' athletic achievements rather than their disability." (The prefix *para* is derived from the Greek word meaning beside or alongside and is not related to *paraplegia.)*

The Paralympic Games are held every four years in the Olympic host city and in the same facilities as the Olympic Games two to three weeks after completion of the Olympiad. The following are the sports in the Paralympic Games:

Summer

- archery
- athletics (track and field)
- boccia
- equestrian
- football 5-a-side
- football 7-a-side
- goalball
- judo
- para-canoe
- para-cycling
- para–table tennis
- para-triathlon
- powerlifting
- rowing
- sailing
- shooting
- swimming
- volleyball (sitting)
- wheelchair basketball
- wheelchair dance
- wheelchair fencing
- wheelchair rugby
- wheelchair tennis

Winter

- Alpine skiing
- biathlon
- cross-country skiing
- ice sledge hockey
- wheelchair curling

As has been the case with many sports organizations for athletes with disabilities, the Paralympic Games grew from the aftermath of World War II. The precursor, known as the Stoke Mandeville Games, held at a rehabilitation facility in a town of that name in England, pitted World War II veterans with spinal cord injuries against one another in 1948. The first international version of the Stoke Mandeville Games was held in Rome in 1960, where 400 athletes participated from 23 countries, and is considered to be the first summer Paralympic Games. Other disability groups were added in Toronto in 1976, and the first Winter Paralympics followed in Sweden in 1976. By 2012, when the games were held in London, they had grown to include 4,200 athletes from 160 countries competing in 20 sports.

The International Paralympic Committee (IPC), headquartered in Bonn, Germany, was founded in 1989 and is the governing body of the Paralympic Games. The IPC is part of the International Olympic Committee. The mission of the IPC is "to enable paralympic athletes to achieve sporting excellence and inspire and excite the world about their sports abilities" (http://www.paralympic.org/TheIPC/HWA/AboutUs). The membership of the IPC is made up of representatives from approximately 170 National Paralympic Committees, 4 International Organizations of Sport for athletes with specific disabilities (the IBSA is the representative for people with visual impairments), 5 regional organizations, and 13 International Sports Federations. Although there are international organizations, the USABA is the governing body of blind sports. USA Track and USA Swimming are the organizations that oversee swimming and track and field competition for blind athletes.

The IPC, as well as the Paralympic Committees for the United States (usparalympics.org) and Canada (www.paralympic.ca), provide a wealth of information on their websites about the Paralympic movement and all of the sports included in the Paralympic Games. The U.S. website provides a general description of each sport, along with information about the performance plan for that sport, which outlines annual sport objectives and performance goals; contains schedules of trials and training camps, educational sessions, and competitions; and provides information about team selection and other news.

INTERNATIONAL BLIND SPORTS FEDERATION (IBSA)

Whereas the IPC aims its efforts at a broad range of disability groups, the International Blind Sports Federation (which uses the acronym IBSA), as its name indicates, focuses only on athletes with blindness or low vision. IBSA carries out its mission to "promote and foster sports for the blind and visually impaired" at an international level by promoting and organizing competitive events, working to develop and finalize the rules and conditions for the sports, raising awareness of the participation of people with visual impairments in sports, and promoting cooperation among its member organizations (www.ibsa.es). The IBSA holds its World Championships every four years, two years after the Olympiad.

The following is a list of sports covered by IBSA:

- Alpine skiing
- archery
- athletics
- futsal (indoor football)
- goalball
- judo
- nine-pin bowling
- Nordic skiing
- powerlifting
- shooting
- showdown (another indoor sport similar to table tennis)
- swimming
- tandem cycling
- ten-pin bowling
- torball (an indoor court game with aspects of goalball and volleyball)

A few of these sports activities, such as futsal, showdown, and torball, are primarily played in Europe.

IBSA was founded in Paris in 1981 and is a member of the IPC. It currently reports 108 country affiliates on five continents. Its priority is placed on those countries that have not developed adequate sports programs. The leadership of IBSA sees sport as an essential medium for the advancement of people who are blind everywhere.

IBSA provides a great deal of information about individual sports, and its website is the best source of the rules of the major sports played by athletes with visual impairments (which appear under the "Technical Department" link). IBSA's website also provides news, announcements of upcoming competitions across the globe, and records attained and top athletes in each sport—a good source of role models for children and youths.

CONCLUSION

When an individual with a visual impairment or deafblindness becomes involved with one of the umbrella organizations discussed in this chapter, or with any of the sport-specific organizations listed in the Resources section of this book, it can put him or her on a pathway that might start with casual recreational activities or weekend games for young people. This path might lead to local, state-level, and national competitions and might even lead to international glory at the Paralympics or World Championship Games. Although it is up to each individual where he or she wants to go, these resources can help that individual along the way.

Information is included in the Resources section to support teachers, vision professionals, physical educators, families, and individuals in creating and sustaining the kinds of physical activities and programs that promote health and fitness, self-confidence, and independence for people with visual impairments or deafblindness. These resources will be helpful to anyone who needs to obtain more information about adapting a particular sport; find equipment for adapting activities for physical education classes, recreational activities, or starting a community sports program; or even find like-minded people to exercise with. It is the authors' profound hope that the information and resources in this volume will supply the tools to increase access to sports, recreation, and fitness activities among children and adults with visual impairments and deafblindness of every age and ability. The opportunities are endless, and the level of competition is as challenging as one desires. The motto at Camp Abilities, the sports camps founded by Lieberman and mentioned in Chapter 1, is "A Loss of Sight, Never a Loss of Vision." No matter the level of visual impairment or deafblindness, each person should have hopes, dreams, and goals related to sport and physical activity.

References

Adelson, E., & Freiberg, S. (1974). Gross motor development in infants blind from birth. *Child Development, 45,* 1–126.

Agency for Health Care Policy and Research. (1993). *Cataract in adults: Management of functional impairment.* Clinical Practice Guideline No. 4. (AHCPR Publication No. 93-0542). Rockville, MD: U.S. Department of Health and Human Services.

Agran, M., Hong, S., & Blankenship, K. (2007). Promoting the self-determination of students with visual impairments: Reducing the gap between knowledge and practice. *Journal of Visual Impairment & Blindness, 101,* 453–464.

Aillaud, C., & Lieberman, L. J. (in press). *Everybody plays: How children with visual impairments play sports.* Louisville, KY: American Printing House for the Blind.

Allen, K. E., & Marotz, L. R. (1994). *Developmental profiles: Prebirth through eight* (2nd ed.). Albany, NY: Delmar.

Alsop, L., Blaha, R., & Kloos, E. (2000). *The intervener in early intervention and educational settings for children and youth with deafblindness.* National Technical Assistance Consortium for children and young adults who are deaf-blind (NTAC) Web site. Retrieved April 18, 2008, from http://www.tr.wou.edu/nftac/documents/spotlight/intervener.htm

American Association of Snowboard Instructors. (2012). *AASI adaptive snowboard guide.* Lakewood, CO: American Association of Snowboard Instructors.

American Blind Bowling Association (ABBA). (2006). *Official Website.* Retrieved April 2, 2007, from http://www.americanblindbowlers.com/index.asp

American Foundation for the Blind. (2006). *Numbers of blind and visually impaired Americans.* Retrieved January 10, 2007, from http://www.afb.org/Section.asp?SectionID=15#num

American Foundation for the Blind (AFB). (2012). Interpreting Bureau of Labor Statistics Employment Data. New York: American Foundation for the Blind. Retrieved 7/4/2012 from http://www.afb.org/section.aspx?SectionID=15&SubTopicID=177

American Foundation for the Blind. (2012). Special report on aging and vision loss. New York: American Foundation for the Blind. Retrieved April 21, 2012, from http://www.afb.org/Section.asp?SectionID=15&TopicID=413&DocumentID=4423

American Printing House for the Blind. (2006). *Distribution of eligible students based on the federal quota census of January 4, 2004* (Fiscal Year 2005). Louisville, KY: Author. Retrieved February 7, 2007, from http://www.aph.org/fedquotpgm/dist05.html

American Psychological Association (APA). (2003). *Guidelines for non-handicapping language in APA journals.* Retrieved January 10, 2007, from http://www.apastyle.org/disabilities.html

Andersen, E. S., Dunlea, A., & Kekelis, L. S. (1984). Blind children's language: Resolving some differences. *Journal of Child Language, 11,* 645–664.

Andrews, B. (n.d.). Basic blind golf techniques. Retrieved 7/4/12 from www.usblindgolf.com/index.php?option=com_content&view=article&id=95&Itemid=108

Anshel, M. H., Freedson, P., Hamill, J., Haywood, K., Horvat, M., & Plowman, S. A. (1991). *Dictionary of sport and exercise sciences.* Champaign, IL: Human Kinetics.

Anthony, T. L. (1993). Orientation and mobility for the young child who is visually impaired. In Blind Children's Center (Ed.), *First steps: A handbook for teaching young children who are visually impaired* (pp. 115–138). Los Angeles, CA: Blind Children's Center.

Anthony, T. L. (1999). When a child in your classroom has a visual impairment. In T. Linder (Ed.), *Read, play, and learn! Storybook activities for young children* (pp. 97–116). Baltimore, MD: Paul Brookes Publishing.

Anthony, T. L., Bleier, H., Fazzi, D. L., Kish, D., & Pogrund, R. L. (2002). Mobility focus: Developing early skills for orientation and mobility. In R. L. Pogrund & D. L. Fazzi (Eds.), *Early focus: Working with young children who are blind or visually impaired and their families* (2nd ed., pp. 326–404). New York: AFB Press.

Anthony, T. L., Lowry, S. S., Brown, C. J., & Hatton, D. D. (2004). *Developmentally appropriate orientation and mobility.* Chapel Hill: FPG Child Development Institute, University of North Carolina.

Arndt, K. L., Lieberman, L. J., & Pucci, G. (2004). Communication during physical activity for youth who are deafblind. *Teaching Exceptional Children Plus, 1*(2), Article 1.

Arnhold, R. W., & McGrain, P. (1985). Selected kinematic patterns of visually impaired youth in spring running. *Adapted Physical Activity Quarterly, 2,* 206–213.

Arnot, R., & Gaines, C. (1984). *Sports talent.* Harmondsworth, United Kingdom: Penguin.

Axelrod, C. (2004). Supporting high quality interactions with students who are deafblind, part one: A summary of current research. *See/Hear* 9(4).

Ayers, A. J. (1983). *Sensory integration and the child.* Los Angeles: Western Psychological Services.

Bailey, A. L., & Hall, A. (1990). *Visual impairment: An overview.* New York: AFB Press.

Barclay, L. (2011). *Learning to listen/listening to learn: Teaching listening skills to students with visual impairments.* New York: AFB Press.

Barker, P. (1996). *Dragon boats: A celebration.* Vancouver, BC: Raincoast Books.

Barnett, L. A., & Webber, J. J. (2008). Perceived benefits to children from participating in different types of recreational activities. *Journal of Park & Recreation Administration, 26*(3), 1–20. Retrieved 7/4/2012 from EBSCO*host* .com.

Barraga, N. (1976). *Visual handicaps and learning: A developmental approach.* Belmont, CA: Wadsworth.

Barraga, N. C., & Erin, J. N. (2001). Movement, exploration, and spatial awareness. In *Visual impairments and learning* (4th ed., pp. 35–46). Austin, TX: Pro Ed.

Beets, M., Foley, J., Tindall, D. W., & Lieberman, L. J. (2007). Accuracy of voice-announcement pedometers for youth with visual impairment. *Adapted Physical Activity Quarterly, 24*(3), 218–227.

Benton, K. (2011). Developing a multisensory outdoor education program. *Insight Journal, 4,* 177–180.

Bentzen, B. L., & Marston, J. R. (2010). Teaching the use of orientation aids for orientation and mobility. In W. R. Wiener, R. L. Welsh, & B. B. Blasch (Eds.), *Foundations of orientation and mobility: Vol. 2. Instructional strategies and practical applications* (3rd ed., pp. 315–351). New York: AFB Press.

Best, C., Lieberman, L. J., & Arndt, K. (2002). The use of interpreters in physical education. *Journal of Physical Education, Recreation & Dance, 73*(8), 45–50.

Biddle, S. J. H., Fox, K. R., & Boutcher, S. H. (Eds.). (2000). *Physical activity and psychological well-being.* New York: Routledge.

Bigelow, A. (1986). The development of reaching in blind children. *British Journal of Developmental Psychology, 4,* 355–366.

Bigelow, A. E. (1992). Locomotion and search behavior in blind infants. *Infant Behavior and Development, 15,* 179–189.

Blas, T. (2011). Getting fit with an accessible rowing machine. Technology for the Blind. Retrieved 7/4/12 from http://blindtechnology.wordpress.com/2011/02/16/getting-fit-with-an-accessible-rowing-machine/.

Blessing, D. L., McCrimmon, D., Stovall, J., & Williford, H. N. (1993). The effects of regular exercise programs for visually impaired and sighted schoolchildren. *Journal of Visual Impairment & Blindness, 87,* 50–52.

Blinde, E. M., & McCallister, S. G. (1998). Listening to the voices of students with physical disabilities. *Journal of Physical Education, Recreation & Dance, 69*(6), 64–68.

Blinde, E. M., & McClung, L. R. (1997). Enhancing the physical and social self through recreational activity: Accounts of individuals with disabilities. *Adapted Physical Activity Quarterly, 14,* 327–344.

Block, M.E. (2007). *A teacher's guide to including children with disabilities in general physical education.* Baltimore, MD: Brookes Publishers.

Boffoli, N., Foley, J. T., Gasparetti, B., Yang, S. P., & Lieberman, L. J. (2011). Enjoyment levels of youth with visual impairments playing different exergames. *Insight: Research and Practice in Visual Impairment and Blindness, 4,* 171–176.

Bourquin, E., & Sauerburger, D. (2005). Teaching deafblind people to communicate and interact with the public: Critical issues for travelers who are deaf-blind. *RE:view, 37,* 109–116.

Bozeman, L., & McCulley, R. (2010). Improving orientation for students with vision loss. In W. Wiener, R. Welsch, & B. Blasch (Eds.), *Foundations of orientation and mobility: Vol. 2. Instructional strategies and practical applications* (3rd ed., pp. 27–53). New York: AFB Press.

Bradsher, J. E. (1997). *Disability among racial and ethnic groups, #10. Disability Statistics Abstract.* University of California at San Francisco. Retrieved September 1, 2006, from http://www.dsc.ucsf.edu

Brambring, M. (2006). Divergent development of gross motor skills in children who are blind or sighted. *Journal of Visual Impairment & Blindness, 100*(October), 620–634.

Brocklehurst-Woods, J. (1990). The use of tactile and vestibular stimulation to reduce stereotypic behaviors in two adults with mental retardation. *American Journal of Occupational Therapy, 44*(6), 536–541.

Brown, C., & Bour, B. (1986). *Volume V-K: Movement analysis and curriculum for visually impaired preschoolers.* Tallahassee: State of Florida Department of Education Bureau of Education for Exceptional Students.

Brown, C. J., Anthony, T. L., Lowry, S. S., & Hatton, D. D. (2004). Motor development and movement. In T. L. Anthony, S. S. Lowry, C. J. Brown, & D. D. Hatton (Eds.), *Developmentally appropriate orientation and mobility* (pp. 347–482). Chapel Hill: FPG Child Development Institute, University of North Carolina at Chapel Hill.

Brown, D. (2007). The vestibular sense. *Deafblind International Review* (January–June), 1–22.

Brown, S. C. (1991). Conceptualizing and defining disability. In S. Thompson-Hoffman & I. F. Storck (Eds.), *Disability in the United States: A portrait from national data* (pp. 1–14). New York: Springer.

Buell, C. E. (1973). *Physical education and recreation for the visually handicapped.* Reston, VA: American Alliance for Health, Physical Education, Recreation and Dance.

Buell, C. E. (1982). *Physical education and recreation for the visually handicapped* (2nd ed.). Reston, VA: American Alliance for Health, Physical Education, Recreation and Dance.

Bundy, A. C. (2008). Facilitating sensorimotor development. In T. Linder (Ed.), *Transdisciplinary play-based intervention* (2nd ed., pp. 29–141). Baltimore, MD: Paul Brookes Publishing.

Burton, D., & Huffman, L. (2007). Exercising your right to fitness: An overview of the accessibility of exercise equipment. *AccessWorld 8* (5), www.afb.org/afbpress/pub.asp?DocID=aw080603

Carello, C., & Turvey, M. T. (2000). Rotational invariance in dynamic touch. In M. A. Heller (Ed.), *Touch representation and blindness* (pp. 27–66). Oxford: Oxford University Press.

Carroll, T. J. (1961). *Blindness: What it is, what it does and how to live with it.* Boston: Little, Brown.

Celeste, M. (2002). A survey of motor development for infants and children with visual impairments. *Journal of Visual Impairment & Blindness, 96*(3), 169–174.

Centers for Disease Control (CDC). (2004). Participation in high school physical education:

United States, 1991–2003. MMWR, *53*(36), 844–847. Retrieved April 2, 2007, from http://www.cdc.gov/mmwr/about.html

Chen, D., Downing, J., & Rodriguez-Gil, G. (2001). Tactile learning strategies for children who are deafblind: Concerns and considerations from project SOLUTE. *Deaf-Blind Perspectives, 8,* 1–6.

Chiang, Y., Bassi, L. J., & Javitt, J. C. (1992). Federal budgetary costs of blindness. *Millbank Quarterly, 70*(2), 319–340.

Clark, A. J. (1991). The identification and modification of defense mechanisms in counseling. *Journal of Counseling & Development, 69,* 231–236.

Cochran, N. A., Wilkinson, L. C., & Furlow, J. J. (1981). *Learning on the move: An activity guide for preschool parents and teachers.* Dubuque, IA: Kendall/Hunt.

Cohen, L. G., Celnik, P., Pascual-Leone, A., Corwell, B., Falz, L., Dambrosia, J., & Honda, M. (1997). Functional relevance of cross-modal plasticity in blind humans. *Nature, 389,* 180–183.

Columna, L., Davis, T., Lieberman, L. J., & Lytle, R. (2010). Determining the most appropriate physical education placement for students with disabilities. *Journal of Physical Education, Recreation & Dance, 81,* 30–37.

Concept2 (n.d.). Rowing and skiing for the visually impaired. Retrieved 5/5/12 from www.concept2.com/us/communities/adaptive/visually_impaired.asp

Conroy, P. (2012). Supporting students with visual impairments in physical education: Needs of physical educators. *InSight: Research and Practice in Visual Impairment and Blindness,* 5(1), 3–10.

Cooper Institute for Aerobic Research. (2004). *The Prudential FITNESSGRAM test administration manual.* Dallas, TX: Cooper Institute for Aerobic Research.

Corbin, C. B., Welk, G., Lindsey, R., & Corbin, W. R. (2004). *Concepts of fitness and wellness: A comprehensive lifestyle approach.* Boston: McGraw-Hill.

Corn, A. L., Bina, M. J., & Sacks, S. Z. (2009). *Looking good.* Austin, TX: Pro-Ed.

Corn, A. L., & Koening, A. J. (1996). *Foundations of low vision: Clinical and functional perspectives.* New York: AFB Press.

Corn, A. L., & Lusk, K. E. (2010). Perspectives on low vision. In A. L. Corn & J. N. Erin (Eds.), *Foundations of low vision: Clinical and functional perspectives* (2nd ed., pp. 3–34). New York: AFB Press.

Cratty, B. J. (1971). *Movement and spatial awareness in blind children and youth.* Springfield, IL: Charles C Thomas.

Cratty, B. J., & Sams, T. A. (1969). *The body-image of blind children.* New York: American Foundation for the Blind.

Cutter, J. (2007). *Independent movement and travel in blind children: A promotional model.* Charlotte, NC: Information Age Publishing.

Dave, C. A. (1992). Effects of linear vestibular stimulation on body-rocking behavior in adults with profound mental retardation. *American Journal of Occupational Therapy, 46,* 910–915.

Davis, R. W., Kotecki, J. E., Harvey, M. W., & Oliver, A. (2007). Responsibilities and training needs of paraeducators in physical education. *Adapted Physical Activity Quarterly, 24,* 70–83.

Davis, T. D. (n.d.). *Adapted physical education national standards.* SUNY Cortland website. Retrieved 3/1/2008, from http://www.cortland.edu/APENS/whatisapens.htm

Deci, E. L., & Ryan, R. M. (1995). Human autonomy: The basis for true self-esteem. In M. Kernis (Ed.), *Efficacy, agency, and self-esteem* (pp. 31–49). New York: Plenum Publishing Co.

Dodds, A. (2006). *A psychologist looks at blindness.* Charleston, SC: Booksurge Publishing.

Duffy, M. A. (2002). *Making life more livable: Simple adaptations for living at home after vision loss.* New York: AFB Press.

Dunn, J. M., & Ponticelli, J. (1988). The effect of two different communication modes on motor performance test scores of hearing impaired children. In D. L. Gill & J. E. Clark (Eds.), *Abstracts of research papers 1988* (p. 246). Reston, VA: American Alliance for Health, Physical Education, Recreation & Dance.

Edman, P. K. (1992). *Tactile graphics.* New York: American Foundation for the Blind.

Emerson, R. W., & Ashmead, D. H. (2008). Visual experience and the concept of compensatory spatial hearing abilities. In J. J. Rieser, D. H. Ashmead, F. F. Ebner, A. L. Corn, (Eds.), *Blindness and Brain Plasticity in Navigation and Object Perception*, pp. 367–380. New York. Lawrence Erlbaum.

Engleman, M. D., & Griffin, H. C. (1998). Deafblindness and communication: Practical knowledge and strategies. *Journal of Visual Impairment & Blindness, 92*(11), 783–798.

Fait, H. (1978). *Special physical education.* Philadelphia: W. B. Saunders.

Farrenkopf, C., & McGregor, D. (2000). Physical education and health. In A. J. Koenig & M. C. Holbrook, (Eds.), *Foundations of education*, Vol. 2: *Instructional strategies for teaching children and youths with visual impairments* (2nd ed., pp. 437–463). New York: AFB Press.

Fazzi, D. L., & Klein, M. D. (2002). Cognitive focus: Developing concepts, cognition, and language. In R. L. Pogrund & D. L. Fazzi (Eds.), *Early focus: Working with young children who are blind or visually impaired and their families* (2nd ed., pp. 107–153). New York: AFB Press.

Fazzi, D. L., & Petersmeyer, B. A. (2001). *Imagining the possibilities: Creative approaches to orientation and mobility instruction with a student with multiple disabilities.* New York: AFB Press.

Ferrell, K. A. (1985). *Reach out and teach: Meeting the training needs of parents of visually and multiply handicapped young children.* New York: AFB Press.

Ferrell, K. A. (1986). Infancy and early childhood. In G. T. Scholl (Ed.), *Foundations of education for blind and visually handicapped children and youth: Theory and practice* (pp. 119–135). New York: AFB Press.

Ferrell, K. A. (1998). *Project PRISM: A longitudinal study of the developmental patterns of children who are visually impaired: Executive summary: CFDA 84.0203C: Field-initiated research HO23C10188.* Greeley: University of Northern Colorado.

Ferrell, K. A. (2000). Growth and development of young children. In M. C. Holbrook & A. J. Koenig (Eds.), *Foundations of education: History and theory of teaching children and youths with visual impairments.* New York: AFB Press.

Ferrell, K. A. (2011). *Reach out and teach: Helping your child who is visually impaired learn and grow* (2nd ed.). New York: AFB Press.

Fitzgerald, H., & Kirk, D. (2009). Identity work: Young disabled people, family and sport. *Leisure Studies, 28*(4), 469–488. doi:10.1080/02614360903078659.

Foley, J., Lieberman, L., & Wood, B. (2008). Teaching strategies with pedometers for all children. *RE:View, 39,* 206–212.

Foley, J., Tindall, D. W., Lieberman, L. J., & Kim, S. (2007). How to develop disability awareness using the Sport Education model. *Journal of Physical Education, Recreation & Dance, 78,* 32–36.

Fraiberg, S. (1968). Parallel and divergent patterns in blind and sighted infants. *Psychoanalytic Study of the Child, 23,* 264–300.

Fraiberg, S., Siegel, B., & Gibson, R. (1966). The role of sound in the search behavior of a blind infant. *Psychoanalytical Study of the Child, 21,* 327–357.

Fraiberg, S. H. (1977). *Insights from the blind: Comparative studies of blind and sighted infants.* New York: Basic Books.

Freedman, D. A. (1971). Congenital and perinatal sensory deprivation: Some studies in early development. *American Journal of Psychiatry, 127*(11), 1539–1545.

Frostig, M., & Masow, A. H. (1972). *Move, grow, learn.* River Grove, IL: Follett.

Gallagher, J. (n.d.). Deafblind or deaf-blind, side bar on terminology. *A-Z to Deafblindness.* Retrieved April 21, 2012, from http://deafblind.com/lagati.html

Garvey, C. (1977). *Play.* Cambridge, MA: Harvard University Press.

Gasperetti, B., Milford, M., Blanchard, D., Yang, S., Lieberman, L., & Foley, J. (2010). Dance Dance Revolution and eye toy kinetic modifications for youth with visual impairments.

Journal of Physical Education, Recreation & Dance, 81, 15–17, 55.

Gilbert, A. (2007). *Rowing World Newsletter,* Volume 1.

Ginsburg, H., & Opper, S. (1969). *Piaget's theory of intellectual development: An introduction.* Englewood Cliffs, NJ: Prentice-Hall.

Gleason, D. J. (2004). *Developmental sequence of auditory localization.* Chapel Hill: Early Intervention Training Center for Infants and Toddlers with Visual Impairments, FPG Child Development Institute, University of North Carolina at Chapel Hill.

Gleser, J. M., Margulies, J. Y., Nyska, M., Porat, S., & Mendelberg, H. (1992). Physical and psychosocial benefits of modified judo practice for blind, mentally retarded children: A pilot study. *Perceptual and Motor Skills, 74,* 915–925.

Goldberg, S. & William Trattler, W. (2012). *Ophthalmology Made Ridiculously Simple,* 5th ed. Miami, FL: Medmaster.

Goldfine, B. D. (1993). Incorporating health-fitness concepts in secondary physical education curricula. *Journal of School Health, 63,* 142–147.

Goodwin, D. L. (2001). The meaning of help in PE: Perceptions of students with disabilities. *Adapted Physical Activity Quarterly, 18*(3), 289–303.

Goodwin, D. L., Lieberman, L. J., Johnston, K., & Leo, J. (2011). Connecting through summer camp: Youth with visual impairments find a sense of community. *Adapted Physical Activity Quarterly, 28,* 40–55.

Graham, G., Holt/Hale, S. A., & Parker, M. A. (2009). *Children moving: A reflective approach to teaching physical education* 8th ed. New York: McGraw Hill.

Graziadei, A. (1998). *Learning outcomes of deaf and hard of hearing students in mainstreamed physical education classes.* Unpublished doctoral dissertation, University of Maryland, College Park.

Greeley, J., & Anthony, T. (1995). Play interaction with infants and toddlers who are deafblind: Setting the stage. *Seminars in Hearing, 16*(2), 185–191.

Griffin, S. (2011). The history of tandem bikes. Livestrong.com. Retrieved 5/5/12 from http://www.livestrong.com/article/366725-the-history-of-tandem-bikes/

Guth, D., & LaDuke, R. (1995). Veering by blind pedestrians: Individual differences and their implications for instruction. *Journal of Visual Impairment & Blindness, 89,* 28–37.

Guth, D. A., & Rieser, J. J. (1997). Perceptions and the control of locomotion by blind and visually impaired persons. In B. B. Blasch, W. R. Wiener, & R. L. Welsh (Eds.), *Foundations of orientation and mobility* (2nd ed., pp. 9–38). New York: AFB Press.

Guth, D. A., Rieser, J. J., & Ashmead D. H. (2010). Perceiving to move and moving to perceive: Control of locomotion. In W. R. Wiener, R. L. Welsh, & B. B. Blasch (Eds.), *Foundations of orientation and mobility* (3rd ed.)*:* Vol. I: *History and theory* (pp. 3–44). New York: AFB Press.

Haibach, P., Lieberman, L. J., & Ritter, J. (2011). Balance in adolescents with and without visual impairments. *Insight: Research and Practice in Visual Impairment and Blindness, 4,* 112–121.

Harris, L. (1998). Americans with disabilities still face sharp gaps in securing jobs, education, transportation, and many areas of daily life. *See/Hear, 3*(4), 32–34.

Hatlen, P. (1996). The core curriculum for blind and visually impaired students, including those with additional disabilities. *RE:View, 28*(1), 25–32.

Hatton, D. D., Bailey, D. B., Burchinal, M. R., & Ferrell, K. A. (1997). Developmental growth curves of preschool children with vision impairments. *Child Development, 68*(5), 788–806.

Hein, G. E. (1991). Constructivist learning theory. Paper presented at *CECA (International Committee of Museum Educators) Conference,* Jerusalem, Israel, 15–22 October. Retrieved 7/4/12 from http://www.exploratorium.edu/ifi/resources/constructivistlearning

Heller, M. A., Ed. (2000). *Touch, representation, and blindness.* Oxford: Oxford University Press.

Henderson, H. L., French, R., & Kinnison, L. (2001). Reporting grades for students with disabilities in general physical education. *Journal of Physical Education, Recreation & Dance, 72*(6), 50–55.

Hill, B., Rotegard, L., & Bruininks, R. (1984). The quality of life of mentally retarded people in residential care. *Social Work, 29,* 275–281.

History of Beep Baseball and the NBBA (n.d.). National Beep Baseball Association Hall of Fame. Retrieved 5/23/12 from http://halloffame.nbba.org/history/index.htm.

Hodge, S., Lieberman, L. J., & Murata, N. (2012). *Essentials of teaching physical education: Culture, diversity, and inclusion.* Scottsdale, AZ: Holcom Hathaway.

Holbrook, E. A., Caputo, J. L., Perry, T. L., Fuller, D. K., & Morgan, D. W. (2009). Physical activity, body composition, and perceived quality of life of adults with visual impairments. *Journal of Visual Impairment & Blindness, 103*(1), 17–29.

Holbrook, E. A., Stevens, S. L., Kang, M., & Morgan, D. W. (2011). Validation of talking pedometers with adults with visual impairments. *Medicine & Science in Sports & Exercise, 6,* 1094–1099.

Holbrook, M. C. (Ed.). (1996). *Children with visual impairments: A parents' guide.* Bethesda, MD: Woodbine House.

Hopkins, W. G., Gaeta, H., Thomas, A. C., & Hill, M. (1987). Physical fitness of blind and sighted children. *European Journal of Applied Physiology, 56,* 69–73.

Houwen, S., Hartman, E., Jonker, L., & Visscher, C. (2010). Reliability and validity of the TGMD-2 in primary school age children with visual impairments. *Adapted Physical Activity Quarterly, 27,* 143–149.

Houwen, S., Hartman, E., & Visscher, C. (2009). Physical activity and motor skills in children with and without visual impairments. *Medicine & Science in Sports & Exercise, 41*(1), 103–109.

Houwen, S., Visscher, C., Hartman, E., & Lemmink, K. A. P. M. (2007). Gross motor skills and sport participation of children with visual impairments. *Research Quarterly for Exercise and Sport, 78,* 16–23.

Houwen, S., Visscher, C., Lemmink, K. A. P. M., & Hartman, E. (2008). Motor skill performance of school age children with visual impairments. *Developmental Medicine and Child Neurology, 50,* 139–145.

Huebner, K. M., Prickett, J. G., Welch, T. R., & Joffee, E. (Eds.). (1995). *Hand in hand: Essentials of communication and mobility for your students who are deafblind, Vol. 2.* New York: AFB Press.

Individuals with Disabilities Education Improvement Act (IDEA) of 2004, H.R. 1350, (2004).

International Association of Athletics Federations. (n.d.). What is athletics? Retrieved 4/3/12 from www.iaaf.org/community/athletics/index.html

International Blind Sports Federation (IBSA). (n.d.). Goalball: General Information. Retrieved 5/23/12 from www.ibsa.es/eng/deportes/goalball/presentacion.htm

International Blind Sports Federation (IBSA). (n.d.). Judo rules, 2009-2013. Retrieved 3/7/12 from www.ibsa.es/eng/deportes/judo/reglamento.htm

Iso-Ahola, S. E. & Park, C. J. (1996). Leisure-related social support and self-determination as buffers of stress-illness relationship. *Journal of Leisure Research, 28*(3), 169–187.

Jacobs, J. E., & Eccles, J. S. (1992). The impact of mothers' gender-role stereotypic beliefs on mothers' and children's ability perceptions. *Journal of Personality and Social Psychology, 63*(6), 932–944.

Jan, J., Robinson, G., Scott, E., & Kinnis, C. (1975). Hypotonia in the blind child. *Developmental Medicine and Child Neurology, 17,* 35–40.

Jankowski, L. W., & Evans, J. K. (1981). The exercise capability of blind children. *Journal of Visual Impairment & Blindness, 75,* 248–251.

Johnson, C. C. (2009). The benefits of physical activity for youth with developmental disabilities: A systematic review. *American Journal of Health Promotion, 23*(3), 157–167. Retrieved 7/4/2012 from EBSCO*host*.com.

Kaplan, M. (1975). *Leisure: Theory and policy.* New York: Wiley & Sons.

Katz, D. (1989). *The world of touch.* (L. E. Krueger, Trans.). Hillsdale, NJ: Lawrence Erlbaum Associates.

Kaye, S. (1997). The status of people with disabilities in the United States. *Disability Watch* (pp. 1–37). Volcano, CA: Volcano Press.

Kenney W. L., Bryant C. X., Humphrey, R. H., Mahler, D. A., Froehlicher, V., Miller, N. H., & York, T. D. (Eds.). (1995). *American college of sports medicine: ACSM's guidelines for exercise testing and prescription* (5th ed.). Baltimore, MD: Williams & Wilkins.

Kilpatrick, M., Hebert, E., & Jacobsen, D. (2002). Physical activity motivation: A practitioner's guide to self-determination theory. *Journal of Physical Education, Recreation & Dance, 73*(4), 36–41.

Kilpatrick, M. W., Bartholomew, J. B., & Riemer, H. L. (2003). The development of orientation in exercise (GOES): A modification of the task and ego orientation sport questionnaire (TEOSQ). *Journal of Sport Behavior, 26,* 121–136.

Kirchner, C., & Diament, S. (1999). Usable data report: Estimates of the number of visually impaired students, their teachers, and orientation and mobility specialists: Part I. *Journal of Visual Impairment & Blindness, 93,* 600–606.

Kirwan, B., & Ainsworth, L. (Eds.). (1992). *A guide to task analysis.* London: Taylor and Francis.

Kobasa, S. (1979). Stressful life events, personality, and health: An inquiry into hardiness. *Journal of Personality and Social Psychology, 37,* 1–11.

Kobberling, G., Jankowski, L. W., & Leger, L. (1989). Energy cost of locomotion in blind adolescents. *Adapted Physical Activity Quarterly, 6,* 58–67.

Kobberling, G., Jankowski, L., & Leger, L. (1991). The relationship between aerobic capacity and physical activity in blind and sighted adolescents. *Journal of Visual Impairment & Blindness, 85,* 382–384.

Koenig, A. J., & Holbrook, M. C. (Eds.) (2000). *Foundations of education* (Vols. 1 & 2, 2nd ed.). New York: AFB Press.

Kowalski, E., Lieberman, L. J., Pucci, G., & Mulawka, C. (2005). Implementing IEP or 504 goals and objectives into general physical education. *Journal of Physical Education, Recreation & Dance, 76*(7), 33–37.

Kozub, F. M., & Oh, H. (2004). An exploratory study of physical activity levels in children and adolescents with visual impairments. *Clinical Kinesiology, 58*(3), 1–7.

Kratz, L. E. (1973). *Movement without sight.* Palo Alto, CA: Peek Publications.

Kukla, D., & Thomas, T. (1978). *Assessment of auditory functioning of deaf-blind/multihandicapped children.* Dallas, TX: South Central Regional Center for Services to Deaf-Blind Children.

Lagati, S. (1995). "Deaf-blind" or "deafblind"? International perspectives on terminology. *Journal of Visual Impairment & Blindness: Special Issue on Deaf-blindness, 89*(3), 305.

Lawson, G., & Wiener, W. W. (2010). Audition for students with vision loss. In W. R. Wiener, R. L. Welsh, & B. B. Blasch, (Eds.). *Foundations of orientation and mobility,* Vol. 1: *History and Theory* (3rd ed., pp. 84–137). New York: AFB Press.

Lawton, M. P. (1994). Personality and affective correlates of leisure activity participation by older people. *Journal of Leisure Research, 26*(2), 138–157.

Lee, M., Ward, G., & Shephard, R. J. (1985). Physical capacities of sightless adolescents. *Developmental Medicine and Child Neurology, 27*(6), 767–774.

Leitner, M. J., & Leitner, S. F. (1996). *Leisure in later life,* 2nd ed. New York: Haworth Press.

Lepore, M., Gayle, G. W., & Stevens, S. (2007). *Adapted aquatics programming: A professional guide.* Champaign, IL: Human Kinetics.

Lewis, S., & Allman, C. B. (2000). Educational programming. In M. C. Holbrook & A. J. Koenig (Eds.). *Foundations of education: History and theory of teaching children and youths with visual impairments.* New York. AFB Press.

Lewis, S., & Wolffe, K. E. (2006). Promoting and nurturing self-esteem. In S. Z. Sacks & K. E.

Wolffe (Eds.), *Teaching social skills to students with visual impairments: From theory to practice* (pp. 122–162). New York: AFB Press.

Lieberman, L. J. (2002). Fitness for individuals who are visually impaired or deafblind. *RE:View, 34*(1), 13–23.

Lieberman, L. J. (Ed.). (2007). *Paraeducators in physical education: A training guide to roles and responsibilities.* Champaign, IL: Human Kinetics.

Lieberman, L. J. (2010). Communication with individuals who are deafblind during physical activity: Eight steps. Paper presented at the Association for Education and Rehabilitation of the Blind and Visually Impaired International Conference, Little Rock, Arkansas. Retrieved 3/12/12 from http://www.aerbvi.org/2010conference/documents/LeibermanAERCommunication.ppt

Lieberman, L. J. (2011). Visual impairments. In J. P. Winnick (Ed.), *Adapted physical Education and Sport* (5th ed.). Champaign, IL: Human Kinetics.

Lieberman, L. J., & Arndt, K. L. (2004). Language to live and learn by. *Teaching Elementary Physical Education, 15*(2), 33–34.

Lieberman, L. J., Arndt, K. L, & Barry Grassick, S. (2010). Promoting leadership for individuals who are deafblind through a summer camp experience. *AER Journal: Research and Practice in Visual Impairment and Blindness*, 3 (Fall), 153–159.

Lieberman, L. J., Butcher, M., & Moak, S. (2001). Preferred guide-running techniques for children who are blind. *Palaestra, 17*(3), 20–26, 55.

Lieberman, L. J., Byrne, H., Mattern, C., & Fernández-Vivó, M. (2006, October). *Physical fitness and youth with visual impairments.* Paper presented at the annual meeting of the North American Federation of Adapted Physical Education Conference, Ann Arbor, MI.

Lieberman, L. J., Byrne, H., Mattern, C., Watt, C., & Fernández-Vivó, M. (2010). Health-related fitness in youth with visual impairments. *Journal of Visual Impairment & Blindness, 104*(6), 349–359.

Lieberman, L. J., & Conroy, P. (in press). Paraeducator training for physical education for children with visual impairments. *Journal of Visual Impairment & Blindness.*

Lieberman, L. J., & Cowart, J. (2011). *Games for people with sensory impairments* (2nd ed.). Louisville, KY: American Printing House for the Blind.

Lieberman, L. J., Haibach, P., & Schedlin, H. (2012). Physical education and children with CHARGE syndrome: Research to practice. *Journal of Visual Impairment & Blindness, 106*(2), 106–119.

Lieberman, L. J., & Houston-Wilson, C. (2009). *Strategies for inclusion: A handbook for physical education* (2nd ed.). Champaign, IL: Human Kinetics.

Lieberman, L. J., Houston-Wilson, C., & Kozub, F. (2002). Perceived barriers to including students with visual impairments and blindness into physical education. *Adapted Physical Activity Quarterly, 19*(3), 364–377.

Lieberman, L. J., Lytle, R., & Clarcq, J. (2008). Getting it right from the start: Employing the universal design for learning into your curriculum. *Journal of Physical Education, Recreation & Dance, 79,* 32–39.

Lieberman, L. J., & MacVicar, J. (2003). Play and recreation habits of youth who are deaf-blind. *Journal of Visual Impairment & Blindness, 97*(12), 755–768.

Lieberman, L. J., & McHugh, E. (2001). Health-related fitness of children who are visually impaired. *Journal of Visual Impairment & Blindness, 95,* 272–285.

Lieberman, L. J., Modell, S. J., Ponchillia, P. E., & Jackson, I. (2006). *Going places: Transition guidelines for community-based physical activities for students who have visual impairments, blindness, or deafblindness.* Louisville, KY: American Printing House for the Blind.

Lieberman, L. J., & Pecorella, M. (2006). Activity at home for children and youth who are deafblind. *Deaf-Blind Perspectives, 14,* 3–7.

Lieberman, L., Robinson, B., Byrne, H., & Fernández-Vivó, M. (2006). *Passing of children*

with visual impairments rates on the Brockport Physical Fitness Test. American Alliance for Health, Physical Education, Recreation, & Dance Conference, Salt Lake City, Utah.

Lieberman, L. J., Robinson, B., & Rollheiser, H. (2006). Youth with visual impairments: Experiences within general physical education. *RE:View, 38*(1), 35–48.

Lieberman, L. J., Schedlin, H., & Pierce, T. (2009). Teaching jump rope to children with visual impairments. *Journal of Visual Impairment & Blindness, 103,* 173–178.

Lieberman, L., & Stuart, M. (2002). Self-determined recreational and leisure choices of individuals with deaf-blindness. *Journal of Visual Impairment & Blindness, 96*(10), 724–735.

Lieberman, L. J., Stuart, M. E., Hand, K., & Robinson, B. (2006). An investigation of the motivational effects of talking pedometers among youth with visual impairments and deaf-blindness. *Journal of Visual Impairment & Blindness, 100*(12), 726–736.

Lieberman, L. J., & Taule, J. (1998). Including physical fitness into the lives of individuals who are deafblind. *Deafblind Perspectives, 5*(2), 6–10.

Liebs, A. (in press). The encyclopedia of sports and recreation for people with visual impairments. Charlotte, NC: Information Age Publishing.

Lin, T. (2012, June 5). Hitting the court, with an ear on the ball. *New York Times,* p. D1.

Linder, T. (1993). Play, assessment, and the transdisciplinary process. In T. Linder (Ed.), *Transdisciplinary play-based assessment: A functional approach to working with young children* (pp. 23–40). Baltimore, MD: Paul Brookes Publishing.

Linder, T. (2008). Cognitive development domain. In T. Linder (Ed.), *Transdisciplinary play-based assessment* (2nd ed., pp. 313–397). Baltimore, MD: Paul Brookes Publishing.

Livneh, H. (1991). A unified approach to existing models of adaptation to disability: A model of adaptation, In R. P. Marinelli & A. E. Dell Orto (Eds.), *The psychological and social impact of disability* (3rd ed., pp. 111–138). New York, NY: Springer.

Lolli, D., Sauerburger, D., & Bourquin, E. A. (2010). Teaching orientation and mobility to students with vision and hearing loss. In W. R. Wiener, R. L. Welsh, & B. B. Blasch (Eds.), *Foundations of orientation and mobility:* Vol. 2: *Instructional strategies and practical applications* (3rd ed., pp. 557–563). New York: AFB Press.

Long, R. C., & Guidice, N. A. (2010). Establishing and maintaining orientation for mobility. In W. Wiener, R. Welsch, and B. Blasch (Eds.), *Foundations of orientation and mobility:* Vol. 1: *History and Theory* (3rd ed., pp. 45–62). New York: AFB Press.

Lowenfeld, B. (1973). *The visually impaired child in school.* New York: John Day.

Lowry, S. S. (2004). *Defined spaces.* Chapel Hill: Early Intervention Training Center for Infants and Toddlers with Visual Impairments, FPG Child Development Institute, University of North Carolina at Chapel Hill.

Lowry, S. S., & Hatton, D. D. (2002). Facilitating walking in young children with visual impairments. *RE:View, 34*(3), 125–133.

Loyens, S. M., Rikers, R. P., & Schmidt, H. G. (2009). Students' conceptions of constructivist learning in different programme years and different learning environments. *British Journal of Educational Psychology, 79*(3), 501–514. Retrieved 7/4/2012 from EBSCO*host*.com.

Marschark, M., Spencer, P. E., & Nathan, P. E. (2010). *Oxford handbook of deaf studies, language, and education* (Vol. 2). New York: Oxford University Press.

McCormick, B. P. (2000). People with disabilities national survey of recreation and the environment. *National Center on Accessibility.* Retrieved retrieved 7/4/2012 from www.ncaonline.org

McGregor, D., & Farrenkopf, C. (2000). Recreation and leisure skills. In A. J. Koenig & M. C. Holbrook, Eds., *Foundations of education, Vol. 2: Instructional strategies for teaching children and youths with visual impairments* (2nd ed., pp. 679–719). New York: AFB Press.

McHugh, E., & Lieberman, L. (2003). The impact of developmental factors on stereotypic rocking of children with visual impairment. *Journal of Visual Impairment & Blindness, 97,* 453–470.

McInnes, J. M. (1999). *A guide to planning and support for individuals who are deafblind.* Toronto, ON: University of Toronto Press.

McKenzie, A. R., & Lewis, S. (2008). The role and training of paraprofessionals who work with students who are visually impaired. *Journal of Visual Impairment & Blindness, 102,* 459–471.

Meek, G. A., & Maguire, J. E. (1996). A field experiment of minimum physical fitness of children with visual impairments. *Journal of Visual Impairment & Blindness, 90,* 77–80.

Merabet, L. V., Pitskel, N. B., Amedi, A., & Pascual-Leone, A. (2008). The plastic human brain in blind individuals: The cause of disability and the opportunity for rehabilitation. In J. J. Rieser, D. H. Ashmead, F. Ebner, & A. L. Corn (Eds.), *Blindness and brain plasticity in navigation and object perception,* (pp. 3–41). Hillsdale, NJ: Erlbaum.

Merriam, S. B., & Caffarella, R. S. (1999). *Learning in adulthood: A comprehensive guide.* San Francisco: Jossey-Bass.

Miles, B., & Riggio, M. (1999). *Remarkable conversations: A guide to developing meaningful communication with children and young adults who are deafblind.* Watertown, MA: Perkins School for the Blind Press.

Millar, S. (2000). Modality and mind: Convergent active processing in inter-related networks as a model of development and perception by touch. In M. A. Heller (Ed.), *Touch representation and blindness* (pp. 99–142). Oxford: Oxford University Press.

Modell, S., Rider, R., & Menchetti, B. (1997). An exploration of the influence of educational placement on the community recreation and leisure patterns of children with developmental disabilities. *Perceptual and Motor Skills, 85,* 695–704.

Morelli, T., Foley, J., Columna, L., Lieberman, L., & Folmer, E. (2010). VI-Tennis: A vibrotactile/audio exergame for players who are visually impaired. In *Proceedings of Foundations of Digital Interactive Games (FDG)* (pp. 147–154). New York: ACM.

Morelli, T., Foley, J., Lieberman, L., & Folmer, E. (2011, May). Pet-N-Punch: Upper body tactile/audio exergame to engage children with visual impairments into physical activity. *Graphics Interface (GI),* 223–230.

Morelli, T., Folmer, E., Foley, J. T., & Lieberman, L. (2011). Improving the lives of youth with visual impairments through exergames. *Insight: Research and Practice in Visual Impairment and Blindness, 4,* 160–170.

Morgan, S. (2001). "What is my role?" A comparison of the responsibilities of interpreters, intervenors, and support service providers. *Deaf-Blind Perspectives, 9*(1), 1–3.

Morgan, S. (n.d.). *Sign language with people who are deaf-blind: Suggestions for tactile and visual modification.* Retrieved March 12, 2012, from http://www.deafblind.com/slmorgan.html

Morris, L., Sallybanks, J., Willis, K., & Makkai, T. (2003). Sport, physical activity and antisocial behaviour in youth. *Youth Studies Australia, 23*(1), 47–52. Retrieved 7/4/12 from EBSCO*host*.com.

Nagi, S. Z. (1991). Disability concepts revisited: Implications for prevention. In Institute of Medicine (Ed.), *Disability in America: Toward a national agenda for prevention* (pp. 309–327). Washington, DC: National Academy Press.

Nakamura, T. (1997). Quantitative analysis of gait in the visually impaired. *Disability and Rehabilitation, 19,* 194–197.

National Association for Sport and Physical Education (NASPE). (2004). Moving into the future: National content standards for physical education. Reston, VA: NASPE.

National Association for Sport and Physical Education (NASPE). (2009). *Appropriate instructional practice guidelines for middle school physical education.* (3rd ed.). Reston, VA: NASPE.

National Association for Sport and Physical Education (NASPE). (2011). *Physical education is critical for a complete education.* (Position Statement). Reston, VA: NASPE. Retrieved February 16, 2012 from http://www.aahperd.org/naspe/standards/upload/Physical-Education-Is-Critical-to-Educating-the-Whole-Child-Final-5-19-2011.pdf

National Association for Sport and Physical Education (NASPE). (n.d.). Is It Physical Education or Physical Activity? Retrieved February 16, 2012 from http://www.aahperd.org/naspe/publications/teachingTools/PAvsPE.cfm

National Center for Health Statistics. (2007). *National health interview survey—disability supplement, 1994 and 1995.* Retrieved February 23, 2007, from http://www.cdc.gov/nchs/nhis.htm

National Consortium on Deaf-Blindness. (2011). *The 2010 national child count of children and youth who are deaf-blind.* Monmouth, OR: The National Consortium on Deaf-Blindness. Retrieved April 21, 2012, from http://nationaldb.org/documents/products/2010-Census-Tables.pdf

National Eye Institute. (2006). *Statistics on blindness in the model reporting area, 1969–70.* (Publication No. [NIH] 73–427).

National Eye Institute and the National Institute on Deafness and Other Communication Disorders. (n.d.). What is Usher syndrome? Washington DC: National Institutes of Health. Retrieved from http://www.ushersyndrome.nih.gov/whatis/fulltext.html

National Institutes of Health. *Usher syndrome.* National Eye Institute and the National Institute on Deafness and Other Communication Disorders. Retrieved April 21, 2012 from http://www.ushersyndrome.nih.gov/

Nielsen, L. (1992). *Space and self: Active learning by means of the Little Room.* Lake City, FL: Vision Associates.

Nowell, R., & Innes, J. (1997). *Educating children who are deaf or hard of hearing: Inclusion.* Reston, VA: ERIC Clearinghouse on Disabilities and Gifted Education. ERIC Digest #E557.

O'Connell, J., Lieberman, L., & Petersen, S. (2006). The effects of trained peer tutors on the physical education of children who are visually impaired. *Journal of Visual Impairment & Blindness, 100,* 471–477.

O'Connell, M., Lieberman, L., & Petersen, S. (2006). The use of tactile modeling and physical guidance as instructional strategies in physical activity for children who are blind. *Journal of Visual Impairment & Blindness, 100*(8), 471–477.

Ohlenkamp, N. (2000). Coaching judo for blind athletes. Retrieved 3/7/12 from www.judoinfo.com/vicoach.htm

Olson, M. R. (1983). A study of the exploratory behaviors of legally blind and sighted preschoolers. *Exceptional Children, 50,* 130–138.

Olympic Studies Centre, Research and Reference Service, International Olympic Committee. (2011). Judo: Participation during the history of the Olympic Games. Retrieved 3/7/12 from http://www.olympic.org/Assets/OSC%20Section/pdf/QR_sports_summer/Sports_Olympiques_judo_eng.pdf

Page, R. M., Frey, J., Talbert, R., & Falk, C. (1992). Children's feelings of loneliness and social dissatisfaction: Relationship to measures of physical fitness and activity. *Journal of Teaching in Physical Education, 11,* 211–219.

Pangrazi, R. P., & Beighle, A. (2009). *Dynamic physical education for elementary school children* (16th ed.). San Francisco: Benjamin/Cummings.

Parks, S., Furono, S., O'Reilly, T., Inatsuka, C. M., Hosaka, C. M., & Zeisloft-Falbey, B. (1994). *Hawaii early learning profile (HELP): HELP (birth to three).* Palo Alto, CA: VORT Corporation.

Pascual-Leone, A., & Hamilton, R. H. (1998). Cortical plasticity associated with braille learning. *Trends in Cognitive Science, 2,* 168–174.

Perkins, K., Bailey, J., Columna, L., & Lieberman, L. J. (2012). *Parental perceptions toward physical activity for their children with visual impairments and blindness.* Paper presented at the American Alliance for Health, Physical Education, Recreation and Dance National Convention, Boston, MA.

Piaget, J. (1952). *The origins of intelligence in the child.* New York: International Universities Press.

Piaget, J. (1981). Intelligence and affectivity: Their relationship during child development. Palo Alto, CA: Annual Reviews.

Piletic, C., Davis, R., & Aschemeier, A. (2005). Paraeducators in physical education. *Journal of Health, Physical Education, Recreation & Dance, 76*(5), 47–55.

Pleis, J. R., & Lucas, J. W. (2009). Provisional report: Summary health statistics for U.S. adults: National health interview survey, 2008. National Center for Health Statistics. *Vital Health Statistics, 10*(242).

Pogrund, R. L., & Fazzi, D. L. (2002). *Early focus: Working with young children who are blind or visually impaired.* New York: AFB Press.

Ponchillia, P. (1995). AccesSports: A model for adapting mainstream sports activities for individuals with visual impairments. *RE:View, 27,* 5–14.

Ponchillia, P. E. (2008). Nonvisual sports and art: Fertile substrates for the growth of knowledge about brain plasticity in people who are blind or have low vision. In J. J. Rieser, D. H. Ashmead, F. Ebner, & A. L. Corn (Eds.), *Blindness and brain plasticity in navigation and object perception* (pp. 283–311). Hillsdale, NJ: Lawrence Erlbaum.

Ponchillia, P. E., Armbruster, J., & Wiebold, J. (2005). The national sports education camps project: Introducing sports skills to children with visual impairments through short-term specialized instruction. *Journal of Visual Impairment & Blindness, 99*(11), 685–695.

Ponchillia, P. E., & Ponchillia, S. V. (1996). *Foundations of rehabilitation teaching with persons who are blind or visually impaired.* New York: AFB Press.

Ponchillia, P. E., Strause, B., & Ponchillia, S. V. (2002). Athletes with visual impairments: Attributes and sports participation. *Journal of Visual Impairment & Blindness, 96*(April), 267–272.

Ponchillia, S. V., Powell, L. L., Felski, K. A., & Nicklawski, M. T. (1992). The effectiveness of aerobics exercise instruction for totally blind women. *Journal of Visual Impairment & Blindness, 86,* 174–177.

Portfors-Yeomans, C., & Riach, C. L. (1995). Frequency characteristics of postural control of children with and without visual impairment. *Developmental Medicine and Child Neurology, 37,* 456–463.

Prechtl, D. M., Cioni, G., Einspieler, C., Bos, A. F., & Ferrari, F. (2001). Role of vision on early motor development: Lessons from the blind. *Developmental Medicine and Child Neurology, 43,* 198–201.

Presley, I., & D'Andrea, F. M. (2009). *Assistive technology for students who are blind or visually impaired: A guide to assessment.* New York: AFB Press.

Professional Ski Instructors of America & American Association of Snowboard Instructors (PSIA-AASI). (2003). *Adaptive snowsports instruction.* Lakewood, CO: Professional Ski Instructors of America & American Association of Snowboard Instructors.

Rapin, I., Korey, S. R., Schick, B., & Kennedy, R. F. (1974). Hypoactive labyrinths and motor development. *Clinical Pediatrics, 12*(11), 922–993.

Reindal, S. (2010). Redefining disability: A rejoinder to a critique. *Nordic Journal of Applied Ethics / Etikk i praksis, 4*(1), 125–135. Retrieved 7/4/12 from EBSCO*host*.com.

Revesz, G. (1950). *Psychology and art of the blind* (pp. 218–222). London: Longmans, Green.

Riddick, C. (1993). Older women's leisure activity and quality of life. In J. R. Kelly (Ed.), *Activity and aging: Staying involved in later life* (pp. 86–98). Newbury Park, CA: Sage.

Rink, J. E. (2009). *Designing the physical education curriculum: Promoting active lifestyles.* New York: McGraw-Hill.

Riordan-Eva, P., & Cunningham, E. (2011). *Vaughan & Asbury's general ophthalmology* (18th ed.). New York: McGraw-Hill Higher Education.

Robinson, B., & Lieberman, L. J. (2004). Effects of visual impairment, gender, and age on self-determination. *Journal of Visual Impairment & Blindness, 98*(6), 351–366.

Rogers, S. J., & Puchalski, C. B. (1984). Development of symbolic play in visually impaired children. *Topics in Early Childhood Special Education, 3,* 57–62.

Rogers, S., & Puchalski, C. B. (1988). Development of object permanence in visually impaired infants. *Journal of Visual Impairment & Blindness, 82,* 137–142.

Roman-Lantzy, C. (2007). *Cortical visual impairment: An approach to assessment and intervention.* New York: AFB Press.

Romiszowski, A. (1999). The development of physical skills: Instruction in the psychomotor domain. In C. M. Reigeluth (Ed.), *Instructional design theories and models: A new paradigm of instructional theory* (pp. 457–479). Mahwah, NJ: Erlbaum.

Rosen, S. (1989). [Gait, balance, and veering tendency in congenitally blind children and youth]. Unpublished raw data.

Rosen, S. (2010). Kinesiology and sensorimotor functioning for students with vision loss. In W. R. Wiener, R. L. Welsh, & B. B. Blasch (Eds.), *Foundations of orientation and mobility:* Vol. I: *History and theory* (3rd ed., pp. 138–172). New York: AFB Press.

Rosengran, L., & Undemar, C. (2001). *Can I play with you? How visually impaired children and young people experience their social situation.* Tomtebode Resource Center, Solna, Report No. 23.

Rousseau, R. (2012). History and style guide of wrestling. Retrieved 4/10/12 from http://martialarts.about.com/od/styles/a/wrestling.htm

Rowland, C. (1984). Preverbal communication of blind infants and their mothers. *Journal of Visual Impairment & Blindness, 78,* 297–302.

Rusotti, J., & Shaw, R. (2004). *When you have a visually impaired student in your classroom: A guide for paraeducators.* New York: American Foundation for the Blind.

Sacks, S. Z., & Silberman, R. K. (1998). *Educating students who have visual impairments and other disabilities.* Baltimore, MD: Paul Brookes.

Sacks, S. Z., & Wolffe, K. E. (Eds.). (2006). *Teaching social skills to students with visual impairments: From theory to practice.* New York: AFB Press.

Sadato, N., Pascual-Leone, A., Grafman, J., Ibañez, V., Deiber M. P., Dold, G., & Hallett, M. (1996). Activation of the primary visual cortex by Braille reading in blind subjects. *Nature,* 380 (6574), 526–528.

Santrock, J. W. (1994). *Child development* (6th ed.). New York: W. C. Brown Communications.

Sapp, W., & Hatlen, P. (2010). The expanded core curriculum: Where we have been, where we are going, and how we can get there. *Journal of Visual Impairment & Blindness, 104*(6), 338–348.

Satchwell, L. (1994). Preschool physical education class structure. *Journal of Physical Education, Recreation & Dance, 65.*

Sathian, K., & Lacey, S. (2008). Visual cortical involvement during tactile perception in blind and sighted individuals. In J. J. Rieser, D. H. Ashmead, F. Ebner, A. L. Corn (Eds.), *Blindness and brain plasticity in navigation and object perception.* Hillsdale, NJ: Erlbaum.

Sauerburger, D. (1993). *Independence without sight or sound.* New York: American Foundation for the Blind.

Schedlin, H., Lieberman, L. J., Houston-Wilson, C., & Cruz, L. (2012). Academic learning time-physical education of students with visual impairments: An analysis of two students. *Insight: Research and Practice in Visual Impairment and Blindness, 5*(1), 11–22.

Scheib, K., & Ponchillia, P. (1999). The Aqualert II: An end-of-lane signaling device. *RE:View, 31,* 32–39.

Schiller, J. S., Lucas, J. W., Ward, B. W., & Peregoy, J. A. (2012). Provisional report: Summary health statistics for U.S. adults: National health interview survey, 2010. National Center for Health Statistics. *Vital Health Statistics, 10*(252).

Scholl, G. T. (1986). Growth and development. In G. T. Scholl (Ed.), *Foundations of education for blind and visually handicapped children and youth* (pp. 23–33). New York: AFB Press.

Schuster, R., Hammitt, W. E., & Moore, D. (2006). Stress appraisal and coping response to hassles experienced in outdoor recreation settings. *Leisure Sciences, 28*(2), 97–113. doi:10.1080/01490400500483919.

Schwartz, T. L. (2010). Causes of visual impairment: Pathology and its implications. In A. L. Corn & J. N. Erin (Eds.), *Foundations of low vision: Clinical and functional perspectives* (2nd ed., pp. 137–191). New York: AFB Press.

Shapiro, D., Moffett, A., Lieberman, L. J., & Dummer, G. (2005). Perceived competence of children with visual impairments. *Journal of Visual Impairment & Blindness, 99,* 15–25.

Sherrill, C. (2004). *Adapted physical activity, recreation and sports: Crossdisciplinary and lifespan* (6th ed.). Boston: McGraw-Hill.

Shindo, M., Kumagai, S., & Tanaka, H. (1987). Physical work capacity and effect of endurance training in visually handicapped boys and young male adults. *European Journal of Applied Physiology, 56,* 501–507.

Short, F. (2011). Individual education plans. In J. P. Winnick (Ed.) *Adapted physical education and sport.* Champaign, IL: Human Kinetics.

Short, F., & Winnick, J. (1986). The influence of visual impairment on physical fitness test performance. *Journal of Visual Impairment & Blindness, 80,* 729–731.

Siri, W. E. (1961). Body composition from fluid space and density. In J. Brozek & A. Hanschel (Eds.) *Techniques for measuring body composition* (pp. 223–244). Washington, DC: Academy of Science.

Skaggs, S., & Hopper, C. (1996). Individuals with visual impairments: A review of psychomotor behavior. *Adapted Physical Activity Quarterly, 13,* 16–26.

Skellenger, A. C., Rosenblum, L. P., & Jager, B. K. (1997). Behaviors of preschoolers with visual impairments in indoor play settings. *Journal of Visual Impairment & Blindness, 91,* 519–530.

Skinner, B. F. (1974). *About behaviorism.* New York: Vintage Books.

Smart, J. (2009). *Disability, society, and the individual* (2nd ed.). Austin, TX: Pro Ed.

Smith, A., & Geruschat, D. R. (2010). Orientation and mobility for adults with low vision. In A. L. Corn & J. N. Erin (Eds.), *Foundations of low vision: Clinical and functional perspectives* (2nd ed., pp. 833–870). New York: AFB Press.

Smith, M., & Levack, N. (1996). *Teaching students with visual and multiple impairments: A resource guide.* Austin: Texas School for the Blind.

Smith, T. B. (2002). *Guidelines: Practical tips for working and socializing with deaf-blind people.* Burtonsville, MD: Sign Media.

Sonksen, P. M., Levitt, S., & Kitsinger, M. (1984). Identification of constraints acting on motor development in young visually disabled children and principles of remediation. *Child Care, Health, and Development, 10,* 273–286.

Spungin, S. J. (Ed.) (2002). *When you have a visually impaired student in your classroom: A guide for teachers.* New York: AFB Press.

Sticken, J., & Kapperman, G. (2010). Integration of visual skills for independent living. In A. L. Corn and J. N. Erin (Eds.), *Foundations of low vision: Clinical and functional perspectives* (2nd ed., pp. 97–110). New York: AFB Press.

Stokes, B. (2002). *Amazing babies: Essential movement for your baby in the first year.* Allenwood, NJ: Move Alive Media.

Strickling, C. A., & Pogrund, R. L. (2002). Motor focus. In R. L. Pogrund & D. L. Fazzi (Eds.), *Early focus: Working with children who are blind or visually impaired and their families* (2nd ed., pp. 287–325). New York: AFB Press.

Strong, D., & LeFevre, D. (2006). Parachute games with DVD (2nd ed.). Champaign, IL: Human Kinetics.

Stuart, M. E. (2003). Sources of subjective task value in sport: An examination of adolescents with high or low value for sport. *Journal of Applied Sport Psychology, 15*(3), 239–255.

Stuart, M. E., Lieberman, L. J., & Hand, K. (2006). Parent-child beliefs about physical activity: An examination of families of children with visual impairments. *Journal of Visual Impairment & Blindness, 100*(4), 223–234.

Sundberg, S. (1982). Maximal oxygen uptake in relation to age in blind and normal boys and girls. *Acta Pediatrica Scandinavia, 71,* 603–608.

Suomi, J., Collier, D., & Brown, L. (2003). Factors affecting the social experiences of students in elementary physical education classes. *Journal of Teaching in Physical Education, 22*(2), 186–202.

Tandem bicycle, The (2010). Retrieved 5/5/12 from www.bikefortwo.com[0]

Taub, D. E., & Greer, K. R. (2000). Physical activity as a normalizing experience for school-age children with disabilities: Implications for legitimization of social identity and enhancement of social ties. *Journal of Sport and Social Issues, 24,* 395–414.

Trief, E., & Shaw, R. (2009). Visual impairment and early development. In E. Trief & R. Shaw, *Everyday activities to promote visual efficiency: A handbook for working with young children with visual impairments.* New York: AFB Press.

Trippe, H. (1996). Children and sports: Encouraging a healthy attitude to exercise should start in primary school. *British Medical Journal, 312,* 199–200.

Tröster, H., & Brambring, M. (1993). Early motor development and blind infants. *Journal of Applied Developmental Psychology, 14*(11), 83–106.

Tröster, H., & Brambring, M. (1994). The play behavior and play materials of blind and sighted infants and preschoolers. *Journal of Visual Impairment & Blindness, 88,* 4, 421–432.

Tröster, H., Brambring, M., & Beelman, A. (1991). The prevalence and situational causes of stereotyped behaviors in blind infants and preschoolers. *Journal of Abnormal Child Psychology, 19,* 569–590.

Tröster, H., Hecker, W., & Brambring, M. (1994). Longitudinal study of gross-motor development in blind infants and preschoolers. *Early Child Development and Care, 104,* 61–78.

Tsai, E. (2005). A cross-cultural study of the influence of perceived positive outcomes on participation in regular active recreation: Hong Kong and Australian university students. *Leisure Sciences, 27*(5), 385–404. doi:10.1080/01490400500227290.

Tudor-Locke, C., Pangrazi, R., Corbin, C., Rutherford, W., Vincent, S., Raustorp, A., Tomson, L., & Cuddihy, T. (2004). BMI-reference standards for recommended pedometer-determined steps/day in children. *Preventive Medicine, 38,* 857–864.

Turkington, C., and Sussman, A. E. (Eds.). (2000). *The encyclopedia of deafness and hearing disorders* (2nd ed., p. 62). New York: Facts on File.

Tuttle, D. W. (1984). *Self-esteem and adjusting with blindness.* Springfield, IL: Charles C. Thomas.

U.S. Census Bureau. (2006). *Survey of Income and Program Participation, 1994–95.* Retrieved September 10, 2006, from http://www.census.gov/hhes/www/disable/dissipp.htm

U.S. Department of Education, Office of Special Education Programs, (2004). *Building the legacy: IDEA 2004.* Retrieved April 18, 2008 from http://idea.ed.gov/explore/home

U.S. Department of Health and Human Services, President's Council on Physical Fitness and Sports. (1999). *Physical activity and health:* A report of the Surgeon General, HE 20.7602. Washington, DC: U.S. Department Of Health And Human Services, Centers for Disease Control and Prevention. Retrieved July 4, 2012, from http://www.cdc.gov/nccdphp/sgr/index.htm

Ulrich, D. A. 2000. *The Test of Gross Motor Development,* 2nd ed. Austin, TX: Pro-Ed.

Umansky, W., & Hooper, S. R. (1998). *Young children with special needs.* Columbus, OH: Prentice Hall.

United States Association of Blind Athletes. (2007). *IBSA visual classifications.* Retrieved March 1, 2008, from http://www.usaba.org/Pages/sportsinformation/visualclassifications.html

Valente, M., & McCaslin, D. L. (2011, March). Vestibular disorders and evaluation of the pediatric patient. *The ASHA Leader.* Retrieved May 2, 2012, from www.asha.org/Publications/leader/2011/110315/Vestibular-Disorders-and-Evaluation-of-the-Pediatric-Patient.htm

Vaughan, D. G., Asbury, T., & Riordan-Eva, P. (1995). *General ophthalmology* (14th ed.). Norwalk, CT: Appleton & Lange.

Wagner, M. & Haibach, P. (2012). *Motor development cirriculum: Children with visual impairments.* American Alliance for Health, Physical Education, Recreation, and Dance Conference, Boston, MA.

Wagner, M., Haibach, P., & Lieberman, L. (in press). Motor skills of children with visual impairments. Adapted Physical Activity Quarterly.

Warnick, R. (2002). Rural recreation lifestyles: Trends in recreation activity patterns and self-reported quality of life and health—an exploratory study. *Journal of Park & Recreation Administration, 20*(4), 37–64.

Warren, D., & Hatton, D. (2003). Cognitive development of children with visual impairments. In I. Rapin & E. Segalowitz (Eds.), *Handbook of neu-*

rophysiology: Vol. 7, Part II. Child Neuropsychology (2nd ed., pp. 439–458). New York: Elsevier.

Watson, D., and Taff-Watson, M. (Eds.). (1993). *A model service delivery system for persons who are deaf-blind* (2nd ed.). Fayetteville: University of Arkansas.

Wehmeyer, M. L., Argan, M., & Hughes, C. (1998). *Teaching self-determination to students with disabilities: Basic skills for successful transition*. Baltimore, MD: Paul H. Brookes.

Wellner, A. S. (1998). Getting old and staying fit. *American Demographics, 20,* 24–26.

Werner, P., & Rini, L. (1967). *Perceptual motor development equipment: Inexpensive ideas and activities.* New York: Wiley.

Wiener, W., & Lawson, G. (1996). Audition in the visually impaired traveler: Fundamentals of sound and audition. In B. Blasch, W. Weiner, & R. Welsh (Eds.), *Foundations of orientation and mobility* (2nd ed., pp. 238–252). New York: AFB Press.

Wikipedia, the Free Encyclopedia, (2008). *Rowing (sport).* Retrieved April 19, 2008, from http://en.wikipedia.org/wiki/Sport_rowing

Wilkinson, M. E. (2010). Clinical low vision services. In A. L. Corn and J. N. Erin (Eds.), *Foundations of low vision: Clinical and functional perspectives* (2nd ed., pp. 238–295). New York: AFB Press.

Williams, C. A., Armstrong, N., Eves, N., & Faulkner, A. (1996). Peak aerobic fitness of visually impaired and sighted adolescent girls. *Journal of Visual Impairment & Blindness, 90,* 495–500.

Winnick, J. P. (1985). Performance of visually impaired youngsters in physical education activities: Implications for mainstreaming. *Adapted Physical Activity Quarterly, 3,* 58–66.

Winnick, J. P., & Short, F. X. (1985). *Physical fitness testing for the disabled: Project UNIQUE.* Champaign, IL: Human Kinetics.

Winnick, J. P., & Short, F. X. (1999). *The Brockport physical fitness test.* Champaign, IL: Human Kinetics.

Wiskochil, B. (2002). *The effects of trained peer tutors on academic learning time in physical education.* Unpublished master's thesis, SUNY Brockport.

Wiskochil, B., Lieberman, L. J., Houston-Wilson, C., & Petersen, S. (2007). The effects of trained peer tutors on academic learning time-physical education on four children who are visually impaired or blind. *Journal of Visual Impairment & Blindness, 101,* 339–350.

Wolfensberger, W. (1972). *Normalization.* Toronto: National Institute on Mental Retardation.

Wright, B. (1960). *Physical disability: A psychological approach.* New York: Harper and Bros.

Wyatt, L., & Ng, G. Y. (1997). The effect of visual impairment on the strength of children's hip and knee extensors. *Journal of Visual Impairment & Blindness, 91,* 40–46.

Zabelski, M. (2007). Start at the beginning: The importance of early intervention. In S. LaVenture (Ed.), *A parents' guide to special education for children with visual impairments* (pp. 37–58). New York: AFB Press.

Zabriskie, R. B., Lundberg, N. R., & Groff, D. G. (2005). Quality of life and identity: The benefits of a community-based therapeutic recreation and adaptive sports program. *Therapeutic Recreation Journal, 39,* 176–190.

Zeller, J. (2009). *Canoeing and kayaking for people with disabilities.* Champaign, IL: Human Kinetics.

Zimmerman, G. J. (1996). Optics and low vision devices. In A. L. Corn & A. L. Koenig (Eds.), *Foundations of low vision: Clinical and functional perspectives* (pp. 124–138). New York: AFB Press.

Zimmerman, G. J., Zebehazy, K. T., & Moon, M. L. (2010). Optics and low vision devices. In A. L. Corn & J. N. Erin (Eds.), *Foundations of low vision: Clinical and functional perspectives* (2nd ed., pp. 192–237). New York: AFB Press.

Zola, I. K. (1993). Self, identity and the naming question: Reflections on the language of disability. *Social Science & Medicine, 36,* 167–173.

APPENDIX

CAMP ABILITIES Activity Assessment

CAMP ABILITIES ACTIVITY ASSESSMENT

Camper ______________________________

Counselor ______________________________ **Date** ______________

Track and Field Assessment Checklist

Skill	Criteria			
	Verbal Cue	Partial Physical Assistance	Total Physical Assistance	Other
Long Jump	Personal Best ______________			
Start with take-off foot				
12–18 strides				
Accelerate to maximum speed				
Knees up and tall in last strides				
Jump up and out				
Drive up knee and opposite arm vigorously				
Curve body like half moon				
Arms above head and behind shoulders				
Close jackknife				
Collapse buttocks to heels upon landing				
Arms thrust forward				
Feet together				
Shot Put	Personal Best ______________			
Wrap four fingers firmly around shot				
Keep shot firm against neck				
Push shot past head				
Punch out				
Think position facing back toward direction of throw				
Hips rotate				
Kick backward with nonsupport leg				

(Continued on next page)

Camp Abilities Activity Assessment 2

Track and Field Assessment Checklist

Skill	Criteria			
	Verbal Cue	Partial Physical Assistance	Total Physical Assistance	Other
Left leg straightens hard, right leg pushes up and out, causing a shooting motion				
Slap and pull				
Discus	Personal Best: ________________			
Hold the discus open-handed with an eagle claw grip				
Release discus, palm down, off index finger				
Keep body in wound-up position until thrown, then shout				
Rotate hips				
End throw with a long pull, head and chest up, facing sector				
Block-push-shoot				
Running				
Body erect, relax face, neck, shoulders, and arms				
Rest thumb on index finger				
Swing arms forward and back				
Open stride				
Strike heel and roll to toe				
Toes straight ahead or slightly out				
Head facing straight ahead				

Beep Baseball Assessment Checklist

Skill	Criteria			
Running Bases	Verbal Cue	Partial Physical Assistance	Total Physical Assistance	Other
Standing at home, turn toward and point to beeping base				
Walk to beeping base with guide				
Walk to beeping base without guide				
Jog to beeping base with guide				
Jog to beeping base without guide				

Camp Abilities Activity Assessment 3

Beep Baseball Assessment Checklist

Skill	Criteria			
Running Bases	Verbal Cue	Partial Physical Assistance	Total Physical Assistance	Other
Fielding the Ball				
Assume a ready stance (feet apart, knees bent, hands ready)				
Go to ground slowly—lie on one side, body bent slightly at the waist, arms and legs outstretched				
Go to ground into fielding position rapidly				
Field a ball rolled gently				
Field a ball rolled with force				
Field a batted ball				
Hitting				
Hold a bat properly				
Swing a bat with smooth, level swing				
Swing bat and hit ball off a tee				
Swing bat and hit pitched ball				

Goalball Assessment Checklist

Skill	Criteria			
Ready Position	Verbal Cue	Partial Physical Assistance	Total Physical Assistance	Other
Face the other team				
Knees bent				
Hands on knees				
Underhand Roll				
Shift weight back and bring ball back with dominant hand				
Step forward with opposite foot				
Shift weight forward				
Release ball in front (ball should drop within 8′ of release)				
Follow through in front				
Falling to a Lying Position				
Ready position				

(Continued on next page)

Camp Abilities Activity Assessment 4

Goalball Assessment Checklist

Skill	Criteria			
Ready Position	Verbal Cue	Partial Physical Assistance	Total Physical Assistance	Other
Determine if ball is to left or right				
Lie on ground with legs together and arms above and in front of head				
Passing				
Realize when you must pass ball to teammate (player already passed 2X in a row)				
Say teammate's name				
Bend down				
Roll ball toward team member				

Tandem Biking

Skill	Day 1	Day 2	Day 3	Day 4
Preparation Skills				
Wear appropriate footwear				
Closed-toe shoes				
Sneakers				
Put on helmet				
Make sure helmet is secure on head				
Straddle seat in ready position				
Push off				
Put feet on pedals				
Dismount Skills				
Put foot on ground				
Maintain balance				
Bring leg around, dismounts bike				
Take helmet off				
Distance				
⅛ mile				
¼ mile				
½ mile				
1 mile				
2 miles				

Camp Abilities Activity Assessment 5

Tandem Biking				
Skill	Day 1	Day 2	Day 3	Day 4
3 miles				
4 miles				
5 miles				
5+ miles				

Gymnastics Assessment Checklist				
Skill	Criteria			
Single Bar				
Grip bar				
Jump to front support				
Forward roll over bar				
Pull over				
Front support, cast				
Cast, back hip circle				
Single leg around				
Single knee swing up to support				
Straight body hang from high bar				
Straight body swing from high bar				
Balance Beam				
Step onto beam				
Step into squat position				
Front support mount				
Front support to straddle sit				
Jump to one-foot squat support				
Stand from a squat position				
Stationary stand				
Stationary stand on one foot				
Squat stance				
Balance on hands and knees				
Sit on beam				
Beam walk on hands and knees				

(Continued on next page)

Camp Abilities Activity Assessment 6

Gymnastics Assessment Checklist

Skill	Criteria			
Slide steps sideward				
Walk sideways				
Walk forward				
Dip steps forward				
Dip steps backward				
¼ turn (straight stand or squat position)				
½ turn (straight stand or squat position)				
One whole turn (straight stand or squat position)				
Walk forward, ½ turn				
Walk backward, ½ turn				
Step off end of beam to straight stand				
Straight jump dismount				
Tuck jump dismount				
Straddle jump dismount				
Rings				
Straight body support				
Tuck support				
Inverted straight body support				
Inverted tuck support				
Straight arm support				
Pike support (L position)				
Dismount (swinging with straight body, land on two feet)				
Side Horse				
Jump to front support				
Jump to single leg straddle support				
Front support, single leg straddle				
Straight body travel, to opposite end of horse				
Single leg circle				
Double leg circle				
Floor Exercise				
V sit				
Knee scale				

Camp Abilities Activity Assessment 7

Gymnastics Assessment Checklist

Skill	Criteria			
One leg scale				
Jump ½ turn				
Jump one whole turn				
Tuck jump				
Pike jump				
Straddle jump				
Log roll				
Tuck forward roll				
Straddle forward roll				
Tuck backward roll				
Straddle backward roll				
Mule kicks				
Handstand				
Cartwheel				
Combination of Floor Skills				
Jump ½ turn, jump one whole turn				
Tuck jump, straddle jump				
Tuck jump, pike jump				
Forward roll, jump ½ turn, backward roll				
Forward roll, straddle forward roll				
Backward roll, jump ½ turn, forward roll				
Backward roll, backward straddle roll				
Handstand forward roll				
Handstand forward roll to a cartwheel				
Handstand forward roll, jump ½ turn or one whole turn				

Camp Abilities Activity Assessment 8

Judo Assessment

Rear Break Fall	Physical Assistance	Verbal Cue	Independent
Tuck chin			
Arms out at 45-degree angle			
Cupped hands			
Slap when belt touches mat			
Legs bent slightly			
Feet together			
Exhale			

Standing Rear Break Fall	Physical Assistance	Verbal Cue	Independent
Cross arms in front of the chest			
Squat down into a tucked position			
Rocking back			
Rear break fall			
Tuck your chin			
Arms at 45-degree angle			
Cupped hands			
Slap when belt touches the mat			
Legs bent slightly			
Feet together			
Exhale			

Right Standing Rear Break Fall	Physical Assistance	Verbal Cue	Independent
Tuck your chin			
Squat with left leg			
Sweep right leg in front of left leg			
Right hand over left, hugging stomach			
Roll down onto right thigh and bottom			
Right ankle and foot up			
Landing on outside of right thigh			
Landing on ball of foot			

Left Standing Rear Break Fall	Physical Assistance	Verbal Cue	Independent
Tuck your chin			
Squat with right leg			
Sweep left leg in front of other leg			

Camp Abilities Activity Assessment 9			
Right hand hugging stomach, left hand over			
Roll down onto left thigh and bottom			
Left ankle and foot up			
Landing on outside of left thigh			
Landing on ball of right foot			

Tai-Sabaki (Body Control)	Physical Assistance	Verbal cue	Independent
Straight body			
Right-handed grip			
Feet shoulder-width apart			
Sound of feet sliding across the mat			
Arms and body loose and relaxed			

Kumikata (Grip) for Right Hand	Physical Assistance	Verbal cue	Independent
Right hand on left lapel			
Left hand on right sleeve (elbow)			
Back straight			
Look up			
Feet shoulder-width apart			

Tai-Otoshi (Body Drop)	Physical Assistance	Verbal Cue	Independent
Right-handed grip			
Right foot in front of opponent's right foot			
Left foot in front of opponent's left foot			
Back to your opponent			
Right foot past your opponent's right foot			
Pull forward and downward with left hand			
Push with right hand in the direction your opponent is moving			
Keep pulling until opponent is on his or her back			
Hold opponent's left sleeve after throw			
Opponent lands on his or her back			

Ostoto-Gari (Larger Outer Reap)	Physical Assistance	Verbal Cue	Independent
Right-handed grip			
Step left foot outside opponent's right foot			

(Continued on next page)

Camp Abilities Activity Assessment 10			
Pull opponent toward you			
Swing right leg past opponent's right leg			
Reap right leg backward			
Hit back of opponent's leg			
Pull down with left arm			
Push back with right arm			
Bow at the waist			
Hold opponent's sleeve after the throw			
Opponent lands on his or her back			

O-Goshi (Large Hip Throw)	Physical Assistance	Verbal Cue	Independent
Right-handed grip			
Right foot in front of opponent's right foot			
Left foot in front of opponent's left foot			
Bend the knees			
Reach around waist with right arm			
Pull opponent onto hips (contact)			
Lift opponent up by straightening the knees			
Pull opponent with left hand and turn upper body to the left			
Hold the opponent's left sleeve after throw			
Opponent lands on his or her back			

Ouchi-Gari (Large Inner Sweep)	Physical Assistance	Verbal Cue	Independent
Right-handed grip			
Pull opponent toward you			
Leave right foot on ground			
Put left foot directly behind right leg			
Slip right leg in behind opponent's left leg			
Bring the back of right knee against opponent's left knee			
Push opponent directly down with both hands			
Hold opponent's left sleeve after the throw			
Opponent lands on his or her back			

Camp Abilities Activity Assessment 11

Orientation & Mobility Assessment

Attending Behavior	Always	Sometimes	Never
Turn toward voice or noise			
Reach or move toward a noise stimulus			
Respond to olfactory information and cues			
Auditory Abilities			
Attend to environmental sounds			
Attend to speech			
Localize a stationary sound			
Track a moving sound			
Identify and label environmental sounds			
Use sounds to orient to the environment			
Apply spatial concepts to sound localization (e.g., water fountain is to my right, traffic is behind me)			
Use echolocation to determine the presence of obstacles (e.g., walls, people)			
Recognize sound shadows and remain orientated			
Move toward a stationary sound			
Laterality, Turns, Directionality			
Demonstrate left and right awareness			
Demonstrate laterality in relation to objects			
Make a quarter or 90-degree turn upon request			
Make a half or 180-degree turn upon request			
Make a whole or 360-degree turn upon request			
Initiate turns as needed in independent travel			
Demonstrate application of directionality in a complex environment			
Recognize directionality in relation to objects			

Basic Skills	Always	Sometimes	Never
Demonstrate the following sighted guide techniques:			
• Proper arm, hand, and body position			
• Correct position without letting go			
• Stopping and going			
• Changing surfaces			
• Going up and down curbs			

(Continued on next page)

Camp Abilities Activity Assessment 12

Orientation & Mobility Assessment

Basic Skills	Always	Sometimes	Never
• Narrow passage techniques			
• Congested area techniques			
• Changing directions (e.g., in dorm lounge area, in crowds, in cafeteria)			
• Going through a closed door (e.g., hold the door, assist)			
• Ascending and descending stairs			
Landmarks and Cues			
Use landmarks for orientation			
Use clues for orientation			
Basic Spatial Awareness			
Name the four compass directions			
Identify the front, back, left side, and right side of a room in relation to the door			
Identify the directional corners of a room (e.g., front right, front left, back right, back left)			
On-Campus Orientation & Mobility			
Become acclimated to changes in lighting			
Identify contrast changes (e.g., carpet, tile) and drop-offs visually			
Avoid contacting objects in path			
Detect stairs			
Go up and down alone			
Locate open and closed doors			
Locate needed areas (e.g., washroom, dorm room)			
Locate outdoor areas of the campus (e.g., track, beep baseball field, tandem biking)			
Locate other buildings on campus (e.g., Tuttle North, Residence, Judo)			
Night Travel			
Become acclimated to changes in lighting conditions (e.g., light to dark, dark to lighted room)			
Detect obstacles in path of travel			
Detect drop-offs			
Use a shadow to gain information			

Resources

This resource listing provides a sampling of organizations that offer information about adapted sports and recreation activities, events and programs, and sources of adapted equipment for people who are blind, visually impaired, or deafblind. Website addresses only are provided for organizations that do not have permanent mailing addresses. For a more comprehensive list of sources in the field of visual impairment and blindness, see the Directory of Services search on the American Foundation for the Blind website, www.afb.org.

NATIONAL ORGANIZATIONS

Visual Impairment, Deafblindness, and Physical Education

The organizations in this section offer information and resources for professionals in the fields of visual impairment, deafblindness, and physical education.

American Association for Physical Activity and Recreation
1900 Association Drive
Reston, VA 20191-1598
(703) 476-3430
Fax: (703) 476-9527
www.aahperd.org/aapar/index.cfm
aapar@aahperd.org

Membership organization for physical activity and education professionals and students, providing information and resources for teaching physical education, physical activity, fitness, exercise, outdoor recreation, and adventure. Offers teacher credentialing, workshops, and webinars in adapted physical education. Councils include the Adapted Physical Activity Council.

American Foundation for the Blind
2 Penn Plaza, Suite 1102
New York, NY 10121
(212) 502-7600 or (800) 232-5463
TDD: (212) 502-7662
Fax: (212) 502-7777
www.afb.org
info@afb.org

National organization serving as an information clearinghouse for people with visual impairments and their families, professionals, schools, organizations, corporations, and the public. Operates a toll-free information hotline; conducts research and mounts program initiatives to promote inclusion of people with visual impairments, especially in literacy, technology, aging, and employment; and advocates for services and legislation. Through AFB Press, its publishing arm, publishes books, pamphlets, DVDs, and electronic and online products including the *Directory of Services for Blind and Visually Impaired Persons in the United States and Canada,* the *Journal of Visual Impairment & Blindness,* and *AccessWorld: Technology and People with Visual Impairments.* Maintains web-based initiatives, including FamilyConnect® (www.FamilyConnect.org), an online, multimedia community for parents and families of children with visual impairments created with the National Association for Parents of Children with Visual Impairments; CareerConnect® (www.CareerConnect.org), a free resource for people who want to learn about the range and diversity of jobs performed by adults who are blind or visually impaired; and VisionAware™, a website providing information, resources, and daily living techniques that can increase independence and enhance quality of life for individuals with vision loss.

American Printing House for the Blind (APH)
1839 Frankfort Avenue
P.O. Box 6085
Louisville, KY 40206
(502) 895-2405 or (800) 223-1839
www.aph.org
info@aph.org

National nonprofit organization that offers educational, workplace, and independent living products and services for persons with visual impairments; administers the Federal Quota Program to provide funds for purchase of educational materials for students with visual impairments; conducts educational research and development; maintains the AFB M. C. Migel Library, a centralized source of materials related to blindness and visual impairment; and administers other programs and services. Adapted physical educational and daily living products include sound-emitting balls and portable sound sources for use in games and sports; and kits for adapted tennis, jump rope, walking and running, and table tennis. The website includes an extensive section on physical education and recreation for children with sensory impairments (www.aph.org/pe), including resources and sources of additional information. Provides on-site workshops on a variety of topics, including physical activity for children with visual impairments or deafblindness.

Canadian Deafblind Association
2000 Appleby Line, Suite 421
Burlington, ON L7L 7H7
Canada
(866) 229-5832
Fax: (905) 319-2027
www.cdbanational.com
info@cdbanational.com

National organization dedicated to promoting and enhancing the well-being of people who are deafblind through awareness, education, advocacy, research, partnerships, and provision of programs and services. Produces *Intervention,* a newsmagazine devoted to deafblindness and parenting issues.

Council for Exceptional Children
2900 Crystal Drive, Suite 1000
Arlington, VA 22202-3557
(703) 620-3660 or (888) 232-7733
TTY: (866) 915-5000
Fax: (703) 264-9494
www.cec.sped.org
www.cecdvi.org
service@cec.sped.org

Professional organization dedicated to improving the educational success of individuals with disabilities and/or gifts and talents. Provides information, resources, and professional development for professionals; advocates for appropriate governmental policies; sets professional standards; and advocates for individuals with exceptionalities; publishes books on special education, journals, newsletters; and holds conventions and conferences. The Division on Visual Impairments focuses on federal, state, and local issues and policies related to education of infants, children and youths with visual impairments.

National Association for Sport and Physical Education
1900 Association Drive
Reston, VA 20191
(703) 476-3410 or (800) 213-7193
Fax: (703) 476-8316
www.aahperd.org/naspe
naspe@aahperd.org

Membership organization of professionals and future professionals in physical education and sport, whose mission is to enhance knowledge, improve professional practice, and increase support for high-quality physical education, sport, and physical activity programs.

National Consortium on Deaf-Blindness
c/o Teaching Research
Western Oregon University
345 North Monmouth Avenue
Monmouth, OR 97361
(800) 438-9376
TTY: (800) 854-7013
Fax: (503) 838-8150
http://nationaldb.org/about.php
info@nationaldb.org

National technical assistance and dissemination center for children and youths who are deaf-blind. Maintains DB-Link, the largest collection of information related to deafblindness, including adapted physical education. Makes resources available to the public by direct requests and through the NCDB website, conferences, and a variety of electronic media.

SPORTS ORGANIZATIONS

The organizations listed provide programs, training, or competition in general or in particular sports; information about rules and adaptations for individuals with visual impairment or deafblindness to participate in sports; sources of equipment; and other information. Other sources of information for local activities include state or regional blind athletes associations affiliated with the United States Association of Blind Athletes or provincial blind sports associations affiliated with the Canadian Blind Sports Association. Information about adaptations, rules, and competitions for individual sports also can be found through national and international sports organizations.

General Sports Organizations

British Blind Sport
Pure Offices, Plato Close
Tachbrook Park
Leamington Spa, Warwickshire CV34 6WE
England
01926 424247
www.britishblindsport.org.uk
info@britishblindsport.org.uk

National organization advocating for people with visual impairments in the United Kingdom and internationally to have the same opportunities as sighted people to access and enjoy sport and recreational activities. Provides information on archery, athletics, cricket, football (soccer), goalball, martial arts, mountain biking, shooting, and ten pin bowling, among other sports.

Canadian Blind Sports Association
325-5055 Rue Joyce Street
Vancouver, BC V5R 6B2
Canada
(604) 419-0480 or (877) 604-0480
Fax: (604) 419-0481
www.canadianblindsports.ca

Organization serving individuals who are blind, visually impaired, deafblind, or are blind and have additional disabilities and their families and other supporters. Serves as the national governing body for goalball in Canada. Provincial and territorial member associations provide support for all Canadians with visual impairments who are involved in a range of sports.

Canadian Paralympic Committee
225 Metcalfe Street, Suite 310
Ottawa, ON K2P 1P9
Canada
(613) 569-4333
Fax: (613) 569-2777

Membership organization of sports organizations that runs programs across Canada to build awareness and educate Canadians about how sport and activity can help people with disabilities fulfill their potential and fully participate in their community. Offers information about sports and competitions and fosters participation in the

Paralympic Games and the Parapan American Games for athletes with disabilities held in conjunction with the Pan American Games.

International Blind Sports Federation
www.ibsa.es

International organization with affiliates in five continents that develops and promotes sports for people who are blind or visually impaired. Organizes competitive events, develops and finalizes rules and conditions for individual sports, and raises awareness of the participation of people with visual impairments in sports. Holds World Championship Games every four years. Provides descriptions of adapted sports, including rules and regulations, and a calendar of upcoming competitions.

United States Association of Blind Athletes
1 Olympic Plaza
Colorado Springs, CO 80909
(719) 866-3224
Fax: (719) 866-3400
www.usaba.org

National organization providing sports opportunities to children, youths, adults, and veterans with visual impairments or deafblindness in sports including, but not limited to, track and field, Nordic and Alpine skiing, biathlon, judo, wrestling, swimming, tandem cycling, powerlifting, and goalball. Offers detailed information about individual sports and adaptations; maintains a calendar of upcoming events and competitions. Sells goalballs and instructional goalball videos.

United States Paralympics Committee
1 Olympic Plaza
Colorado Springs, CO 80909
(719) 866-2032
Fax: (719) 866-2029
www2.teamusa.org/US-Paralympics.aspx

Division of the U.S. Olympic Committee responsible for selecting and managing the U.S. teams that compete in the Paralympic Games. Offers information such as game rules and schedules, and general resources for competitors.

Organizations for Specific Sports and Activities

Adventure Travel

Wilderness Inquiry
808 14th Avenue, SE
Minneapolis, MN 55414-1516
(612) 676-9400 or (800) 728-0719
Fax: (612) 676-9401
www.wildernessinquiry.org
info@wildernessinquiry.org

Operates more than 100 integrated multi-day trips to locations around the world and offers day-long programs, training sessions, and other events in which people who do not have disabilities travel with others who do as equals and peers. Activities include backpacking, canoeing, dogsledding, hiking, horsepacking, kayaking and sea kayaking, safari, skiing, and white water rafting.

Archery

See listing for British Blind Sport

Athletics (Track & Field)

Achilles International
42 West 38th Street, Suite 400
New York, NY 10018
(212) 354-0300
Fax: (212) 354-3978
www.achillestrackclub.org
info@achillesinternational.org

Provides information, training, and programs for runners with physical or visual disabilities. The Achilles Kids program provides training, racing opportunities, and an in-school program for children throughout the United States. The Freedom Team of Wounded Veterans program brings training, access to specialized equipment, and marathon opportunities to disabled U.S. military veterans.

Beep Baseball

National Beep Baseball Association
5175 Evergreen Drive
North Olmsted, OH 44070
(440) 779-1025
www.nbba.org

Assists, promotes, encourages, and develops amateur beep baseball programs throughout the United States and internationally. Offers a description of the game, rules and regulations, and a calendar of events on its website as well as sources of beep baseballs, bases, and blindfolds.

Beep Kickball

Beep Kickball Association
c/o Judy Byrd
4323 Big House Road
Norcross, GA 30092
(770) 317-2035
www.beepkickball.com
judybyrd@gmail.com

Promotes and sponsors beep kickball, a new sport for children and adults with visual impairments. Promotes beep kickball competitions, and sells beep kickballs.

Bowling

American Blind Bowlers Association
www.abba1951.org

Holds tournaments for bowlers with visual impairments across the United States. Publishes *The Blind Bowler,* which includes articles submitted by members and information about tournament events and standings, and supplies guide rails for bowling lanes.

Camps

Camp Abilities

Runs developmental sports camps with sports and recreation activities adapted and modified for children with blindness, visual impairments, or deafblindness, such as aquatics, track and field, goalball, gymnastics, tandem biking, beep baseball, Power Showdown, bocce, horseback riding, bowling, dancing, rollerblading, fishing, rowing, and rock climbing. Additional independent camps are patterned after the original in Brockport, New York.

Camp Abilities-Brockport, New York
The College at Brockport
State University of New York
350 New Campus Drive
Brockport, NY 14420
(585) 395-5361
Fax: (585) 395-2771
www.campabilitiesbrockport.org

This website also provides links to instructional materials about how to teach sports and recreation to children with visual impairments or deafblindness.

Camp Abilities Alaska
Alpine Alternatives
2518 E. Tudor Road, Suite 105
Anchorage, AK 99507
(907) 561-6655 (Local)
Fax: (907) 563-9232
www.campabilitiesalaska.org/index.html
alpine4kids@arctic.net

Camp Abilities Boston
Perkins Outreach Services
175 North Beacon Street
Watertown, MA 02472
(617) 972-7867
Fax: (617) 972-7586
www.perkins.org/news-events/news/camp-abilities-boston.html
Kelly.Cote@Perkins.org

Camp Abilities Connecticut
Board of Education and Services for the Blind
184 Windsor Avenue

Windsor, CT 06095
(860) 602-4222
Robbin.Keating@ct.gov

Camp Abilities Long Island
P.O. Box 363
Long Beach, NY 11561
(516) 567-8898
www.campabilitieslongisland.org/Contact-Us.php
campabilitieslongisland@yahoo.com

Camp Abilities PA
306 Sturzebecker HSC
West Chester University
West Chester, PA 19383
(610) 436-2516 (Local)
www.campabilitiespa.org
campabilitiespa@aol.com

Camp Abilities Tucson
P.O. Box 87227
Tucson, AZ 85745
(520) 770-3204 (Local)
www.campabilitiestucson.org
campabilitiestucson@gmail.com

Camp Abilities, Maryland @ Lions Camp Merrick
690 Planters Wharf Road
Lusby, MD 20657
(301) 395-4695
campabilitiesmaryland.com
campabilitiesmaryland@live.com

Lions Camp Merrick
3650 Rick Hamilton Place
P.O. Box 56
Nanjemoy, MD 20662
(301) 645-5616
www.lionscampmerrick.org
campmerrick@aol.com

Offers camps (including Camp Abilities) where children and youths with special needs can participate in outdoor activities such as canoeing, a challenge course, archery, fishing, nature walks, swimming, storytelling by the campfire, basketball, baseball, softball, and arts and crafts. Hosts an annual special camp for blind adults.

National Camps for Blind Children/National Camps for the Blind
Christian Record Service
4444 South 52nd Street
Lincoln, NE 68516-1302
(402) 488-0981
Fax: (402) 488-7582
www.blindcamps.org
info@christianrecord.org

Offers free summer and winter camps in the United States and Canada for children and adults who are legally blind. Summer camps are open to people from 9 to 65 years of age and offer a variety of activities, including horseback riding, waterskiing, swimming, hiking, rappelling, canoeing, backpacking, archery, go-carts, beep baseball, and talent night. Winter camps are designed to give youths with visual impairments (ages 14 to 30) the opportunity to participate in winter activities, including skiing, sleighing, snowmobiling, and tubing.

Sports Education Camps

Offer short-term sport and recreation experiences to introduce children from 8 to 19 years of age to basic physical activity, health promotion, and fitness based on the model developed by Western Michigan University and the United States Association of Blind Athletes. Activities taught include aerobic exercise, archery, beep baseball, bowling, canoeing, kayaking, goalball, gymnastics, horseback riding, ice skating, judo, kick boxing, powerlifting, rock climbing, roller blading, rowing, showdown, swimming, tandem cycling, track and field, and wrestling. Campers participate in interactive sessions on healthy eating, exercise, sports adaptations, and self-advocacy.

Colorado Sports Education Camp
Colorado Springs, CO
c/o Donna Keale
(719) 330-7387
dkeale@csdb.org

Lakeshore Foundation Sports Education Camp
Birmingham, AL
c/o Cliff Cook
(205) 313-7426
cliffc@lakeshore.org

Missouri Sports Education Camp for Blind and Visually Impaired Youth
c/o Lighthouse for the Blind
10440 Trenton Avenue
St. Louis, MO 63132
ayorke@lhbindustries.com
jpotts@usaba.org
trackcoordinator@usaba.org

New England Blind Athletic Association Sports Education Camps
c/o Mark Sinclair
11 Veazie Street
Veazie, ME 04401
(207) 831-5229
www.nebaamaine.org
NEBAA03@aol.com

Western Michigan University Sports Education Camp
Kalamazoo, MI
c/o Scott and Leanne Ford
(231) 715-1732
michigansec@gmail.com

Cricket

See listing for British Blind Sport

Goalball

See listings for Canadian Blind Sports Association, International Blind Sports Federation, and United States Association of Blind Athletes

Golf

American Blind Golfers Association
www.Americanblindgolf.org

Promotes golf for people with visual impairments and holds a national championship.

International Blind Golf Association
www.internationalblindgolf.com/about

Governs, sanctions, and provides funding for international open blind golf events.

United States Blind Golf Association
www.blindgolf.com

Offers information on adaptations and coaching and other information. Holds regional golf tournaments. Publishes *The Midnight Golfer,* a quarterly newsletter.

Ice Sports

Ice Owls Hockey Team
Agincourt Recreation Centre
31 Glen Watford Drive
Scarborough, ON M1S 1A1
Canada
www.iceowls.ca

Provides information on adapting hockey for people with visual impairments.

Judo

Blind Judo Foundation
24145 NE 122nd Street
Redmond, WA 98053
(425) 444-8256
www.blindjudofoundation.com

Promotes judo for people who are blind or visually impaired by identifying head instructors and their dojos interested in working with people who are blind or visually impaired and offers professional development activities, information, and educational resources for coaches on how to work with visually impaired students. Provides funding to students for training.

Outdoor Recreation and Skiing

See also Adventure Travel; Camping; Sports Education Camps

Adaptive Sports Association
125 E. 32nd Street
Durango, CO 81301
(970) 259-0374
Fax: (970) 259-2175
www.asadurango.org/
info@asadurango.com

Provides outdoor programs for people with all disabilities, including blindness, deafblindness, and low vision. Offers a summer program that includes activities such as rafting; flatwater, canoeing, and kayaking; and overnight camping. The winter program includes skiing, snowboarding, and a variety of "sit-ski" instruction for people with disabilities. Lessons are typically one-on-one.

American Blind Skiing Foundation
8100 Foster Lane #310
Niles, IL 60714-1159
(312) 409-1605
www.absf.org
absf@absf.org

Offers an educational skiing program for persons who are blind or visually impaired.

Blind Outdoor Leisure Development
Challenge Aspen
P.O. Box 6639
Snowmass Village, CO 81615
(970) 923-0578
Fax: (970) 923-7338
www.challengeaspen.com

Offers skiing, snowmobiling, ice skating, and many summer activities such as hiking and rock climbing for people with disabilities. Hosts daily adaptive ski and snowboard programs and camps for people with any physical or cognitive disability.

Breckenridge Outdoor Education Center
P.O. Box 697
Breckenridge, CO 80424
(970) 453-6422 or (800) 383-2632
(970) 453-4676
www.boec.org
boec@boec.org

Offers skiing, riding, year-round camping, snowshoeing, wilderness programs, a climbing wall, a ropes course, canoeing, kayaking, rafting, group leadership development and team-building programs, and customized programs for people with all disabilities, including blindness, deafblindness, and low vision.

National Sports Center for the Disabled
Winter Park Resort
P.O. Box 1290
Winter Park, CO 80482
and
Sports Authority Field at Mile High
1801 Mile High Stadium Circle, #1500
Denver, CO 80204
(303) 316-1540 or (970) 726-5514
www.nscd.org

Offers winter and summer sports and activities for people with many types of disabilities, including blindness and low vision. Activities include rafting, kayaking, canoeing, special camps, mountain biking, camping, rock climbing, horseback riding, Nordic and Alpine skiing, snowboarding, Nordic hut trips, and ski racing.

New England Blind and Visually Impaired Alpine Ski Festival
c/o Maine Adaptive Sports and Recreation
8 Sundance Lane
Newry, Maine 04261

info@NEVIFest.org
www.nevifest.org

Conducts a national ski festival for skiers of all levels with visual impairments and training for guides.

Ski for Light
1455 West Lake Street
Minneapolis, MN 55408
(612) 827-3232
www.sfl.org
info@sfl.org

Conducts a week-long event in which adults who are blind or mobility impaired are taught the basics of cross-country skiing by pairing them with an experienced, sighted, cross-country skier who acts as ski instructor. Events are offered in areas across the United States by regional affiliates as well as in Canada and Japan. Some affiliates also offer summer programs called Sports for Health.

Vermont Adaptive Ski and Sports
P.O. Box 139
Killington, VT 05751
(802) 786-4991
Fax: (802) 786-4986
www.vermontadaptive.org
office@vermontadaptive.org

Offers access to and instruction in sports and recreational opportunities, including alpine skiing, snowboarding, kayaking, canoeing, sailing, cycling, hiking, rock climbing, tennis, horseback riding, and more, for people with physical, cognitive, and emotional disabilities.

Skiing

See Outdoor Recreation

Soccer

See listing for British Blind Sport

Swimming

USA Swimming Disability Committee
1 Olympic Plaza
Colorado Springs, CO 80909
(719) 866-4578
www.USAswimming.org

Encourages people with disabilities to participate in the sport of swimming as a division of USA Swimming, the national governing body for the sport of swimming in the United States. Maintains a resource section of information on its website.

Tandem Cycling

The Rush-Miller Foundation
www.rushmillerfoundation.org

Assists children with visual impairments from 5 to 17 years of age to obtain their first bike.

U.S. Blind Tandem Cycling Connection
http://bicyclingblind.org/

Promotes participation of individuals who are visually impaired or blind in the sport of tandem cycling.

Water Sports

Blind Ambition
P.O. BOX 40110
Portland, OR 97240
www.blindambition.info

Recreational paddling club for people who are blind.

Blind Sailing International
www.blindsailing.org

Offers a description and history of blind sailing and information about recreational and competitive sailing for people who are blind or visually impaired, adaptive equipment, and international racing rules.

Handicapped Scuba Association/HSA International
www.hsascuba.com
hsa@hsascuba.com

Conducts diver training for divers with disabilities and plans, coordinates, and conducts diving vacations.

International Rowing Federation-Adaptive
www.worldrowing.com/rowing/adaptive

Provides information about regulations and competitions for adaptive rowing in international events and the Paralympics from the world governing body for rowing.

USA Water Ski/Water Skiers with Disabilities
1251 Holy Cow Road
Polk City, FL 33868
(863) 324-4341
Fax: (863) 325-8259
www.usawaterski.org/pages/divisions/WSDA/main.htm

Promotes waterskiing by people with disabilities and hosts a national championship water-ski event. Offers the *IWSF Disabled Rule Book* and the *IWSF Disabled Competition Handbook* on its website.

SOURCES OF PRODUCTS AND ADAPTED EQUIPMENT

Abilitations Integrations Catalog
P.O. Box 922668
Norcross, GA 30010-2668
(800) 850-8602
www.integrationscatalog.com

Offers products for people with sensory processing disorder, learning differences, attention and focus issues, behavioral concerns, and autistic spectrum disorder.

Adolph Kiefer and Associates
1700 Kiefer Drive
Zion, IL 60099
(800) 323-4071
www.kiefer.com
info@kiefer.com

Sells prescription swim goggles.

American Blind Bowlers Association
www.abba1951.org

Sells bowling guard rails.

American Printing House for the Blind

See listing under National Organizations

Buddy Bike
(786) 489-2453
http://buddybike.com/index.html

Manufactures and distributes an alternative tandem bicycle for cyclists with special needs.

Concept 2
105 Industrial Park Drive
Morrisville, VT 05661
(802) 888-7971 or (800) 245-5676
Fax: (802) 888-4791
rowing@concept2.com
www.concept2.com

Manufactures rowing machines with accessible controls.

GlowProducts.com
(877) 233-4569
Fax: (250) 383-9989
http://glowproducts.com
glow_sticks@glowproducts.com

Offers a variety of glow and light-up products, including light-up or glow-in-the-dark soccer balls, baseballs, golf balls, and Frisbees.

Gopher
2525 Lemond Street SW
P.O. Box 998
Owatonna, MN 55060-0998
(800) 533-0446
Fax: (800) 451-4855
220 24th Avenue NW

P.O. Box 998
Owatonna, MN 55060-0998
www.gophersport.com

Distributes products for fitness, athletics, recreation, physical education, and health, including high-contrast activity balls and hoops; colored volleyballs, nets, headbands, mats, medicine balls, scooter boards, pinnies, jump ropes, and bean bags; parachutes; blindfolds; high-contrast cones and markers; and gym floor tape.

Independent Living Aids
200 Robbins Lane
Jericho, NY 11753
(516) 937-1848 or (800) 537-2118
Fax: (516) 937-3906
www.independentliving.com
can-do@independentliving.com

Distributes products for individuals who are visually impaired or blind, including sports and recreation balls with beepers, colors, or bells; sound-emitting locator devices; goalballs; and regulation soccer balls with bells.

Maxi-Aids
42 Executive Boulevard
Farmingdale, NY 11735 USA
(631) 752-0521 or (800) 522-6294
www.maxiaids.com

Sells products for people with visual, hearing, and mobility disabilities. Sells high-contrast balls and balls with beepers and bells.

Northern Lites Industries
117 Industrial Drive
Medford, WI 54451
(800) 360-5483 (Factory)
(715) 499-9167 (Mobile)
www.northernlites.com
snowshoe@northernlites.com

Source of Quicksilver line of snowshoes with reliable stay-on easy-on, easy-off bindings.

Rousettus LLC
(866) 990-8496
www.rousettus.com

Manufactures and distributes a yoga mat with tactile markings for people who are visually impaired.

Targe Innovations
P.O. Box 456
Kemptville, ON K0G 1J0
Canada
(613) 258-4888 or (866) 408-2743
www.targe.ca

Develops and distributes equipment for goalball and rugby and for Paralympic athletes, including goalballs, goalball pads, visors, and rugby training balls.

United States Association of Blind Athletes

See listing under general Sports Organizations

Wii Fit
www.vifit.org

Describes how games on the Wii system can be used by people with visual impairments for physical activity. Offers computer downloads for Wii Tennis, Wii Bowling, and Pet-n-Punch.

Wolverine Sports
745 State Circle
Ann Arbor, MI 48108
(800) 521-2832
Fax: (800) 654-4321
www.wolverinesports.com

Offers a full range of sports equipment including pinnies, mats, whistles, clocks and watches, balls, and gymnasium equipment.

Index

Page references in italics indicate figures.

A

abdominal muscular endurance, 73–74
AccesSports Model, 137, 146–152, 153–154t, 265, 318
adapted physical education, 48–49, 64–65
adapting games/sports/activities, 135–156
  AccesSports model, 137, 146–152, 153–154t
  activity goals and IEP goals, 145–146
  benefits, 136–138
  boundaries, adapting, 149–150
  closed vs. open skills, 139, 145
  competition vs. cooperation, 138–139
  disability awareness instruction, 152, 154–156
  functional abilities' impact on, 140–146, 144t
  guidelines, 140–146
  purpose of, 135–136, 156
  rules, adapting, 150–151
  rules of competition, 140
  sports designed for people with visual impairments, 139–140
  structuring the curriculum, 138–139
  targets/goals, adapting, 147–149
  See also modifying instruction
adolescents/adults. *See* sports activities
aerobics, *77*, 327–329
airplane (play), 179
albinism, 36–37
Albone, Dan, 256
Alpine skiing. *See* skiing, downhill
American Blind Bowling Association, 300
American Canoe Association, 310
American Foundation for the Blind (AFB), 58, 291
American Manual Alphabet, 118–119, *119*
American Printing House for the Blind (APH), 70, 322
American Sign Language (ASL), 117–118
analogies, use of, 108
APH (American Printing House for the Blind), 70, 322
aquatics, 103
  See also swimming
archery, 141, 154t
ASL (American Sign Language), 117–118
assessment
  Camp Abilities Activity Assessment Checklist, 75–76
  in elementary physical education, 190–191
  for fitness, 315
  measuring physical activity, 75
  measuring sports skills, 75–76
  of physical education for students, 71–77
  purpose, 72
  rubrics for, 76–77, *77*
  testing fundamental movements, 72–73
  testing physical fitness, 73–75
attitudinal barriers to physical activity, 18–20
audition. *See* hearing
autonomy, 221

B

babies. *See* play/movement in early childhood
balls, throwing/chasing, 179
baseball, 220, 221t
  See also beep baseball
basketball, 101
beep baseball
  bases, 279
  description, 278–279
  history, 220, 278
  modifications for students with deafblindness, 283–284
  rules, 279–282
  target adaptations, 279
  teaching tips, 282–283
bicycling
  for fitness, 323–324
  independently, 324
  for recreation, 302–304
  stationary, 324
  See also tandem cycling
blindness
  defined, 29–30
  as a physical disability, 32
  simulating, 154–155
  sports identified with (*see* beep baseball; goalball)
  See also deafblindness; legal blindness
Blind Sailing International, 306
boating
  dragon boating, 262–265
  kayaking/canoeing, 308–310
  rowing, 260–262
  sailing, 306–307
body composition, 73–74
body concepts, 9
body-on-body play, 179

bold-line maps, 103–104
boundaries, adapting, 149–150
bowling, 300–302
BPFT (Brockport Physical Fitness Test), 73–75, 315–316
braille cell, 103
braille output devices, 119
Braille Sports Foundation, 278
brain plasticity/cross-modal brain reorganization, 42–45
Brockport Physical Fitness Test (BPFT), 73–75, 315–316
Buell, Charles and Josephine, 340

C

calling, 239–240, 320–321
Camp Abilities Activity Assessment Checklist (CAAAC), 75–76
Canadian Blind Sports Association (CBSA), 339, 341
canoeing, 308–310
cardiovascular fitness, 73–74
carpet squares for step-by-step instruction, 113–116
  instruction plans using, 126–134
  orientation to, 126–128
  See also step-by-step instruction
Carroll, T. J., 17–18
cataracts, 34–35
CBSA (Canadian Blind Sports Association), 339, 341
cerebral palsy, 166–167
CHARGE syndrome, 12, 37, 169
classification of athletes, 32–33, 235–236
closed vs. open skills, 139, 145
cochlear implants, 46–47
cognitive mapping, 9
command-style teaching (direct instruction), 194
communication's role in modified instruction, 95–96
competence, 221
competition
  rules of, 140
  vision classification for, 236
  vs. cooperation, 138–139
  See also Paralympic Games, sports activities, United States Association of Blind Athletes, *and specific sports*
complex equipment, describing, 97–102
complex movement skills, methods of teaching, 106–116
  carpet squares, 113–116, 126–128
  issues, 106
  parachutes, 113
  physical guidance, 109–111
  step-by-step instruction, 111–116, 129–134
  tactile modeling, 108–110
  verbal instruction, 107–108
concept development, and early vision loss, 7–12
contrast and visibility, 39–40
Cook, Char, 264
Cooper, Bonnie, 264
Copeland, Arthur and Helen, 340
cross-modal brain reorganization/brain plasticity, 42–45
cycling. *See* bicycling; tandem cycling

D

dance/movement exploration, 195
deafblindness
  benefits of physical education, 63–64
  causes/types, 12, 37–38
  defined, 29–31
  demographics, 34
  modifying instruction for students with (*see* modifying instruction)
  as a physical disability, 32
  physical education for students with (*see* physical education)
  sound beacons with, 46
  See also learning/development, visual impairment/deafblindness's impact on; visual impairment/deafblindness, overview of
deafness
  causes/types, 12
  as a culture, 46
  early-onset, impact on learning and development, 12–13
Dean, Jamie, 261
denial, 15
development. *See* learning/development, visual impairment/deafblindness's impact on
diabetic retinopathy, 36
direction, defined, 10–11
disability
  awareness of, 152, 154–156
  categories, 32–33
  environmental/functional models, 20–21
  experiencing, 154–155
  exposure to, 154
  medical model, 20
discus throwing, 237, 242
Dodds, A., 18
dragon boating, 262–265

E

early childhood. *See* movement/play in early childhood
eccentric viewing, 35
echolocation, 176
effort concepts, 11–12
electronic exercise games, 329–330
elementary education programming, 187–226
  active participation, 198–200
  adapting common games, 215–216t, 215–220, 219–220t
  assessment, 190–191
  baseball, 220, 221t
  basic locomotor skills, 205–213
  class organization/instructional approach, 193–196
  curriculum, 190
  equipment, 200
  explanations/concepts, clear, 198–199
  galloping, 210, 213
  hopping, 210, 211
  jumping, 207–210
  jump rope, 199, 217–219, 219t
  leaping, 210, 213
  motivating students, 220–222

object control skills, 200–205
one-to-one instruction, 196–197
planning activities, overview, 191–192
relay races, 219–220, 220t
running, 206–207
scooter activities, 216–217, 216t
skipping, 210, 212–213
sliding, 210, 213
step-by-step instruction for basic skills, 200–213
tag, 215–216, 215t
throwing skills, 202–205
time for learning, 193
time for teaching, 192–193
training paraeducators, 196–197
training peer tutors, 197–198
whiffle ball, 220, 221t
whole-part-whole instruction, 199–200
See also parachutes
equipment
adapted, 200
for snow sports, 294–295
support for, 69–70
exercise balls, 333–336
exercise machines, 330–332
See also rowing machines
extension, 11
See also spatial awareness/concepts
eye, cross-section of, *35*
eyeshades, 267
aversion to, 276–277, 283
description, 272–273

F

Federal Quota Program, 70
FISA (International Rowing Federation), 260–261
fitness, 312–337
accessing activities, 316–317
aerobics/jazzercise, 327–329
assessment, 315–316
benefits, 24–25, 314–315
bicycling, 323–324
electronic exercise games, 329–330
and employment, 315
exercise balls, 333–336
exercise machines, 330–332
goal setting/evaluation, 318–319
at home, 334, 336
jumping rope, 333 (*see also* jump rope)
programming for, 317–318
rollerblading, 323, 323t
running, 319–323 (*see also* running)
swimming, 324–327 (*see also* swimming)
trampoline for, 332–333
walking, 318, 319–323
weightlifting, 330
yoga, 333
Fitnessgram Test, 73
flexibility, 73–75
flow, 11
force, 11
functional abilities, 140–146, 144t
functional vision defined, 29

G

galloping, 210, 213
general space, 10–11
Gilbert, Aerial, 261–262
Gillette, Elexis, 244
glare, 36–37, 39
glaucoma, 35–36
goalball
for beginners, 276–277
blocking, 270
competitive, 272
the court, 269–270
description, 268–269
equipment, 272–272
history, 268, 340
modifications for students with deafblindness, 268, 283–284
penalties, 271
rules, 269
rule violations, 271–272
scoring, 270
starting activity/program, 277–278
substitutions/time out, 271
teaching tips, 275–277
throwing, 270
touch used in, 42–43, 45
Gokey, Steve, 240
golf, 153t, 304–306
grid pattern search, 103
guided discovery (question approach), 194
guide runners, 140, 238–239
See also human guides
guide wires, 240, 319

H

hammock play, 179
Hatlan, P., 62
hearing
auditory adaptations, 45–46
cochlear implants, 46–47
impairment/loss, 13–18, 14–18 (*see also* deafblindness; deafness)
as substitute for vision, 44–45
hearing aids, 46
heart-rate monitors, 322–323
high jump, 237, 244–245
high school physical education. *See* middle school/high school physical education
hopping, 210, 211
human guides, 105, 319–320
See also guide runners
hyper-/hypotonicity, 166–167

I

IBGA (International Blind Golf Association), 306
IBSA. *See* International Blind Sports Federation
ice skating, 292, 293t, 299–300
IDBF (International Dragon Boating Federation), 263
IDEA. *See* Individuals with Disabilities Education Act
IEP. *See* Individualized Education Program
IFSP (Individualized Family Service Plan), 165
illumination, 39
incidental learning, 7

Individualized Education Program (IEP), 47
- activity goals and IEP goals, 145–146
- components, 65, 71
- creating/revising, 65–66
- first, 181
- goals/objectives, 66–69
- inclusion vs. separate instruction, 192
- in physical education, 64–69
- sample form, 82–88
- statement of participation in regular settings, 70–71

Individualized Family Service Plan (IFSP), 165
Individualized Plan for Employment (IPE), 49–50, 290
Individuals with Disabilities Education Act (IDEA), 47, 55, 64–65, 71, 164–165
infants. *See* play/movement in early childhood
International Blind Golf Association (IBGA), 306
International Blind Sports Federation (IBSA), 33, 235–236, 253, 272, 339, 343
International Cycling Union (UCI), 257
International Dragon Boating Federation (IDBF), 263
International Judo Federation, 253
International Olympics Committee, 342
International Paralympic Committee (IPC), 339, 342–343
International Paralympic Movement, 341
International Rowing Federation (FISA), 260–261
interpreters/interveners, 49, 120, 123–124
IPC (International Paralympic Committee), 339, 342–343
IPE (Individualized Plan for Employment), 49–50, 290
isolation, 63

J

Jankowski, L. W., 25
Jazzercise, 327–329
judo, 252–255
jumping, 207–210
- *See also* high jump; long jump

jump rope
- adaptations, 217–219, 219t
- for fitness, 333
- and IEP goals, 145–146
- whole-part-whole instruction, 199

K

Kano, Jigoro, 252
kayaking, 308–310
kinesthetic learning/muscle memory, 41–44
kinesthetic sense, 168

L

language use, precision in, 107–108
leaping, 210, 213
learner description, 98, 101
learning/development, visual impairment/deafblindness's impact on, 3–26
- acquired vision/hearing loss, 12–18
- attitudinal factors, 18–20
- consequences of limited physical education, 21–25
- early-onset deafness, 12–13
- early vision loss, 7–12
- environmental/functional models of disability, 20–21
- fitness's health benefits, 24–25
- and lack of professional training, 21
- medical model of disability, 20
- and overcoming barriers, 25–26
- physical activity, defined, 5
- physical activity, other barriers to, 18–21
- physical activity, school-related barriers to, 21
- physical activity's benefits, 5–6
- and physical skills, 23–24
- reaction/adjustment to loss, 14–18

legal blindness, 29, 32, 33–34
leisure. *See* recreation
level (space awareness), 10–11
Livneh, H., 15–18
location, defined, 10–11
locomotor skills
- space awareness concepts needed for, 10
- teaching basic, 205–213
- testing, 73
- *See also* motor skills

long jump
- adaptations/demonstration, 242–244
- in competition, 237
- the pit, 97–98, 100–101
- running, 210
- standing, 207–210

Lorenzen, Hanz, 268
low vision
- defined, 29–30, 38
- environmental modifications, 38, 41
- and eyeshades, 283
- as a physical disability, 32
- simulating, 155

M

macular degeneration, 35
Malloy, Patrick, 304
map concepts, 9
Marshall, Ray, 282
Mastro, James, 250
McReady, Bill, 256
medical conditions that affect physical activity, 144t
- *See also specific conditions*

Merren, Tyler, 274
middle school/high school physical education, 227–235
- content, 228–229
- effects of curriculum on students with visual impairments/deafblindness, 234–235
- high school curriculum, 231–234
- middle school curriculum, 231
- middle school vs. high school students, 228–229

NASPE standards, 229–231
See also sports activities
modifying instruction, 91–126
assisting students in moving from place to place, 104–105
basic skills instruction plans, 126–134
communicating with students with deafblindness, 117–119, *119*, 121–122
communication's role, 95–96
for complex movement skills (*see* complex movement skills, methods of teaching)
describing a room or activity area, 102–104
describing complex equipment, 97–102
educational team for students with deafblindness, 123–125
interpreters/interveners, 120, 123–124
learner description, 98, 101
modification vs. adaptation, 92–93
part-to-whole learning, 93, 95
for students who are deafblind, overview, 116–117
for students with visual impairments, overview, 96–97
tips for teaching students with deafblindness, 116–117
tips for teaching students with visual impairments, 94–95
Morgan, D. W., 322
motivation, 220–222
motor development, 162–172
motor skills
early vision loss, and development of, 7
object control, 200–205
vision in, 165–166
See also locomotor skills, motor development
movement concepts, 10, 22–23
movement/play in early childhood, 159–186
constructive play, 177–178
development of play, 173–181
dramatic play, 178
early motor development, 162–173, 163t
effects of hearing loss on motor development, overview, 169
effects of visual impairment on motor development, overview, 164–165
to encourage physical activity, 184–186
exploratory/sensorimotor play, 174–176
functional/relational play, 176–177
games with rules, 180–181
interpersonal play, 174
muscle tone, 166–170
object permanence, 170–173
postural tone, 170
preparing for preschool and beyond, 181–183
reaching to sound, 172
rough-and-tumble play, 178–180
starting early, 160–162
transition movements, 168
vision in motor skills, 165–166
muscle memory/kinesthetic learning, 41–44
muscle tone, 166–170
music, moving/dancing to, 179

N

NASPE (National Association for Sport and Physical Education), 55–56, 229–231
National Association of Amateur Oarsmen, 260
National Beep Baseball Association (NBBA), 278
National Consortium on Deaf-Blindness (NCDB), 34, 37, 58
National Sports Education Camps (USABA), 340
NBBA (National Beep Baseball Association), 278
NCDB. *See* National Consortium on Deaf-Blindness
No Child Left Behind Act (2004), 196
Nordic skiing. *See* skiing, cross-country

O

object control skills, 73, 200–205
object permanence, 8–9, 170–173
object-to-object concepts, 9–10
obstacle courses, 179
occluders. *See* eyeshades
occupational therapists, 49–50
Olympic Games, 235, 341
See also Paralympic Games
O&M (orientation and mobility) specialists, 48, 50
one-to-one instruction, 196–197
open vs. closed skills, 139, 145
operative language, 114
organizations of special interest, 338–339, 343–344
See also CBSA; IBSA; Paralympic Games; USABA
orientation and mobility (O&M) specialists, 48, 50
visual impairment/deafblindness, overview of, 27–51
categories of disabilities, 32–33
classification for sports competition, 33
compensating for vision loss, 38–48
deafblindness defined, 29–31
demographics, 33–34
environmental modifications, 38
hearing as substitute for vision, 44–45
influence of terminology/language, 31
personnel in educational settings, 47–49
personnel in rehabilitation settings, 49–51
touch as substitute for vision, 41–44
See also deafblindness, visual impairment

ownership (involvement with students with visual impairments), 155–156

P

palm writing, 119
parachutes for teaching basic skills, 113, 214–215
paraeducators, 49, 80, 196–197
Paralympic Games, 341–343
  athletics (track and field), 236–245
  cycling at, 256–257
  goalball, 272
  history, 342
  judo, 252–254
  long jump at, 244
  summer/winter events, 342
  swimming at, 245–246
  and USABA, 235, 342
  See also specific sports
part-to-whole learning, 93, 95
pathway (space awareness), 11
pedometers, 75, 322–323
peer tutoring, 80, 195, 197–198
perceived competence, 61–62
perimeter search, 103
personal adjustment training, 49–50
person-first language, 31
personnel support, 69
photophobia, 36–37, 39
physical education, 52–81
  assessment, 71–77 (*see also* assessment, elementary education programming)
  benefits, 53–54, 60–64
  blind sports, 79
  collaboration between teachers and physical educators, 58–59
  curriculum, 78–79
  defined, 55–57
  discrete/continuous skills, 79
  equipment via federal quota program, 70
  instructional modification, 79
  and the law, 64–71
  least restrictive environment, 64
  NASPE standards, 56
  one-to-one teams, 79–80
  open/closed skills, 78–79
  perceived competence via, 61–62
  planning a program, 77–80
  qualified personnel, 64–65
  resources/information, 58
  self-determination via, 62
  skills taught, by school level, 56–57
  socialization via, 62–64
  stamina/fitness improvements via, 61 (*see also* fitness)
  statement of participation in regular settings, 70–71
  for students with deafblindness, benefits of, 63–64
  supplementary aids/services, 69–70
  and transition services, 81
  See also elementary education programming, Individualized Education Program, middle school/high school physical education
physical guidance, 109–111
pole vault, 237
Ponchillia, Paul, 9–10, 103, 146, 309
Ponchillia, Susan, 9–10, 103, 309
postural fixing, 169
postural tone, 170
preschool teachers, guidance for, 182–183
print on palm, 119
Professional Ski Instructors of America and the American Association of Snowboard Instructors (PSIA-AASI), 298
professional training, lack of, 21
proprioceptive sense, 168
psychological defense mechanisms, 15

Q

qualified personnel, 64–65

R

races
  cross-country, 237
  distance, 237, 239
  dragon boat, 262–265
  hurdle, 237, 239
  middle distance, 237, 239
  relay, 219–220, 220t, 240–241
  road, 237
  rowing, 260–261
  sprints, 237, 239–240
  swim, 245–249
  tandem cycling, 256–257
raised-/bold-line drawings, 98–99
reaching to sound, 172
ready position, 111, 129–132
recreation, 286–311
  adaptations, overview, 291–292
  benefits, 288–290
  bicycling and tandem cycling, 302–304
  bowling, 300–302
  defined, 288
  goals in education and vocational rehabilitation, 289–291
  golf, 304–306
  kayaking/canoeing, 308–310
  sailing, 306–307
  snow sports, 292–293t, 292–299
  tennis, 291
  therapeutic, 288
  waterskiing, 307–308
recumbent bikes, 303
reference points, 103
regression, 15
Reindl, Sepp, 268
relatedness, 221
relative-distance modification, 40
retinitis pigmentosa, 35
retinopathy of prematurity (ROP), 36
rollerblading, 323, 323t
room familiarization, 102–103
rowing, 260–262
rowing machines, 261, 331–332
rules, adapting, 150–151
running
  adaptations, 238–241, 319–322
  in elementary education, 206–207
  with pedometers/heart-rate monitors, 322–323
  on a treadmill, 321–322
  without assistance on a track, 321
  See also races
Rush-Miller Foundation, 303

S

sailing, 306–307
scale models, 98, 100
Scheppe, Kris, 306
scooter activities, 216–217, 216t
sculling, 260
  See also rowing
sedentary lifestyles, 24–25
  See also fitness
self-determination, 62
self-to-object concepts, 9–10
Shinholster, April, 307
shot put, 237, 241–242
sign language, 117–119, *119*
Simon Says, 179
size and visibility, 40–41
skiing
  cross-country, 292, 292t
  downhill, 292, 292t, 296–298
  guides, 294–298
  water, 307–308
skipping, 210, 212–213
sliding, 210, 213
snowboarding, 292, 293t, 296–298
snowshoeing, 292, 293t, 298–299
snow sports, 292–293t, 292–299
  See also skiing
soccer, 141–142, 153t
soccer, scooter, 216
socialization, 62–64
sound cues/beacons, 45–47, 105, 148
spatial awareness/concepts, 9–11, 22–23
spinning, 324
sports activities, 235–265
  athletics (track and field), 236–245
  dragon boating, 262–265
  judo, 252–255
  rowing, 260–262
  running adaptations, 238–241
  swimming, 245–250
  tandem cycling, 254, 256–260
  vision classification for competitions, 236
  wrestling, 250–252
  See also middle school/high school physical education, sports designed for people with visual impairments, *and specific sports*
sports concepts, 10
sports designed for people with visual impairments, 139–140
  See also beep baseball; goalball
stamina/fitness, improving, 61
  See also fitness
Stargardt disease, 35
stations for task-teaching, 195
step aerobics, 328
step-by-step instruction for basic skills, 111–116, 200–213, 129–134
  hopping, 211
  jumping jacks, 133–134
  ready position, 129–132
  skipping, 212–213
  standing long jump, 208–209
  throwing, 202–205
  See also carpet squares for step-by-step instruction
step machines, 330–331
Stoke Mandeville Games, 342
sunglasses, 39
supplementary aids/services, 69–70
surrey bikes, 303
swimming
  adaptations, 246–249, 325–327
  by beginners, 325
  competitive, 245–246
  counting laps/distance, 327
  for fitness, 324–327
  flotation devices, 325
  lap, 325–326
  teaching tips, 249–250
  trailing, 326–327
  treading water, 325
  turning, 326

T

tactile ability. *See* touch
tactile graphics, 98–99
tactile maps, 103–104
tactile modeling, 108–110
tag, 215–216, 215t
tag, scooter, 216–217
tandem cycling, 254, 256–260, 302–304, 323
targets/goals, adapting, 147–149
task analysis, 111–113, 195–196
task teaching, 195
teachers of students with visual impairments, 48
tennis, 291
Test of Gross Motor Development, second edition (TGMD-2), 72–73, 191
tethers, 238, 320
Theryoung, Robin, 274
throwing
  of balls, generally, 179
  discus, 237, 242
  events, 237, 240
  in goalball, 270
  step-by-step instruction, 202–205
  See also shot put
tickle games, 179
time (effort concept), 11
touch as substitute for vision, 41–44
track and field (athletics), 236–245
  See also long jump; races
trampoline, 332–333
transition movements, 168
treadmills, 321–322
Tuttle, D. W., 18

U

UCI (International Cycling Union), 257
unified model of adjustment, 15–18
United States Association of Blind Athletes (USABA)
  athlete classification by, 235–236
  competitions held by, 33, 298, 339–340
  goalball promoted by, 268, 272
  goals, 339–340
  history, 340
  military veterans served by, 341
  overview, 235, 339
  skiing promoted by, 298
  sports camps/clinics, 340
  sports governed/promoted by, 79, 339, 342
  swimming promoted by, 246
  website, 340–341

United States Rowing Association (US Rowing), 260
upper-body muscular endurance, 73–74
USA Swimming, 246, 248–249, 342
USA Track, 342
U.S. Blind Golf Association (USBGA), 304
U.S. Census Bureau, 33
Usher syndrome, 12, 37, 169
U.S. Paralympic Committee, 235, 246, 253

V

verbal descriptions/instruction, 105, 107–108
vestibular sense, 168–169
VI Fit, 330
visibility, improving, 38–40
vision classification for competitions, 236
vision loss, reaction/adjustment to, 14–18
  See also learning/development, visual impairment/deafblindness's impact on; visual impairment/deafblindness, overview of
vision rehabilitation therapists, 50–51
visual acuity, 30, 32, 34–35, *35*
visual disability defined, 30
visual field, 30, 35–36
visual impairment
  causes, 34–37
  cortical visual impairment (CVI), 36
  defined, 29–30
  early-onset, 7–12 (*see also under* play/movement in early childhood)
  and learning/development (*see* learning/development, visual impairment/deafblindness's impact on)
  modifying instruction for students with (*see* modifying instruction)
  photophobia, 36–37, 39
  physical education for students with (*see* physical education)
  resources for introducing students to athletes with, 155
  simulating, 154–155
  See also blindness; deafblindness; legal blindness, vision loss, visual impairment/deafblindness, overview of
visors, 39, 294, 307
vocational rehabilitation, 290–291
volleyball, 138–139, 151–152

W

walking, 318, 319–323
waterskiing, 307–308
water sports
  See also boating; swimming
Watson, Andre, 253
weightlifting, 330
wheelchair aerobics, 328
whiffle ball, 220, 221t
Whitsell, Karissa, 257
whole-part-whole instruction, 199–200
Wilson, Arthur James, 256
withdrawal, 15
Wolfe, Thomas Patrick, 298
wrestling, 250–252

Y

yoga, 333

Z

Zorn, Trischa, 246

About the Authors

Lauren J. Lieberman, Ph.D., is Distinguished Service Professor in the Department of Kinesiology, Sport Studies and Physical Education, The College at Brockport—State University of New York. An acknowledged expert in the physical education of students with visual impairments and deafblindness, in 1996 she founded Camp Abilities, a sports camp for children who are visually impaired, blind, or deafblind, with 16 affiliates in other states and countries. Dr. Lieberman has authored or co-authored numerous books, including *Games for People with Sensory Impairments* (2nd ed.), *Going PLACES: A Transition Guide to Physical Activity for Youth with Visual Impairments, Strategies for Inclusion* (2nd ed.), *A Paraprofessional Training Guide for Physical Education, Sports for Everyone: A Handbook for Starting Sports Camps for Children with Visual Impairments,* and the forthcoming *Everybody Plays: How Children with Visual Impairments Play Sports.* She has also published numerous peer-reviewed articles and presented widely on similar topics. The former chair of the Adapted Physical Activity Council of the American Alliance for Health, Physical Education, Recreation and Dance, Dr. Lieberman is the winner of the 2012 Access Award from the American Foundation for the Blind and the 2012 Professional of the Year Award from the Adapted Physical Activity Council of the American Alliance for Health, Physical Education, Recreation and Dance and is on the board of directors of the U.S. Association for Blind Athletes.

Paul E. Ponchillia, Ph.D., is Professor Emeritus and former Chair of the Department of Blindness and Low Vision Studies at Western Michigan University, Kalamazoo. A former vision rehabilitation therapist, Dr. Ponchillia was a plant nematologist with a doctorate in plant pathology before losing his vision in an accident. With Susan Ponchillia in 1988 he founded and directed the Michigan Sports Education Camp for Students with Visual Impairments, which developed into a national project and the creation of 22 similar camps around the country. He is the co-author with Susan Ponchillia of *Foundations of Rehabilitation Teaching with Persons Who Are Blind or Visually Impaired,* the first text to document the knowledge base of the discipline of rehabilitation teaching, now known as vision rehabilitation therapy, which won the 1998 Warren Bledsoe Award from the Association for Education and Rehabilitation of the Blind and Visually Impaired (AER), and was co-author with Lauren Lieberman and others of *Going PLACES: A Transition Guide to Physical Activity for Youth with Visual Impairments.* Dr. Ponchillia has authored and co-authored many journal articles on sports education for people with visual impairments, rehabilitation, and orientation and mobility, as well as plant biology, and has recently written on sports, art, and brain plasticity in people who are blind or have low vision. A former associate editor of the *Journal of Visual Impairment & Blindness,* he has received numerous awards, including the Michigan Council of the Blind and Visually Impaired 2007 Distinguished Service Award, the 1999 George Card Award from the American Council of the Blind, and the 1997 Western Michigan University Distinguished Service Award for outstanding service to the university and the community, and he shared with Susan Ponchillia the 1990 Bruce McKenzie Award for distinguished service to rehabilitation teaching from Division 11 of AER. Dr. Ponchillia was enshrined in the Michigan Athletes with Disabilities Hall of Fame September 28, 2000, and was an Olympic Torch runner for the 1996 Atlanta Olympic Games. He is also an accomplished sculptor and stone carver in the Inuit tradition.

Susan V. Ponchillia, Ed.D., now deceased, was Professor in the Department of Blindness and Low Vision Studies at Western Michigan University (WMU), Kalamazoo, where she taught for 28 years. A former certified rehabilitation teacher, Dr. Ponchillia was renowned for her work with the indigenous people of Tlicho, a nation in subarctic Canada, who have a genetic predisposition to rare forms of retinitis pigmentosa, producing the documentary film, *Sing Me a Fish: Tlicho People of Subarctic Canada Living with Vision Loss,* which detailed her experiences with this population. Dr. Ponchillia was co-founder of the Michigan Sports Education Camp for Students with Visual Impairments and co-author of *Foundations of Rehabilitation Teaching with Persons Who Are Blind or Visually Impaired,* which won the 1998 Warren Bledsoe Award, and she published widely on visual impairment and diabetes, sports and physical education, and rehabilitation teaching. Dr. Ponchillia was a former member of the Educational Advisory Board of the *Journal of Visual Impairment & Blindness.* She was awarded the WMU College of Health and Human Services' Teaching Excellence Award in 2002 and shared with Paul Ponchillia the 1990 Bruce McKenzie Award for distinguished service to rehabilitation teaching.

Tanni L. Anthony, Ph.D., is the Director of the Program Instruction/Related Services Team in the Exceptional Student Services Unit; State Consultant on Blindness/Low Vision; and Project Director, Colorado Services for Children and Youth with Combined Vision and Hearing Loss Project, Colorado Department of Education, Denver. A recognized authority on young children with visual impairments with and without multiple disabilities, she was one of the editors of *Developmentally Appropriate Orientation and Mobility.* Dr. Anthony has taught courses, contributed numerous book chapters, and presented widely in areas such as early development, orientation and mobility, early intervention, and assessment.

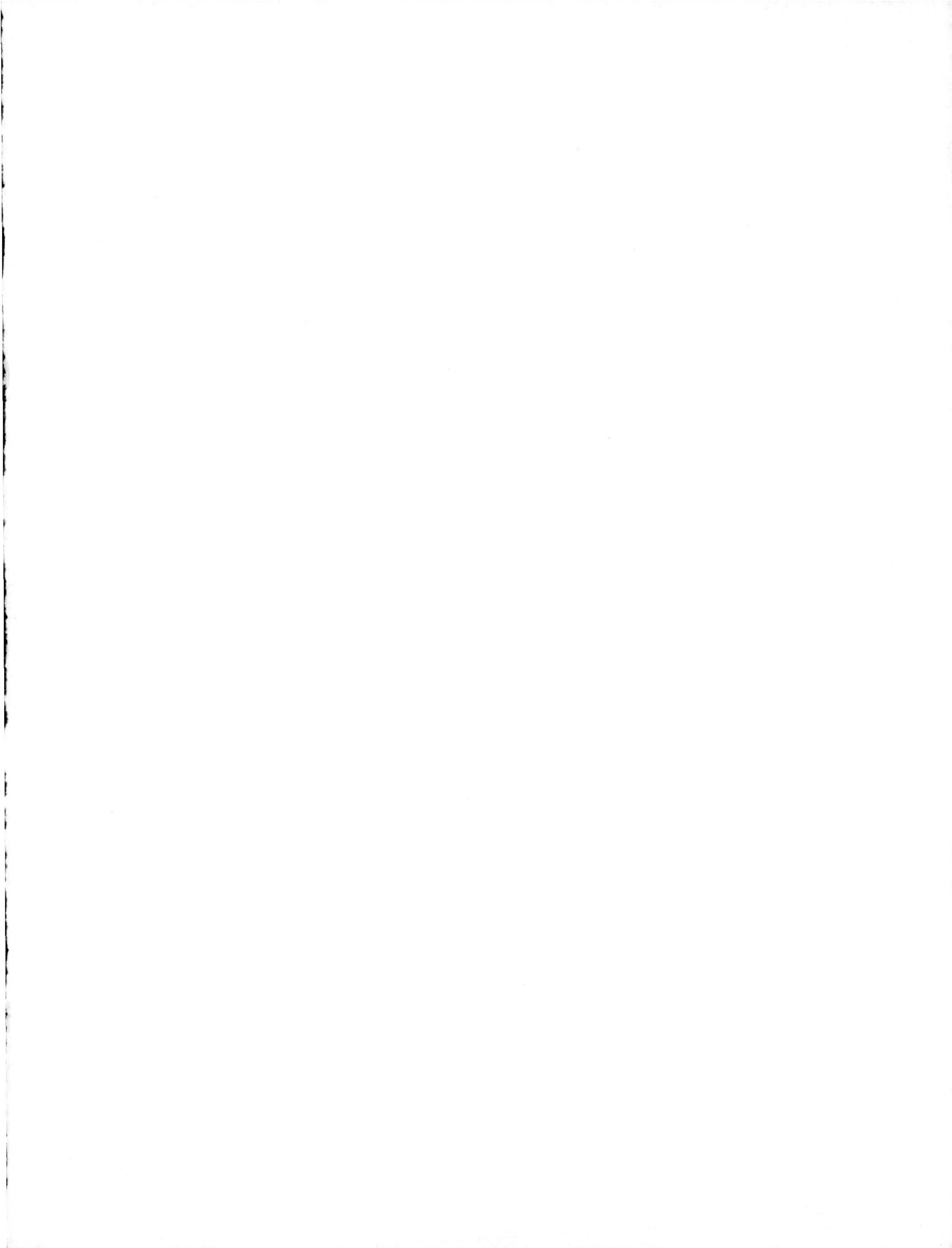

CPSIA information can be obtained at www.ICGtesting.com
Printed in the USA
LVOW09s2050051115

461279LV00003B/3/P